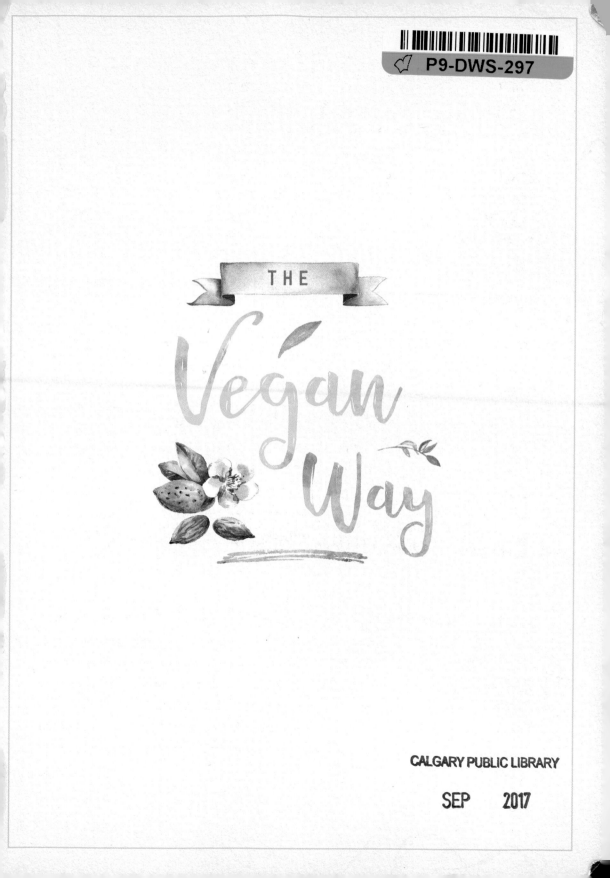

THE
Vegan Way

JACKIE DAY

THE
Vegan
Way

21 Days to a Happier, Healthier,

Plant-Based Lifestyle That Will

Transform Your Home,

Your Diet, and You

ST. MARTIN'S GRIFFIN NEW YORK

THE VEGAN WAY. Copyright © 2016 by Jacqueline Day. All rights reserved. Printed in the United States of America. For information, address St. Martin's Press, 175 Fifth Avenue, New York, N.Y. 10010.

www.stmartins.com

Design by Laura Klynstra
Illustrations by Creative Market and Shutterstock

The Library of Congress Cataloging-in-Publication Data is available upon request.

ISBN 978-1-250-08771-3 (trade paperback)
ISBN 978-1-250-08772-0 (e-book)

Our books may be purchased in bulk for promotional, educational, or business use. Please contact your local bookseller or the Macmillan Corporate and Premium Sales Department at 1-800-221-7945, extension 5442, or by e-mail at MacmillanSpecialMarkets@macmillan.com.
First Edition: October 2016

10 9 8 7 6 5 4 3 2 1

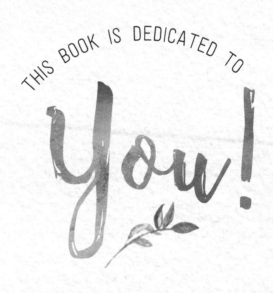

THIS BOOK IS DEDICATED TO

You!

Contents

INTRODUCTION 1

My Road to Vegan
Discover the author's path to becoming vegan. 5

Setting a Date
Figure Out the Best Time to Start. 13

The 21-Days-to-a-Vegan Road Map
Understand how the 21-day process works, and that it's flexible, easy, and fun. 19

Day 1: Finding Your Muse
Identify your source of inspiration. 29

Day 2: Creepy Crawlies in Your Food, Oh My!
Evaluate your pantry, refrigerator, and freezer. Identify, separate, and sort. 39

Day 3: Finding Your Vegan Oasis
*Research/list the best places to buy vegan groceries near you—
stores, farmers' markets, etc.* 55

Day 4: Let's Get Nutty!
Substitute a plant-based milk for dairy. 67

Day 5: Eggs Make Babies, Not Breakfast
Experiment with egg replacements while cooking and/or baking. 79

Day 6: I Smell Something Fishy!
Select a meal that normally contains fish and transform it into a delicious vegan meal. 93

Day 7: Mystery Meat
Replace meat with delicious plant-based options. 101

Day 8: But I Love Cheese (Too Much!)
Learn how to use and create delicious options in place of dairy cheese. 119

Day 9: Fast, Cheap, and Easy
Practice cooking with limited time and a tight budget. 127

Day 10: Culinary "Arts"
Experiment with textures and colors while preparing meals. 147

Day 11: Because Bunnies Don't Have Tear Ducts
Understand animal testing and cruelty-free options. Evaluate your cosmetics/toiletries. 177

Day 12: I Spy with My Vegan Eye
*Check all household items for animal products—
from under the kitchen sink to bed pillows.* 189

Day 13: The Skeletons in Your Closet
Look at labels on clothes, shoes, and accessories—separate, donate, etc. 195

Day 14: Excuse Me, Waiter, There's a Fish in My Beer!
Learn which beers and wines are vegan. 205

Day 15: Keeping the Happy in the Holidays
*Figure out where you'll be and what you'll eat in advance,
while trying not to offend anyone.* 211

Day 16: Vegan Wanderlust
Plan ahead for when you're on the road—hotels, restaurants, fast-food places, etc. 223

Day 17: Now, *That's* Entertainment!
*Try out some cruelty-free entertainment such as a day trip to a fun vegan event, a sanctuary,
bird watching, or animal-free circus, etc., instead of the zoo/animal circus/aquarium.* 235

Day 18: Adopt, Don't Shop
*Learn how to make a compassionate choice when you want a companion animal—
pet stores/puppy mills vs. shelters/rescue groups.* 245

Day 19: Help! Vegan 911!
Tips and tricks to stay on the vegan wagon. 251

Day 20: Planting Seeds of Compassion
Learn easy, everyday ways to spread the word and make a difference! 259

Day 21: Vegan for the WIN!
It's not just you; learn how the entire world is going vegan, too! 271

ACKNOWLEDGMENTS 281
RESOURCES 283
NOTES 291
INDEX 299

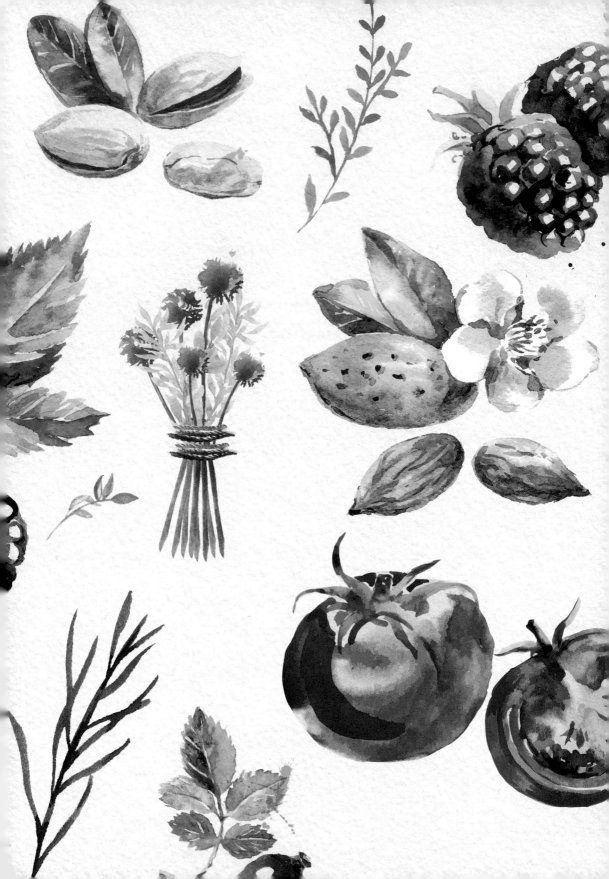

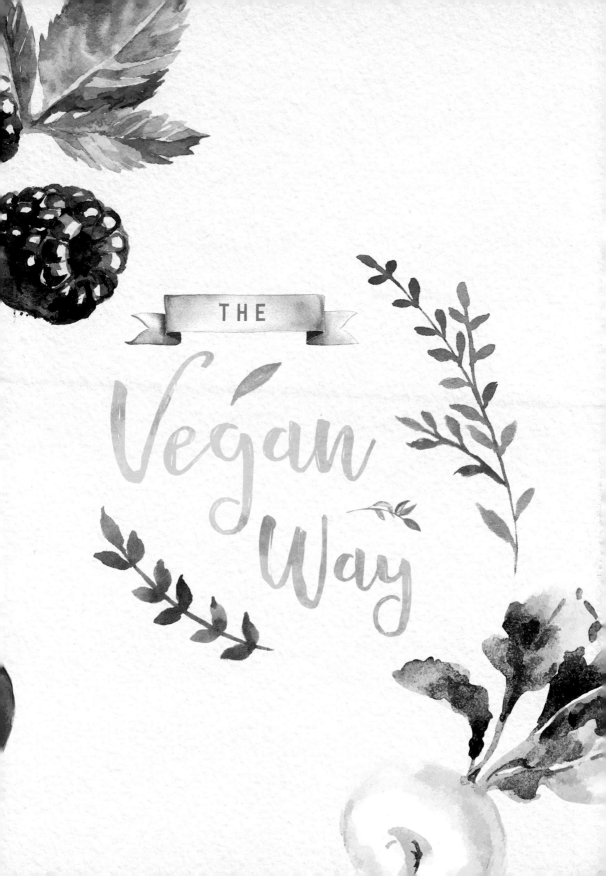

THE

Vegan
Way

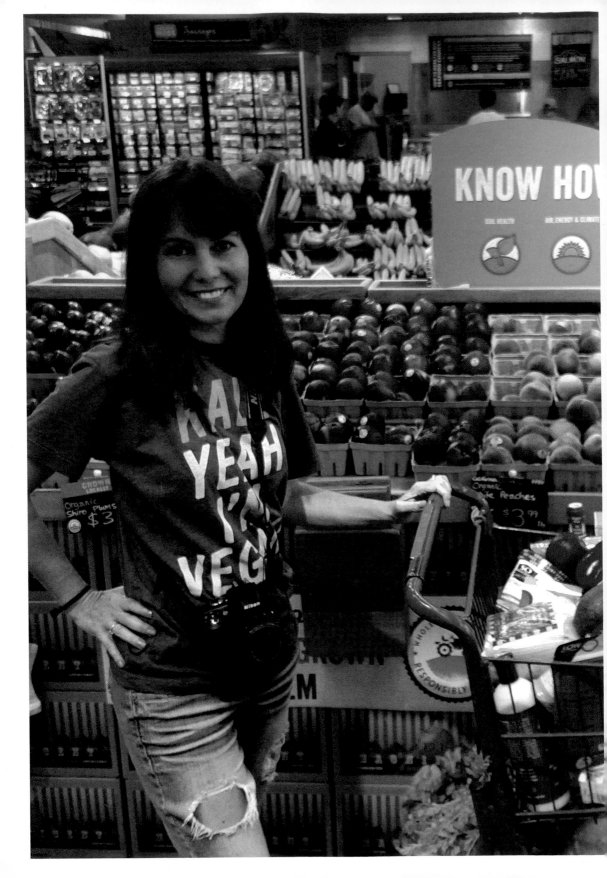

Introduction

"You are free to choose, but you are not free from the consequences of your choice."
—UNIVERSAL PARADOX

If you were stranded alone on a deserted island with nothing to eat but animals, would you eat them? Don't answer that. I bet you won't be stranded on a deserted island any time soon. Here's a better question. If you were given the power to singlehandedly make the world a much better place, for yourself and those around you, simply by eating delicious foods, wearing cool clothes, using fantastic products, and exercising thoughtfulness, would you? There's no catch. It's truly that wonderful, and that simple. You hold the power—on your fork with every bite you eat, and in your pocketbook with every dollar you spend. And with *The Vegan Way* in hand, in 21 days you'll have all the tips and inspiration you need to embrace that untapped power and change the world.

There are so many uncertainties in our universe but this I know to be true: we're all here, right now—living, breathing, thinking, and interacting with the world around us. We're like water drops splashing on the ocean, creating endless ripples, far beyond our sight. This we can all agree on. And I, for one, want to make sure that during this brief, wondrous period of certainty, when I am fully aware of my actions and can make my own decisions, that I live my life compassionately. Therein lies the foundation of being vegan: we strive to cause as little harm as possible. We continually expand our circle of compassion, empathy, and wellness as wide as we possibly can. Here's why:

BECAUSE WE LOVE OUR BODIES

Let's face it; we've only got one, so we better treat it well. Our bodies are ground zero for all that we do, whether we're helping others or helping ourselves. Degrees, family, wealth, fame, career: all are 100 percent meaningless to us if we're dead. But sadly, heart disease, type 2 diabetes, strokes, and cancer, most of which are caused by poor lifestyle choices, are killing over 50 million people every year. *Why?* Often because saturated fat–filled, cholesterol-laden, hormone- and antibiotic-infested animal products are so darn cheap and accessible. Thanks to junk, mistakenly called "food," we've created the first generation of adults who won't live as long as their parents. We'll talk more about the dark side of the food industry as we progress.

So, does a vegan diet ensure good health? No. And I'd be wary of anyone who tells you otherwise. Some vegans gorge on Cookie Dough Oreos, Unglazed Pop Tarts, and Spicy Sweet Chili Doritos and wash it all down with a high-fructose, phosphoric acid–packed Coke. *Vegan?* Shockingly, yes; all of it. However, unhealthy vegans are the *exception*. In fact, for many folks, the desire to go vegan begins with a stern warning from their doctor: switch to a healthy, whole food, plant-based diet, or have a heart attack. The incentive is the gift of good health, and it makes good sense! So stay tuned, because in Days 1 through 10, I'll walk you through the wonderful world of healthy vegan food, *step by step*, and show you how to make the switch from eating meat, eggs, and dairy to enjoying affordable, delicious, healthy, easy-to-make vegan cuisine.

BECAUSE WE LOVE ANIMALS

Some folks initially explore becoming vegan for health reasons, but at age twenty-three, and fresh out of college, good health was the last thing on my mind. For me, it was all about the animals. As you'll read in just a bit, my "road to vegan" was spurred by a fortuitous encounter that led me to learn how animals are used and abused on factory farms.

Although I was already a vegetarian, I was unknowingly hurting so many animals simply by eating their by-products. I hadn't thought about what happens to the chickens after they can no longer lay eggs. Nor the dairy cow mothers once they can no longer give milk. Or to the newborn male calves who can't give any milk at all. Most people believe that as long as the animal doesn't die to produce the product then all must be well—after all you're *just* having an egg, a glass of milk, or a slice of cheese, not a hamburger.

You won't find any graphic images in this book—we'll keep the journey as positive as possible—but I won't skirt the truth. I'll present the hard facts and set the record straight. The treatment of animals for our food, clothing, household products, cosmetics, and entertainment is nothing short of a horror story, and one that must be told. And it provides more than enough fodder for many to go vegan. In fact, most who go vegan and *stay* vegan do so for the animals. After all, if we can live a happy, healthy life without hurting them, why wouldn't we?

BECAUSE WE LOVE THE ENVIRONMENT

When I was twelve I tagged along with my girlfriend on a youth group camping trip. I wasn't religious, but any excuse to go to explore the woods worked for me. We went for a hike and as we were trotting down the trail, the minister asked us to stop and gather around to behold the beauty of an enormous mushroom. We had never seen anything like it before. It looked so sturdy and soft as velvet; the type you'd see in a children's fairy tale, one nice enough to be a home to a band of little elves. After admiring it for a few minutes, he said, "That's really something, isn't it?" and then gave it a big kick with his boot as he walked away.

The image of that perfect mushroom breaking into pieces as it was thrust into the air broke a little part of me as well. I know it was just a mushroom, but for me it was the first time I had ever witnessed, and internalized, the senseless and unnecessary destruction of our environment.

If you need resources from nature in order to have shelter, clothing, transportation, food, or any absolute necessities, that's understandable. After all, we need certain basics from our environment in order to survive. But to ruin the environment for no reason other than greed, selfishness, or apathy makes no sense at all. It's this same awareness of the senseless destruction of our environment caused by factory farming that inspires so many to go vegan. As we progress, we'll learn how eating animal products impacts our water, soil, air, oceans, rain forests, climate, and biodiversity. If you care about our environment, you'll really love how being vegan helps protect it, far more than driving an electric car or taking shorter showers.

There's a lot to think about here, but don't worry, this isn't a sprint; it's a marathon, with comfy shoes, yummy food, and plenty of time to rest and reflect. Over the next 21 days, you'll be getting new tips, tricks, and ideas to enable you to make super-easy daily changes that will blossom into wonderful lifelong habits. And you won't be alone. I'll be your mentor and your cheerleader every step of the way! No guilt, no shame, just positive advice and healthy energy to guide you through. And you couldn't have picked a better time to start.

From vegan festivals and cruelty-free cosmetics to vegan grocery stores and cruises, you've got it good. There's never been a better time to go vegan! Vegan sushi, vegan mayo, vegan hair salons, vegan magazines, vegan celebrities, vegan Doc Martens, vegan cupcakes, vegan restaurants in airports, vegan pumpkin lattes, vegan dating sites, vegan wedding planners, all-you-can-eat vegan buffets, vegan doctors, vegan beer, vegan nail polish; there's even vegan meringue for a vegan key lime pie! If you're thinking you're going to be alone and bored at home eating a slab of plain white tofu, you are in for a *big* surprise! It's no wonder so many of the folks I've helped have been able to make the switch. Vegan everything is everywhere!

So why should you trust little ole, five-foot, ninety-eight-pound me? Sure, I've got degrees and awards, but that's not enough. Far more important, over my twenty-eight-plus years of being vegan, I've kept an open mind, and an open ear. I've learned a lot about what helps and what *hinders* people who want to be vegan. You want positive reinforcement, not buckets of blame. You want simple suggestions, not complicated recipes or hard-to-find ingredients—all that you can figure out on your own, if and when you want. You want to be fit and healthy, and have an occasional sweet treat once in a while, too. You want to know what the best vegan foods are for special occasions, but also what's most affordable for every day. You want to learn from others who are already happy and healthy vegans, rather than be misguided by those who are neither. You don't want to start from scratch, scrambling around on the Internet trying to figure everything out all alone. Whether you live in vegan hot spots like Portland or Los Angeles, or in a small town in the middle of Tennessee, you want someone to guide you through, in the easiest possible way. If you fall, you want someone to say, "Hey, it's OK. Dust your knees off. Tomorrow's a new day!" And that's why I've written this book: to tell you everything there is to know about going vegan, exactly how *you* want to hear it, and how to put it into action—now!

Whether it's for your health, the animals, the environment, or a combo of all three, going vegan is affordable, easy, and fun. And you're not alone. Over 8 million Americans have already made the switch! Are you ready to get started? Follow me and let's go!

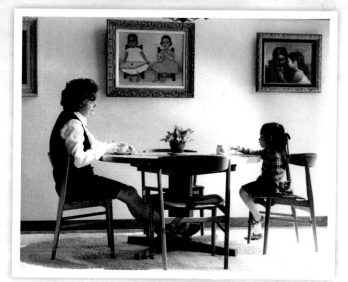

MY
Road to Vegan

We all traverse different paths throughout life's adventures, be it our careers, relationships or life goals. Some folks seem to meander effortlessly with grace (or so it seems), while for others, reaching what they want is akin to swimming through thick mud, in a winter parka, with boots on. Well, kick back, get comfortable, maybe grab a warm beverage or some fresh lemonade, and I'll start by sharing how I became vegan, and how I arrived right here: writing a book dedicated to you.

I never really thought about the importance of good food growing up. I just ate whatever my mother made and served to our small family. There were no Twinkies or Wonder Bread in the cupboards, no colas or orange pop in the fridge, and with the exception of one memorable occasion, never a TV dinner in the freezer. I was lucky in that sense. All meals were cooked from scratch and with great care, and until I became a teenager, I truly enjoyed them.

My mother was British and a master of traditional English fare: Yorkshire pudding, Shepherd's pie, roasted meats, creamy sauces, and other European recipes passed down through the generations. My Croatian father had an outsized sweet tooth, second only to my own. He was a ship captain during WWII and, since meat and fresh greens were limited at sea, he developed a preference for light-colored foods such as breads, potatoes, halibut, eggs, and pasta with butter. My mother always took this into account when cooking, and so although our meals were always tasty, they generally looked like food you'd find in a British Pub: heavy, with ribbons of brown and white.

As a child, my mother's comfort food was more than fine with me. I grew up in the small coastal town of Pacific Grove, California, where we were socked in with fog for most of the year. Locals are known for joking "I never knew a winter as cold as a summer in Pacific Grove," so any food that was warm and filling fit the ticket. Then one chilly evening our little West Highland terrier nudged my leg under the table hoping to coax me into tossing him a bit of meat from my dinner plate. This sneaky maneuver was nothing new; Angus knew he'd get a treat from me. But for some reason, this nudge was different; it triggered my mind to spin unlike ever before. I began to think, "How can it be OK to pet our dog under the table, while stabbing my fork into a cow atop it?" Why was I feeding a dog, while eating cow? How was this fair? Who made this rule? And most important, why did I follow it blindly?

And remember that one and only occasion when my mother bought a supply of TV dinners? A few days later I ate one and bit into a piece of chicken, and there it was: a bright purple-blue stringy vein. My teeth had snapped it and left a piece hanging on the bone. It hit me; this food called "chicken" was actually a real chicken, a once-living, breathing, with-a-heart-that-beat chicken. It was then that my thirteen-year-old brain also realized that liverwurst was actually made from someone's liver and that Thanksgiving dinner was celebrated around a dead bird. So many things my mother fed us had once been alive; I had just never fully processed it. Until then, I simply hadn't made the connection.

And so it was 1977, I was thirteen years old, and I didn't want to eat animals anymore. I didn't have any vegetarian friends or family, nor did I know of any vegetarian celebrities, athletes, or politicians, but it didn't matter; my mind was made up. I just ate the "sides" that were served with our family meals, and slowly but surely, realizing this wasn't just a phase, my mother made more meatless meals for me to eat. She knew not to use the meat spoon to stir anything I was eating, and baking my meal alongside or within a meat dish was a big no-no, too. I wasn't about to pick out my vegetables from a beef stew. And somehow a British meat-eating mother, a ship captain father who had a penchant for plain white meals and pastries, and their budding vegetarian daughter all managed to share in dinner together at the table every evening.

Our Westie's nudge also led me to question the status quo at school. My mother made me a lunch each day, so meals were never a problem, but in my freshman science class we studied genetics by raising our own little batch of fruit flies. We kept them in tiny baby food jars in the back of the classroom where we painstakingly documented the ratio of red eyes to white. On the last day of the experiment, my teacher instructed us to grab our jars and said he was going to pass around a rag wet with ether for us to place tightly over the opening of each jar. I didn't understand the purpose, so I asked him to explain, and he replied, "This is how we kill the flies; we're done with them." As I watched my fellow students take turns following his instructions, I became increasingly nervous as the rag made its way to my corner of the room. I decided to let my teacher know that I was going to let my fruit flies go outside instead. He told me, sternly, that if I did that, I'd be releasing my scientific experiment into the world, and I'd be responsible for adversely affecting our entire environment by letting them escape and that I did not have permission to leave the classroom. I returned to my desk for a few minutes while my classmates looked on. I was visibly upset and they were wondering what I was going to do. I, however, knew exactly what I was going to do. I waited patiently until no one was looking, and I snuck outside to set them all free, and I'm pretty sure the world isn't any worse off for it. A pattern of questioning those more powerful, while following my own moral compass, was starting to take shape.

Then it was off to UC Berkeley, where I would study the History of Science with more like-minded folks and where vegetarian food wasn't a novelty; it was a staple. There were none of the vegan bakeries and vegan specialty stores so abundant today, but there were more than enough vegetarian restaurants and food trucks to make me happy. During an elective for the California Public Interest Research Group (CALPIRG), I even created a pamphlet of all the healthy food sources in the city so that other students could easily find them.

Looking back, one would think I'd become vegan in Berkeley, but I didn't. At twenty-three, I moved to Los Angeles and became a substitute teacher. This choice gave me the freedom to make my own schedule while I tried to figure out which career I wanted to pursue. It also freed up my time and allowed me to participate in a few peaceful protests throughout the city, which led me to my second, and most fortuitous, enlightenment. A demonstration I attended at UCLA was winding down, and a girl who was visiting from Canada asked me if I wouldn't mind giving her a ride to her friend's house. I don't normally give strangers a lift home, but she seemed nice enough and had just spent the entire day marching and chanting to free cats from brain experiments, so I took my chances and obliged.

We hopped in my tiny '76 Honda Civic and I started to drive, making casual chit-chat along the way. We talked about why we love animals so much and why we don't eat them, and then she asked me something no one had ever asked me before: "Do you drink milk?" I had no idea where she was heading with the question, but I answered truthfully, "Yes. Don't you?" She then proceeded to tell me that by drinking milk, I was actually harming the animals just as much as by eating a burger, as the male dairy calves are sold to the veal industry where they spend their short, miserable lives in small metal crates, and the dairy mothers are ultimately killed after they can no longer give milk.

This friendly stranger continued to tell me about each animal product, and why she didn't eat any of them. She even told me she didn't eat honey. What could possibly be wrong with eating honey, I thought. She explained that her uncle had a bee farm in Canada and she saw firsthand how the bees were squished each time they put the giant lids back on the hives and that there was no avoiding it. By eating honey, she reasoned, we're killing bees, and we don't need to. "And that's why I'm vegan," she said. And by the time I dropped her off thirty minutes later, I was vegan, too. I said good-bye to the only vegan I had ever met or knew of, and I never saw her again. As my tiny car door closed, a new world opened.

From that point forward, I wanted to learn all that I could about the link between animals and our diet. I bought books, wrote to animal rights organizations for pamphlets, and went to libraries to do research. In the late '80s, like most folks, I didn't have Internet at home, so I'd use the Medline Database at medical school libraries to read journal abstracts. They were dense with medical terms, but I muddled through them. And the more I learned, the more I realized that my diet and lifestyle impacted so much more than my personal health and the animals. It also affected the environment, the economy, and social justice issues, too. I knew, and still believe, that by becoming vegan, I was helping everyone. It was the butterfly effect and I was more than ready to help it flutter onward.

After a brief time teaching high school history in East Los Angeles, I realized that although I enjoyed studying history in college, teaching it was another matter. If someone was facing an early death because they ate poorly, or consumed toxic water thanks to factory farms, historical facts in textbooks would be of little significance. I became convinced that understanding how to take care of oneself and the surrounding world should be the foundation of education. Once these basics were mastered, students could learn whatever they want. First and foremost, however, was to learn to be well.

Fueled by a newfound desire to become a high school health teacher, I went to the Los Angeles County Board of Education and studied their health books, took an exam, and earned a teaching credential in health sciences. Ironically, I was in the midst of a breakup and had stopped eating. Far from a role model of good health, and at only seventy-eight pounds, I was certain I'd never score a position as a health teacher, but my will was strong, and my mission great, and somehow I beat out the competition and landed a job at a local high school. Most of the students lived in poverty, either in nearby projects or were bused in as overflow from inner-city schools, and needless to say, the school had its share of chaos. My list of unhappy moments include having to run for help when I saw someone step out of a car on campus with a gun (and a baby in the backseat), and putting my hand in feces on my classroom doorknob. If there was ever a school that needed a few extra seeds of respect and compassion, it was there.

I started each day by writing the word *RESPECT* on the chalkboard and reminded students that health was about respecting your bodies, inside and out. It wasn't just important to eat well and exercise, but to also respect the natural environment and people surrounding them as well. I covered up all the drab surplus gray-green paint with purple, replaced the old food pyramid charts with plant-based posters, and decorated my podium with over a dozen inspirational bumper stickers, with "Speak your mind, even if your voice shakes" front and center. I was determined to have my classroom be a center of freedom of thought and creativity, where one could become inspired to make the world a better place.

I tried to illuminate the really fun aspects of being vegan, too. I took my students on a field trip to The Gentle Barn, an animal sanctuary where they could meet, pet, and hug the kind of animals that adults had told them to eat. I bought a wok for the classroom so

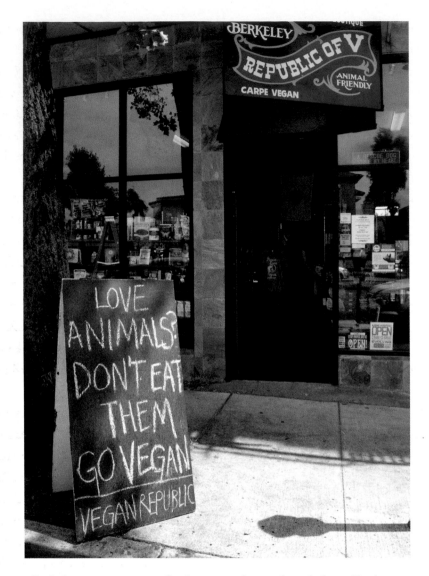

when I talked about a new vegan food item, such as tofu or kale, we'd whip up samples and enjoy them. And we even planned and held a vegan Earth Day Health Festival in the spring for the entire campus and community.

My work on food policy garnered local, national, and international interest, and I soon found myself traveling across the state and country to attend conferences and to share my thoughts on healthy living, always trying to encourage folks to consider going vegan along the way. Even when I received the national Healthy School Hero Award in Washington, D.C., sponsored by the National Dairy Council, I took the one thousand dollar award and gave it to the Physician's Committee for Responsible Medicine's campaign to get dairy milk out of public schools. (Thanks for the dough, Big Ag!)

Shortly thereafter, People for the Ethical Treatment of Animals asked if I would lead their education department, and I accepted. I packed the car with my cats and a few belongings and drove from Los Angeles to Norfolk, Virginia. I soon found myself absorbed in animal rights more than ever before. From begging a school board to rescue a pig at the county fair in Miami to speaking on the evening news on behalf of fish in Malibu, I was determined to be a voice for the voiceless and change the world.

Unfortunately, my father died the day I arrived in Norfolk, and within a few weeks, I received a call from my significant other of five years that he was no longer following me to Virginia. Yep, by phone. My life turned upside down, and only got worse—much worse—after that. I decided to head back to California, where I was surrounded by familiar faces, but my life was at its lowest low, somber fodder for another book, another day. I was completely lost and was forced to restructure my life entirely. I immersed myself in law school, started writing *My Vegan Journal*, and began a Facebook page where I could inspire and help people transition to becoming vegan across the world. Just as when I entered that interview at seventy-eight pounds, I was determined to get my life back on track, and help others while doing so.

My life has had its ups and downs, but I've never doubted my decision to become vegan. In fact, I'm not even sure I can call it a decision anymore. I'm vegan because I've evolved. Just like Cro-Magnons evolved into Homo sapiens. It's just who you are; it's who I am. I'm vegan and I can't imagine knowingly hurting an animal ever again. But I do know what it's like to face those hard situations, where you feel like you're all alone, and no one understands what being vegan is all about. I've had to tell my doctor on more than one occasion what a vegan diet entails. I've been the only vegan at celebrations. I've fallen in love with someone who ate meat (and married him!). And I've had to sit down at dinner and see those disappointed faces when I let my in-laws know I wouldn't eat the meal they worked so hard to "veganize" because although they used dairy-free butter, it still contained oil from fish.

Uncomfortable situations? No doubt. But would I change a thing? No way. Feeling alone or misunderstood is a small price to pay in order to help reduce the horrific suffering in the world. I can't complain. I'm happy, healthy, energetic, and so gladdened to see that veganism is more visible than ever before. But most important, I am ready to inspire *you* to take the plunge yourself! It's not a challenge; it's an adventure. So, let's go!

Thought FOR THE Day

There are about 795 million people in the world who are hungry. That's 1 in 9 people . . . more than the *entire* population of the United States, Canada, and the European Union combined. The grain we feed to animals could feed nearly 350 *billion* people. If we stop raising animals for meat, and give people the grain instead, everyone would have plenty of food. 'Tis true. People can feast or famish; it's up to me, and you.

Setting a Date

You can be successful going vegan no matter when you start, but boy, can you make your life a whole lot easier if you pick the right time! Can you imagine being a big meat eater and deciding to go vegan the week of Thanksgiving, or right before a wedding? Is it *possible*? Of course! Easy? Probably not. How about going vegan just before Christmas, and finding yourself forced to look happy when you unwrap that woolen cable knit sweater from Aunt Marge? Or opening that box of See's Candy and having to eat that obligatory "*Mmmm!* Thank-you!" piece. Yikes.

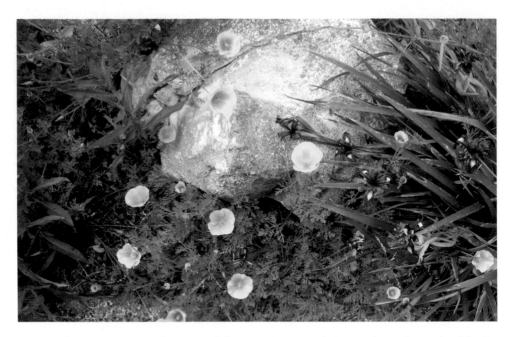

Don't get me wrong. In terms of the environment, the animals, and your health, the best time to go vegan is right this second. If I had my druthers, I'd waive a magic wand. Poof! You're vegan! But try to think of this as a relationship you want to nurture; one that will last forever. You don't want a quick romp in the sack, or a two-week fling. You want *true love*, not a flash in the pan. So let's make a plan, Stan! Just keep these things in mind:

THERE IS NOT, NOR WILL THERE EVER BE, A *PERFECT* DATE TO START.
It's true; if you're waiting for the perfect time, you'll likely be waiting forever. There's a good, great, right, better, and even an absolutely phenomenally fantastic time to go vegan. However, if you're waiting for the *perfect* something or other it's usually just a thinly veiled excuse to avoid it. *There is no perfect time.* I experienced this while writing, or rather *attempting* to write, this book. I'm so incredibly grateful and excited to have the opportunity to write, but boy, did I spin around in circles waiting for the *perfect* time to start. I first blamed my procrastination on my crappy coffee (who can write while sipping a weak cup of Joe?), then it was my computer (who can type with annoying Windows 8?), then it was my five-dollar, secondhand chair (stop making me fidgety, ya stupid, cheapo chair!). I kept replacing one thing after another, creating excuse upon excuse, assuring myself that I couldn't possibly write a book until I had all the proper tools, supplies, snacks, beverages, lighting, clothes, ambient noise, and weather.

Turns out it wasn't any of these things that was holding me back; it was my "mind-set." I'm still sitting on my crappy chair, but it has a comfy old folded blanket on it, and alas, I'm writing. As Harvard School of Education professor Lisa Lahey points out, "The mind-set is the thing that has to change in order to alter the behavior." And the same is true when you're transitioning to a healthy vegan lifestyle. You really don't need much other than a little advice, a pinch of inspiration, and most important *the will* to do it. All the gizmos, gadgets, space, time, and money won't get you from "excuse-itarian" to full-fledged vegan if you don't have the proper mind-set: you want to be vegan, and darn it, you're making it happen. And I'm writing this book. My mind is set! As Canadian author and environmental activist Margaret Atwood said, "If I waited for perfection, I would never write a word." So, let's do this!

Bottom Line: You don't need "stuff" or perfect circumstances to go vegan. If you *really* want to go vegan, you can and *will* go vegan, so drop your excuses off right here, right now—thump! There's a one-bag limit on this trip, and you're filling it up with yummy food!

OK, grab your handy-dandy calendar. If you don't have one you want to scribble on, you can easily print a free one online or use the one on your computer. Let's start flipping through the dates and figure out the best day for you to start.

- Take note of all the holidays, weddings, and any other grandiose festivities that center around food. You'll likely want to avoid starting on your new adventure on those dates, including a few days after them, too. Tempting leftovers will be lurking, begging you to come hither.

- Take note of any business trips or vacations you'll be taking. I'll show you how to stay vegan while traveling; it's a cinch, but for the first few days, it will be easier if you're close to home sweet home.

- Any big exams, interviews, or super-important meetings around the bend? Let's not mix the first few days of our beautiful new lifestyle with events that are likely to be highly stressful.

- Coming down with the flu? Day one of your period? Let's skip those days, too. Sure, you can go vegan when your uterus is contracting or you're sneezing your head off, but I suggest letting any preexisting storms pass. Our vegan cruise wants to leave the dock with a rosy forecast of sunshine and smooth sailing. All aboard!

OK, so we've crossed out a lot of rocky start dates on our calendar. Now let's look at some appealing ones that will inspire you to get started on the right foot!

NEW YEAR'S DAY: Yep, it's an oldie but goodie! Make a New Year's resolution to go vegan. A new year, a new you!

EARTH DAY: I can't think of a better present you could give her. By going vegan, you'll be saving so much of our planet's natural resources! Earth Day is April 22, and what's so cool is that there are hundreds of Earth Day celebrations throughout the world that week, which often have lots of fantastic vegan food and activities.

VALENTINE'S DAY: The day of love. In the words of children's author Ruby Roth, "Vegan is love." And it's true. When you're vegan, you're showing how deeply you care about animals and the environment. And when you ditch eating animal products, you're likely to ensure that big, loving heart of yours is a healthy one, too!

THE WEEKEND: For most, Saturday and/or Sunday is a day off from work or school, but if you have an untraditional schedule, try to pick a day where you have the least amount of commitments. More free time usually means less stress, and provides extra time to dash out to the grocery store if you want to, or to look up fun vegan stuff on the Internet, or to simply have extra time to kick back and relax reading this book! Your day "off" is a great time to start!

OK, so did you pick a good date to start? Great! Write it down! Now let's seal the deal. Here are a few tidbits just to make sure you're off to a solid kickoff:

PUT SOME THOUGHT INTO WHETHER OR NOT ANNOUNCING THAT YOU'RE GOING VEGAN WILL BE AN ASSET, OR A DETRIMENT.
Take a moment to reflect and figure out if you reach goals easier with a little outside pressure, or if you're best left alone. We're all different. I generally work best under pressure, especially if I feel like others are counting on me to do something. If you're like me, you'll want to memorialize your commitment to going vegan and perhaps announce that you're going vegan to someone who will be supportive of you. In 2015 a Dominican University study showed that those who shared their goals with a friend were 33 percent more successful than those who didn't.[1] The data also demonstrated a positive effect on those who felt accountable, so you might want to let a friend know that you're going to

send them a short e-mail or text each day to let them know how you're doing; or time permitting, you can have a quick chat. If you don't have a friend or family member whom you think will be supportive, check out some of my support group suggestions in the "vegan resources" section. And you can always write to me, too!

Although there may be some benefit to sharing your new vegan adventure with a good friend, announcing it to the masses might be a bad thing. According to NYU psychology professor Peter Gollwitzer, those who kept their intentions private were more likely to achieve them than those who made them public and were acknowledged by others. The theory goes that once you've told people of your intentions, it gives you a "premature sense of completeness."[2] NBA champion John Salley, who switched to a vegan diet because he wanted his "body and libido back" to how he felt in his younger years[3], thinks it's easier to become vegan if you *don't* announce it to anyone and advises folks to just "focus on yourself . . . being conscious of your surroundings, body, and food addictions first."[4] So, for some folks, keeping things on the down low gives them a leg up.

But hey, this is the age of unabashed selfies and video broadcasts of our each and every move. If you think you'll be more accountable if you blurt out "I'm going vegan!" to the world, by all means, post it as your Facebook status, "tweet" it to your followers, or write a blog post about your experience, day by day, for all to read and enjoy. Just know that once it's out there, it's *out there*. You might also get a few notoriously irritating "*Mmmm*, bacon!" responses, but that's OK. I've been vegan for over twenty-eight years and I still get those boring, wake-me-up-when-you-say-something-original remarks, but I handle them gracefully now, and you'll be able to as well. No sweat. So stay tuned; I've got your back.

Bottom line: We're all different, so pause, think, and do what you think will work best for you!

DON'T WORRY; BE HAPPY.

Going vegan is fun; it truly is! For the most part, the vegan people that I know are the happiest, most interesting, energized, welcoming folks I've ever met. And our conversations often revolve around cute animals, new restaurants, and scrumptious food! What's not to love about *that*? Yes, there are a few cranky pants and Debbie downers out there who seem to bicker over everything, but hey, every group of people has them. You'll find that most vegans are super supportive and more than happy to help you if you ask. And you know what? What's the worst thing that could happen if you fall off the vegan wagon and grab a little chunk of ole' dairy cheese? Or cave in to Aunt Millie's deviled eggs? You'll probably feel a bit guilty, but that's about it.

Bottom Line? Don't stress. You're going to be fine!

KNOW THAT I LOVE YOU.

Yep, it's a little mushy—OK, it's *a lot* of mushy—but it's true. I love you. I can barely watch the news these days because there is so much sadness in this world and, more often than not, I end up teary-eyed, and look away. But just knowing that someone, *somewhere*, is out there trying their best to transition to a compassionate lifestyle gives me so much hope, and I love you for that. You're the pen to my paper, the peanut butter to my jelly, the nutritional yeast to my vegan mac 'n cheese. Allowing me to have this wondrous opportunity to help guide you on your new adventure makes me so very happy. Even if *just one of you* decides to live your life in a kinder, gentler way, I will be overjoyed. Know that I'm so appreciative for each and every little step you take over the next 21 days, even if they're sprinkled with stumbles. You rock my vegan socks, and I am smitten.

Bottom Line? You've got company, chickadee! You're not alone. I'm covering you up in a soft, warm, cruelty-free blanket of unconditional love, so snuggle up!

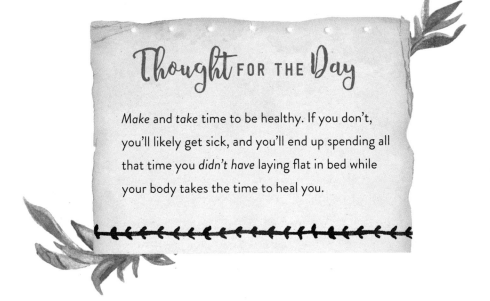

Thought FOR THE Day

Make and *take* time to be healthy. If you don't, you'll likely get sick, and you'll end up spending all that time you *didn't have* laying flat in bed while your body takes the time to heal you.

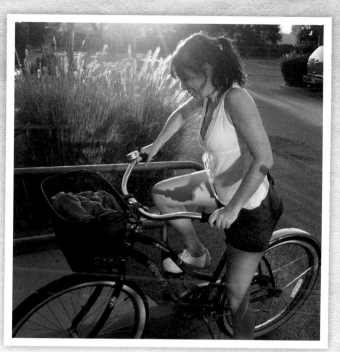

THE 21-Days-TO-A Vegan Road Map

The 21-day plan to becoming vegan is a pretty straightforward one. I've already begun planting little seeds of compassion in the past few chapters, and they're about to grow and flourish. As you read on, you'll find all sorts of information and inspiration to help you get into the vegan groove. I've tossed in a few easy recipes, too. However, this *isn't a cookbook*; it's a game changer. It's a medley of vegan food for thought, and all the tips and tools you'll need to get into the proper mind-set to change your life, and change the world, in a very easy and enjoyable way.

Now that you've picked your start date, all you need to do is read one chapter each day, and do three things:

- Complete the Goal for the Day.
- Write in your journal.
- Review your daily checklist at the end of each chapter.

The goal for the day is always explained clearly at the beginning of the chapter, and it's very simple and brief. We'll start off by taking a peek in our pantry, fridge, and freezer and organize things a bit. Heaven knows they could probably use a cleaning whether or not you want to go vegan, right? Mine sure do. Then we'll replace the simplest of things in our food, like ditching dairy cream in our morning coffee or smoothie, and gradually learn how to switch out meat, eggs, and fish, replacing them with much healthier fare. Then it's off to look around our home to ensure it reflects comfort and kindness for all. We'll turn on the closet light, too, because we all know cruelty is never in fashion. Our bubble baths, showers, and mani-pedis will all become relaxing indulgences that pamper without harm. And then we'll make sure our entertainment and holidays inspire joy to the world, rather than dark despair. You'll also find a few extra words of compassion and tips sprinkled throughout from my vegan friends, just to keep things extra "vegantastic." All it takes is 21 days. You can do it!

As you get into the swing of things, you'll be encouraged to enhance the voyage by writing about each day in your vegan journal. It can be a paper journal that you keep by your bedside, or if you prefer, an electronic version—jotting notes on an iPad will work well, too. It can even be as simple as a dozen pieces of binder paper stapled together. You don't need anything fancy. Whatever you decided to use, just know that you don't have to worry about presentation; no one will see if your sentences are complete or accurate, so just write freely and often. Even just a little list of thoughts each day will be helpful. Here are a few things to keep in mind as you write in your journal:

GOALS

If you're struggling with something as you transition to becoming vegan, writing it down will help you articulate exactly what it is, and will help you focus on improving whatever is hindering you. Getting into an easy routine by writing a little something each day usually helps folks with accountability, no matter what they're trying to accomplish.

PROGRESS

Writing each day helps you see just how far you've come, especially if you hit a bump in the road. You might stumble a bit one day, but hey, there's probably many days that were wonderful successes, and by writing them down, you'll have them all at your fingertips to read over; and they'll remind you of how great you're doing in the big scheme of things. A journal can help you stay positive, and that's important. You'll also be able to document difficulties so you don't repeat them, such as "Note to self: Do *not* walk down that candy aisle again; next time, straight to the grains and produce!"

THE "WHY" OF IT ALL

Writing down all the reasons *why* you're doing something really helps remind you of the purpose behind the action, and that will help propel you along. As you read this book, if you come across something that makes you sad (such as how animals are treated) or something that makes you angry (such as how you've been duped by certain government agencies and companies), or really surprises you (there's *fish* in my orange juice?) writing down a few facts or thoughts about it will help set things in stone, so that you'll remember *why* the simple steps you're taking are so darn important. You'll likely find a few inspirational quotes that you'll want to jot down, too, and perhaps share with others one day as you plant seeds of compassion of your own.

IT'S HEALTHY

It's no secret that most health educators ask that their students keep a food journal at some point so they can see exactly how healthy, or more likely, *unhealthy*, they're eating. Keeping a log of daily events helps you see your habits and create healthy changes. And for those who want to lose weight, a journal can help with that, too! A recent Kaiser Permanente study showed that those who kept a journal on what they ate lost twice as much weight as those who didn't.[1] It was the process of reflecting on what they eat that helped them become aware of their habits, enabling them to transition to a healthier diet, with more fruits and vegetables. Makes sense, right? With a journal, it's easy to keep track of all sorts of health issues like weight, energy, stamina, acne, etc. You're likely going to have loads of wonderful news to report on how you're feeling, so go ahead and write all those good things down.

I think this is perhaps the *most* important reason to keep a vegan journal. You're about to learn about so many new and yummy foods, ways to cook, places to shop, websites to visit, books to read, and fun things to do and you'll need a place to jot them all down. You'll also want to scribble down a few things you want to avoid. What if you're in the store reading an ingredients list and you can't remember the sneaky little word food manufacturers use for beaver butt? Or you forget the name of that cruelty-free shampoo you wanted to try out, or the day and time of your local farmers' market? Rather than dragging this book around, just jot down the important things you want to remember in your little journal and take that along with you. It can hold your recipes and grocery lists, too, because goodness knows, it's no fun getting home only to find you forgot the oats for your overnight oats, or worse, that tub of cashew milk ice cream for your movie night. Don't let it happen. Take your journal. And here are a few morsels of advice, based on my twenty-eight-plus years of being vegan:

꩜ Know that you can never be a perfect vegan, so don't be too hard on yourself.

If you've grown accustomed to scoring *perfect* work reviews, earning *perfect* scores on exams, having *perfect* organizational skills, or can nail a high E flat like the finest coloratura soprano on any given day—congrats! I am kale green with envy! Just know it's *impossible* to be 100 percent vegan. I repeat: it is impossible to be 100 percent vegan. That's both good and bad. It relieves a bit of the pressure (*whew!*), but it's also a bummer because, ideally, it would be great if there was a way to avoid harming anyone and everyone, *all the time*, wouldn't it? Sadly, there are animal products in our car tires and computer screens, and mice and gophers are inevitably destroyed while harvesting our grain. A chunk of our income tax goes toward antiquated animal research, as well as toward the subsidy of corn and soy for Big Ag to grow and sell to factory farms. We inadvertently kill bugs and butterflies as we drive, as we bike, and as we walk. One day you will accidentally buy and eat an animal product in a meal you *thought* was vegan, and in the flurry of a medical emergency, you might even be willing to do whatever the surgeon suggests to save your life. So as you transition to a compassionate lifestyle, just remember, being vegan means you're doing the very best you can do to cause the *least* amount of pain and suffering to others. Being vegan *doesn't* mean you're ending *all* suffering, because, sadly, at this moment in time, it's impossible. I'm not perfect; you're not perfect; no one is perfect. So if you normally take pride in being a Perfect Patty, don't drive yourself batty here. OK? Just do your *best*. And if anyone ever finds a planet where we can actually all be *perfect* vegans, you better save me a ticket on the first rocket ship out.

∾ Know that every new moment provides an opportunity to do better than the last.

Going vegan is easy; you *can* do this. But, if by chance, you have a little "whoops" moment with a bit of non-vegan food, don't fret. You don't need to wait until next month, next week, or even the next day to get back on track. The opportunity to start anew awaits you at the very next meal. I'm not trying to give you an easy out, or forgive you here. Mistakes are mistakes, and when it comes to harming animals, the environment, or your own health, mistakes can *really* hurt. Just know that a weak moment of willpower or the curse of the crazy can hit even the best of us. I remember being at my best friend's Halloween party about fifteen years ago after a really horrible breakup, and I didn't know up from down. In the lingo of wellness expert Kris Carr, my doomed relationship was my "shit pickle" and I was a mess. I had already been vegan for over a decade, but I was so angry and upset with myself and the world that the crazies set in and I grabbed a big bowl of Reese's Peanut Butter Cups intended for trick-or-treaters and I gobbled them all up. Did I throw in the towel, right then and there and give up on being vegan? Heck no! I dried my tears, pulled myself together, and I've never eaten a crappy antibiotic-infused cow-boob-juice chocolate peanut butter cup again. So if you get into a pickle, it's no big dill (hee-hee), just dust off your knees, and start anew. There's a lesson to be learned in our mistakes, so take note, adjust accordingly, and move on.

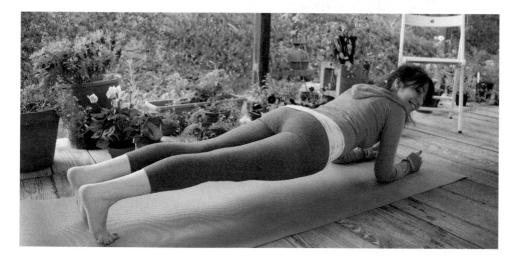

ᐕ Know that the road to the happiest, healthiest you goes far beyond being vegan.

As you begin to enjoy delicious vegan food and embark on a beautiful compassionate lifestyle, don't forget that being healthy and happy is a result of taking good care of yourself—far beyond the foods you eat and the clothes you wear. Most folks notice a huge difference in their energy, alertness, and stamina pretty quickly once they switch to a healthy plant-based diet. After just a few months, singer songwriter Jason Mraz went as far as saying eating a plant-based diet not only made him stronger, fitter, healthier, and more productive, it even made him "a lot better in bed."[2] Hey, now. But here's the reality: a lot of important factors contribute to our wellness. As we meander together through the 21 days, if you find that you're not quite as happy or healthy as you thought you would be, consider perusing the following list and adjust accordingly.

THE HAPPY HEALTHY LIST

SLEEP Make sure you're getting enough, which, according to the National Institutes of Health, is seven to eight hours each night for most adults.[3] Studies show that the lack of sleep not only makes us cranky, but can make folks gain lots of unwanted weight and be more susceptible to catching a cold.[4] Sound, adequate sleep makes us feel better and stay healthier. Get those extra z's, please.

RELATIONSHIPS Let go of the unhealthy ones. After all, you can't make room for the good ones if the bad ones are sucking up all of your time and energy. It's easier said than done, I know, but life is too short to be with poopie people. *Let them go.* Surround yourself with folks who are supportive, make you laugh, and inspire you to be the best you can be.

EXERCISE Exercise reduces our stress and anxiety, increases our energy, and just fifteen minutes a day has been shown to increase life expectancy by three years.[5] You don't need a gym membership or fancy running shoes; just move around. Movement can be as simple as walking up and down a flight of stairs, doing jumping jacks, dancing to your favorite tunes, or jogging around the block. Just wiggle around and get that body moving.

CAREER Eating well won't turn crappy coworkers into saints, nor ho-hum work into your dream job. If you're in a rut and miserable at work, take a beat and look into new opportunities. It's never too late to go back to school, or to follow your heart when it comes to your career. Do what you love, and if you can't do it right this second, make a plan to get there. Just knowing you're in the process of making a positive change will help you feel better.

COMMUNITY Get involved and connect with others. When folks don't feel like they're part of a community, they can feel alone, depressed, and uninspired. If you feel isolated, consider volunteering, joining a meet-up group, being part of a book club, or joining an online support group with those who share a common interest. Consider taking a community college course, or checking out free events at the public library. A sense of community involvement motivates us and lifts our spirits.

SOLITUDE Unplug and unwind. I can't emphasize this one enough. In this hectic rush-rush world that just seems to keep spinning us faster and faster, it's imperative that we detach from stress every now and then and just spend some time alone. Consider taking a break from social media a few times a year, too. You'll be pleasantly surprised by how good it feels. Take a few minutes each day to sit alone outside and simply take it all in: the beauty and wonder of it all. Every day may not be good, but there's something good in every day; you just need to make time to find it and enjoy it. Sit still. Breathe in the good. Exhale the bad. And relax.

OK, sweet peas, here are a few things to look forward to!

A HEALTHIER DIET Know that the better you eat, the more you'll crave foods that are good for you. In the beginning of your transition to becoming a happy, healthy vegan you might find yourself enjoying lots of highly processed and packaged vegan foods, and that's OK. Just know that the more you eat fresh fruits, veggies, legumes, nuts, seeds, and grains, the more you'll want them. It may take a little while, but one day down the road, a crispy, sweet apple will likely become more desirable than a sugary candy bar. You'll soon want a bag of cashews or almonds over a bag of salty MSG-coated chips. And a perfect avocado (ooh la la!) will make your mouth water as much as any chunk of cheese ever has. I know it sounds crazy, but I don't even miss cheese. I kid you not. As time goes on, if you eat good food, you'll *keep* eating good food, and you'll want more of it, so don't be afraid to branch out and try new whole foods, even those you used to loathe as a kid. I couldn't stand Brussels sprouts; now I love them. My husband used to hate beets and zucchini; now he can't get enough. And we eat tomatoes from the farmers' market in the car like we just scored a big bag of Halloween candy, before we even leave the parking lot. There's such an abundance of fresh, nutritious, whole foods to enjoy. Go out there and gobble them up.

THE JOY OF HOME COOKING Know that cooking at home will make your transition to becoming vegan easier *and* healthier. There's just something about being in control of the food you're eating that makes it extra good, for your taste buds *and* your health, even if you're not a master chef. And here's why:

- **INGREDIENTS**: When you cook at home, you control the exact ingredients in the meal. You don't have to worry about someone using fish sauce without telling you, or a chunk of mystery meat falling into your burrito. You can make your vegan Thai iced tea without yellow dye #6 and you don't have to worry about "today's special" being food that was spoiling the day before. You also get to season to taste, and use healthier sugars that you enjoy. My sweet tooth loves to cash in on this benefit! Who knows exactly what's in that bowl of soup at the Main Street diner? Or how long it's been sitting in the pot. Seize the stove, and whenever possible, whip it up yourself.

- **PROPORTIONS**: When you cook at home, you control the proportions in your meal. This is really helpful for those who are trying to lose weight, or for those who want extra nutrients. For example, you can sprinkle B_{12} fortified nutritional yeast on just about anything savory at home, or add flaxseeds to smoothies for those important omega-3s. You can make your plate heavy on the fresh greens, and lighter on the processed pasta or bread. You can also reduce, or skip, the oil and salt. Many chefs don't care what's healthy; they just serve it up, as instructed, with what's on hand. When *you're* in the kitchen, you can make sure every snack and meal is a healthy one.

- **ORGANIC VERSUS CONVENTIONAL**: When you cook at home, you control which produce is organic and which is conventional. For example, I try to avoid conventional apples, peaches, strawberries, and tomatoes because they're notorious for being heavily contaminated with pesticides (you'll find out more on Day 3!). Unless a restaurant is 100 percent organic, which is rare, you're stuck eating produce that you might normally avoid if eating at home.

- **OPPORTUNITIES TO INSPIRE**: When you cook at home, you have the opportunity to inspire loved ones to join in on the experience, and get healthy! If you're the only one in your home that's going vegan, seize the opportunity to have family members or significant others help you out in the kitchen. Consider guiding kids safely through the cooking process, too! When kids are involved with the cooking, researchers found they not only increased their consumption of fruits, vegetables, and dietary fiber, but developed a greater willingness to try new foods.[6] Perhaps invite your kids to measure ingredients, wash produce, and hand-mix batters and sauces. Bring in your significant other to help out with the chopping, baking, and stovetop cooking. Just think of how much time you'll have to enlighten them on all the benefits of going vegan as they're washing those leaves of romaine. Make the kitchen your creative classroom, have some fun, and get healthy together!

☙ **CLEAN FOOD**: When you cook at home, you can control how sanitary your environment is, and that's important. According to the Centers for Disease Control, roughly 1 in 6 Americans get sick from a food-borne illness annually. That's about 48 million people, and a heck of a lot of toilet paper. Food-borne illnesses account for a whopping 128,000 patients being hospitalized each year, and 3,000 deaths, too! I got what was likely food poisoning at a food expo a few years back, and awoke at 3:00 A.M. the next morning with severe stomach pains. As you can probably imagine, the next hour or so in the bathroom was pretty ugly, and we'll leave it at that. I swore I'd never go back to that food expo again, but you get to sample hundreds of vegan products making their debut, so I still go and take my chances. Free vegan food? Count me in! But now I'm far less excited about dining out at restaurants that serve animal products. Most food-borne illnesses come from the mishandling and consumption of raw meat, and considering a *single* hamburger can contain the body parts of over 100 different cows—who lived in horrifically unsanitary conditions—it's easy to understand why meats host so many pathogens.[7] Sure there's always a chance you'll bring produce that's contaminated with animal feces into the house, but when you cook at home, you have far more power to make sure your kitchen is clean. Or, in my kitchen, that would be "clean enough."

A LIFESTYLE THAT'S AS AFFORDABLE AS IT IS HEALTHY Know that you don't need to have a lot of money to be vegan. If I had a nickel for every time I heard someone say, "It's just too expensive to be vegan," I'd probably have enough moolah to buy about three dozen vegan cupcakes. Celebrities often have vegan chefs, vegan recipes often call for pricey ingredients from specialty stores or items that have to be shipped from far away, and vegan restaurants often cater to the foo-foo shoo-shoo crowd. Well, listen up: you don't need to be rich to be vegan, in fact you don't even have to be in the "shrinking middle class." You can be a starving student, or on unemployment, or just flat-out broke, and *still* be vegan. So sit tight, and when we get to Day 9: Fast, Cheap, and Easy, I'll show you how to enjoy the best of what being vegan has to offer, whether you travel by foot or by yacht, live in a penthouse or the projects. Going vegan doesn't take a lot of money; it's what's in your heart that counts, not your pocketbook.

Thought FOR THE Day

Life is full of twists and turns. If there's one thing that's certain, it's that *nothing* is certain. Just follow your heart, and see where you land. It's the journey that matters, not the destination.

DAY 1

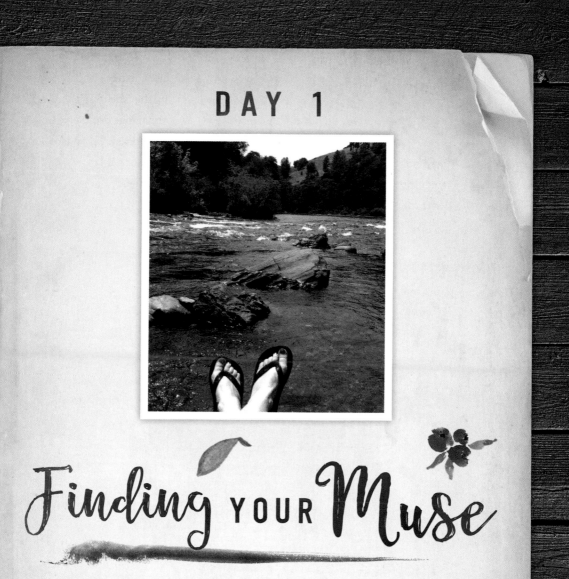

Finding YOUR Muse

GOAL FOR THE DAY: Discover and memorialize
what inspires you to become vegan.

Fifteen years ago when Twitter Cofounder Biz Stone took his wife to visit Farm Sanctuary in upstate New York for her birthday, he "stared right into the eyes of one of these big beautiful cows" and said, "Whoa, you're like a real life earthling." He made the connection and from that moment on, he and his wife have been "happy vegans." She cooks their vegan meals while he reads the classics to her in the kitchen. They're in it for the animals.

Titanic and *The Terminator* series director, James Cameron, and his wife Suzy Amis Cameron, transitioned to a plant-based diet after watching the documentary *Forks Over Knives*. Suzy said the "major eye-opener" for them was "the connection between food and the environment." They had always felt strongly about protecting the environment, but after watching the film and learning how much water, grain, and land it takes to produce animal products, they realized "you can't call yourself an environmentalist if you're still consuming animals. You just can't." They're in it for the environment.

John Robbins, whose uncle cofounded Baskin-Robbins Ice Cream, went vegan after seeing the results of eating lots of, you guessed it: ice cream. He noticed that his family was neither healthy, nor happy, and this inspired his desire "to find a different way of living that was more respectful of his body." Robbins walked away from his inheritance and his family's ice cream cone–shaped swimming pool, moved to the mountains and decided to enjoy a healthy vegan lifestyle instead. He leaped in for the health benefits.

No matter what you're in it for, being vegan is more important now than ever before. As the global population balloons toward a predicted 9.1 billion people by 2050, the consensus is that the Standard American Diet, appropriately abbreviated SAD, is *not* sustainable. We, as a species, simply cannot survive on our current course. Even the United Nations is urging a "substantial worldwide change, away from animal products" to save the world from hunger, poverty, and massive environmental destruction.[1]

The USDA, historically known for *supporting* the meat and dairy industries via billion-dollar subsidies, recently ditched the antiquated food pyramid and replaced it with a food *plate*, which recommends that people eat *less animal products*, and more food from plants in order to promote wellness. It's no surprise considering the state of our nation's health. Approximately 12.7 million kids and 78.6 million adults in the U.S. are obese. Not just overweight, but *obese*. Much of this excess weight is caused by gorging on a daily spread of saturated fat–filled, cholesterol-laden animal products. Folks have been suckered in for decades by manipulative and misleading ads that bombard our TVs, billboards, radio stations, Internet, grocery stores, fast-food joints, and magazines at each and every turn. Diabetes, cardiovascular disease, hypertension, and many cancers also flourish with our SAD diet, but all of these killers can be reduced and often *reversed* by eating a whole foods plant-based diet.[2]

And if avoiding an environmental catastrophe, or preventing an early trip to your final resting place isn't enough impetus to go vegan, compassion most certainly is. The most comfortable pillow is that of a clear conscience. We can live a happy, healthy life without causing harm to others. And there's certainly nothing *humane* about needlessly taking the life away from someone who doesn't want to die. The knife in the open meadow is just as sharp as the blade on the factory farm. Other animals feel pain and love just as people do. As extra incentive, researchers are now finding that being compassionate doesn't just improve the lives of others; it helps our *own* well-being, too. The secret to lasting happiness doesn't lie in the things we buy or achieve, but rather in what we give of ourselves, quite simply: the gifts of time, love, and thoughtfulness. Caring about others distracts us from intense self-focus. When we think of the suffering of animals and strive to help them, it puts our bad day in traffic or long wait at the post office into perspective. When we focus on living a life in a way that eases the pain of others, we become energized and our attention is diverted to helping those in need, rather than festering on the little thorns in our side.

Everyone needs a source of inspiration when they embark on a life goal, and going vegan is no exception. In this chapter, you need to identify who, or what, will light that fire and keep you moving forward even when you want to abandon ship. Maybe it's a famous environmental activist who, against all odds, prevailed in their goal to create a better world, such as Julia Butterfly Hill. Julia lived in a 1,500 year-old, 180-foot redwood tree named "Luna" for over two years so that loggers wouldn't chop it down. Two years *in the tree*, to save the tree! Sure makes chowing down on a juicy marinated portobello burger to spare a cow seem rather easy in comparison. Or perhaps a vegan celebrity, such as Mayim Bialik aka "Amy" from *The Big Bang Theory*, can inspire you. Did you know that the blueberry pies in Season 6's hysterical pie-eating contest are all vegan? Or perhaps strong and steadfast vegan, TV journalist Jane Velez-Mitchell, who knows peace for the world starts "on your plate."[3] Or maybe funny guy Steve-O floats your boat. He's one fearless vegan! And there's the incredibly fit world champion ice-skater, Meagan Duhamel. Did you know she wears non-leather ice skates, too?

Perhaps someone closer to home provides that drive, a special loved one who is already vegan, or someone who you want to stay healthy for (although your good health might be motivation enough by itself!). Or maybe someone you're dating can inspire you. I remember years ago, when I was studying for the Law School Admissions Test, I was dating a supersmart law student named Kenny, who my friend referred to as "out of my league," because he was "JFK, Jr. hot!" I was such a procrastinator and wiggle worm when it came to studying, and then I got to thinking, "What would Kenny do? He'd study!" And that became my mantra; I put it everywhere! I had a big sign taped to the inside of my front door that said, "What would Kenny do?" so I wouldn't keep running out to the coffee shop, a "What would Kenny do?" sticky note on my computer so I wouldn't surf the Internet, and a "What would Kenny do?" on the fridge and bathroom mirror so I wouldn't dillydally! And you know what? It worked. I aced the exam! As for Kenny, he just up and quit being a powerhouse attorney last month, sold all his belongings, moved to Brooklyn and bought a bar. That's what Kenny did! I'm not doing that.

Need help finding *your* muse? That's the first item up to bat. Don't worry, we'll be talking food and fun in no time; we just have to fill up with a bowl of vegan brain food first. Trust me—it will help make your journey easier, so take a look at the menu and pick whatever sounds good to you. Ready? Let's do this. . . .

1. *Find your inspiration:* Here are five sources of inspiration that will put a little pep in your first vegan step. Pick those that sound good to you and jot them down. Here we go!

   ❧ *Look to the Future:* Envision something far into the future that you really want to do or see. Perhaps it's finding true love, or growing old with someone you've already met. Maybe it's that carefree trip to Europe with your best friends, or starting that supercool business you've always dreamed of. Or maybe you simply look forward to enjoying quiet sunsets on your porch, with your thinning gray hair and a face well wrinkled from a lifetime of laughter. Well, you'll have a *far* greater chance of reaching your goal if you eat a healthy vegan diet. Some folks, like record mogul Russell Simmons, strive to be vegan—not just for their own well-being but also because they feel responsible for leaving the world a better place for their kids, "I am a father. I want my children and their children to have a healthy Earth to live on for many years to come." So, hop in that nifty tele-porter, flash to the future, and take a moment to gather your thoughts. Did you think of something you're really looking forward to? If so, *write it down*.

   ❧ *Get a Checkup:* I'm not a medical professional, so I can't give medical advice, but I think it's pretty obvious that everyone should get a checkup now and then just to make sure everything in your body is A-OK, even if you feel great. Your doctor can check your blood pressure, body mass index, heart rate, and a huge range of vital body functions and elements with a full blood panel. Not only are blood tests a great way to figure out what's wrong when you're not feeling well, they also give a solid "baseline" for doctors to go back to for comparison if you ever feel sick. Let's say you go vegan, and a few months later, you get a blood test result that indicates you're low in iron. How would you know if you're low in iron because of something new you're doing *now*, as opposed to some underlying problem that started *long ago*? If you're flat broke and don't have health insurance, do a little research online to find a free health clinic; they're out there. It's good to get a clean bill of health before starting this adventure, but if by chance you find out you're not in great shape due to your poor diet, you know what to do with the new information: *write it down*.

‡ *Read a Book:* Where to begin? Oh my goodness, there are so many fantastic books out there. John Robbins's *Diet for a New America* sealed the deal for me in 1987. It's filled with so many compelling reasons to enjoy a vegan lifestyle; you'll have no problem finding an example in there that you can look back on to keep you on track. It covers the full gamut: animals, health, and the environment. Or you might want to consider reading a book that focuses on one aspect of being vegan that you don't know much about. For example, if

LET GOOD HEALTH BE YOUR MUSE!

"The future of health care will involve an evolution toward a paradigm where the prevention and treatment of disease is centered, not on a pill or surgical procedure, but on another serving of fruits and vegetables."

—*The Permanente Journal*, Kaiser Permanente, Perm J 2013 Spring; 17(2):61–66
[largest managed-care organization in the United States]

According to medical professionals at Kaiser Permanente, physicians should consider recommending a healthy plant-based diet to all patients. It's no surprise considering the array of potential health benefits:

‡ Lower cholesterol levels
‡ Lower risk for type 2 diabetes
‡ Lower blood pressure
‡ Prevention, or reversal, of heart disease
‡ Less need for medications
‡ Reduction in obesity
‡ Reduction of certain cancers
‡ Reduction in rheumatoid arthritis pain
‡ Reduction of toxins in the environment

you're already committed to going vegan to help the environment, consider reading a book that focuses on the health benefits of a plant-based diet. If you're already jazzed about improving your health, then perhaps read a book that focuses on the animals. Expanding your knowledge base will really help you stay the course. If you're interested in reading about everything all at once, Kris Carr's *Crazy Sexy Diet*, Alicia Silverstone's *The Kind Diet*, and Kathy Freston's *Veganist*, all focus on diet and nutrition, but also do a good job exploring our impact on animals and the environment, too. Check out the books I've listed in the resource section. If you choose to read a book, and find your golden nugget of inspiration splashed on a page, *write it down in your journal.*

❧ *Watch a Film:* Again, so many great ones to choose from, however, one does seem to stand out from the crowd. When I ask folks what film helped them make the transition to being vegan, many say *Earthlings* was the kicker. *Earthlings*, narrated by fellow vegan Joaquin Phoenix, documents the abuse of animals for food, pets, research, clothing, and entertainment. It's only about ninety minutes in length, and you can watch it for free on YouTube.[4] No need to go to a theater and fork over the price of a movie ticket; watch it at your convenience whenever and wherever you want to; just make sure to have tissues handy. If you really want to go vegan, this film seems to pave the quickest and clearest path to compassionate living.

Another film, executive produced by Leonardo DiCaprio, that's changing quite a few minds and hearts these days, is *Cowspiracy: The Sustainability Secret*. The film follows Kip Anderson, an environmentalist, on his quest to find out what's accelerating global warming, dead zones, water depletion, deforestation, and the destruction of species, and he finds an illusive, but certain, culprit: animal agriculture. I'd have your journal nearby for this one, as it's packed with hard-hitting information you'll likely want to jot down. And thanks to Leo, it's now streaming globally on Netflix. Start the popcorn and cue it up.

Like James and Suzy Cameron, Russell Brand switched to a plant-based diet after watching *Forks Over Knives* in 2011, and I can certainly understand why: the hard facts uncovered are extremely powerful, and really pack a punch for those who need an extra nudge when it comes to improving their diet. When Russell finished watching the film, he tweeted: "I'm now vegan. Good-bye eggs, hello Ellen." After many years of being a vegetarian, he gave animal products the big boot! *Forks Over Knives* traces the personal journey and research of two doctors: Dr. T. Colin Campbell, a nutritional scientist at Cornell University, and Dr. Caldwell Esselstyn, a surgeon and head of the Breast Cancer Task Force at the Cleveland Clinic. Campbell conducted research on how to go about producing "high-quality" animal protein to give to malnourished people in the third world, but when he went to the Philippines, he was shocked to find that the wealthiest people, who ate the *highest* amounts of animal-based foods, were more likely to get liver cancer, and instead, those who ate more plants were healthier! After studying 6,500 adults, and hundreds of variables, the conclusion was clear: "People who ate the most animal-based foods got the most chronic disease" and "people who ate the most plant-based foods were the healthiest."[5] Dr. Esselstyn came to a similar conclusion from his independent nutritional research on coronary artery disease in severely ill patients. Many of the diseases he routinely treated, such as heart disease, type 2 diabetes, and some cancers were virtually *unknown* in parts of the world where they ate mostly plants. These two docs know their stuff!

Although a lot of folks who watch *Forks Over Knives* go vegan, and *stay* vegan, flash forward a few years, and here we are: Russell Brand is eating eggs and cheese again (whoops!) and pleading to his YouTube fans for "advice from vegans on how to do it well." Well, Russell, I've said it before and I'll say it again: most folks seem to *stay* vegan when they think about things from the animals' perspective. Sure, we care about our health, but we don't have an ingrained image in our brain of our chest being carved open for a pulmonary bypass surgery, nor have we ever seen ourselves lying dead in a coffin (creepy, I know!), so although we totally get that good health is important, the "come hither" of that ooey-gooey melted dairy mozzarella stick can get the best of us. If you're looking for your muse in a film and choose *Forks Over Knives* (top-notch when it comes to nutrition—seriously, watch it!) just follow it up with a quick video or film that reminds you why being vegan is *good for the animals and environment, too.*

> **DID YOU KNOW?**
> Based on a survey of over 8,000 vegans, 42 percent said they became vegan after watching an educational film, movie, or video.[6]

Short on time? Check out *Meet Your Meat* or *From Farm to Fridge*, both of which run around 12 minutes each and are easy to access on YouTube.

۩ *Spend Mindful Time with Animals:* I know it sounds silly; after all most of us spent plenty of time as kids visiting zoos and animal circuses, and enjoyed hours on end playing with our furry friends. So really, spending time with animals is nothing new for most. What I'm talking about here, however, is spending *mindful* time with animals. What does "mindful" mean? It's when you're very focused, in the present moment, and really aware of what's going on. Be quiet and patient, letting the action or inaction of the animal draw you in to their little world. Observe a bird, cow, horse, pig, goat, or any type of animal you choose. Watch how they interact with other animals and observe how skilled they are at finding food or building a nest, and how sweetly they care for their young. Watch them play, and bathe, and rest. If you mindfully watch an animal, you'll soon discover something that most folks go an entire lifetime without understanding: nonhuman animals are *just like us.* Sure they come in different shapes, colors, and sizes, but people do, too. Despite our superficial differences, we all have a common core of feelings we experience: love, fear, pain, loneliness, happiness, and an *incredible will to live life free from harm.* I've observed this by spending hours watching the nesting habits of mourning doves within inches of my old inner city apartment's front door, and years later by watching beautiful scrub jays raise their young in my Northern California countryside yard. Animals are everywhere, just waiting to teach us. All we have to do is watch. If you do so, *mindfully*, they can be your muse. If you find that something they do inspires you to go vegan, *write it down.*

2. *Surround yourself with friendly reminders*: Take whatever words of inspiration you found, and transfer them to signs or sticky notes, and plaster them around the areas you spend time. You don't have to write really long sentences; just something simple to remind you. Stick them on the fridge (for when you want to eat your partner's non-vegan pizza), on your car dashboard (for when you're driving past that sushi bar), in your wallet (for when you're tempted to buy those shearling boots and matching cashmere sweater), inside the cover of your iPad (for when you're tempted to buy that wool coat you saw online) and anywhere else you might need a friendly reminder as to the *supergood reasons* why you're going vegan, dang it. And no matter what happens to those notes, just remember, the knowledge is now *in your brain.* You've got an arsenal of information to help inspire you should you hit a bump on

your road to vegan. And you've got me. I'm here, and ready to carry you along. OK, let's get this compassion show on the road!

Over the years, when I've asked folks who are struggling with the transition to becoming vegan "What's the biggest obstacle?" here's what they told me. Some of these reasons might hit close to home, but don't you worry! We're gonna kick 'em *all* out of the park.

- They worry they won't be healthy.
- Are concerned about the cost of food and cruelty-free products.
- Don't understand what unfamiliar words mean on ingredient lists.
- Feel overwhelmed because they won't ever be a "perfect" vegan.
- Are lacking of support from friends, family, and coworkers.
- Feel like they don't have access to vegan food and cruelty-free products because they live in a remote area.
- They miss the taste of a certain animal product or a traditional meal they love.
- Feel like the world is doomed and they can't make a difference.
- They don't know how to prepare tasty vegan food (i.e. what cooking techniques or spices and seasonings to use).
- Feel like they don't have enough time to prepare vegan meals.
- They can't go from a Standard American Diet to a healthy plant-based diet overnight and give up.
- Non-vegans hurt their feelings.
- They don't want to offend others who cook for them at celebrations and family gatherings.
- The temptation at home is just too much because they live with non-vegans and have non-vegan food around them.
- They dine out frequently and don't know what to eat.
- Have difficulty finding warm clothes and well-made vegan shoes and accessories.
- They don't like to call special attention to themselves when eating out.

And now that you've read them, kiss 'em all good-bye. *Muah!* Worries be *gone!*

Checklist

☐ Did you find a dash of inspiration?

☐ Did you put a few notes around to remind you why you're going vegan?

☐ Did you consider getting a checkup?

☐ Did you find another good book to read, or an informative film to watch?

☐ Did you make a plan to spend a little mindful time with animals?

Thought FOR THE Day

To stand up for the well-being of animals does not imply you love human beings any less. When you're vegan, your circle of compassion simply expands as you discover your heart holds enough love for everyone.

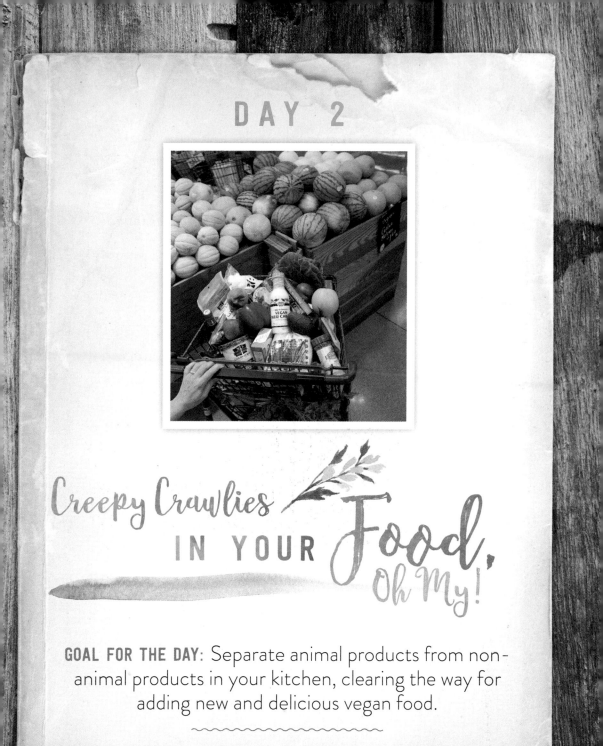

Creepy Crawlies IN YOUR Food, Oh My!

GOAL FOR THE DAY: Separate animal products from non-animal products in your kitchen, clearing the way for adding new and delicious vegan food.

Some foods clearly contain bits and pieces of animals, but would you ever think to check your jar of Planters Dry Roasted Peanuts? I picked up a jar recently and noticed the peanuts were coated with boiled hooves, bones, and tendons: aka gelatin! And who would ever think something other than fruit would be in Tree Top Apple Fruit Punch, especially with a big "100% Juice" on the label? What could they *possibly* sneak in there? It's colored with carmine: aka squished bugs! And what about that beer and wine, surely no animal products wind up in booze, right? Wrong. Many use egg products during the filtering process, or even isinglass: aka fish bladders!

So what's the big deal? A few bugs. A little fish residue. It's not like we're eating an egg from an abused chicken, or a hamburger from a slaughtered cow, right? Well, before we go any further, I want to let you know there are two vegan schools of thought on whether or not we should avoid the itsy-bitsy, teeny-weeny bits and pieces of animals, and their by-products, in our food. After all, sometimes the amount is *so* small, that you can't even see, smell, or taste it, and in proportion to the food or beverage item itself, it might only be the equivalent of a few grains of salt. Some folks—I'll call them the "let it slide" folks —believe that by making a big stink over seemingly trivial amounts of animal products, we're propelling the myth that being vegan is too complicated and burden-some. They worry folks will give up on being vegan before they even give it a try, and as a result, by turning people "off" with a giant laundry list of non-vegan items, we're actually hurting the animals and the overall wellness of the world. They believe that in terms of suffering, the production of tiny by-products pales in comparison to the pain and abuse caused by eating meat, dairy, and eggs. The "let it slide" folks don't think we should ask the waiter if the complimentary dinner rolls were glazed with egg whites, nor ask if the falafel balls were fried in the same oil with the fish sticks. Likewise, a little castoreum— aka beaver butt—in a "naturally" flavored raspberry candy, is no big deal. After all, as I mentioned in the last chapter, one can never *truly* be 100 percent vegan, so why be so picky about one little thing, and not another. "Just stop being so picky!" they say. As my friend and executive director of The Good Food Institute, Bruce Friedrich put it, being obsessed with every minuscule ingredient "makes it seem like we're in a cult."

On the other hand, some folks, I'll call them the "politely picky vegans" avoid all animal products, even the little ones, *as best as they can*. Yes, they know they'll never be a *perfect* vegan, but if there's a way to avoid an animal product, and it's not *too* incredibly difficult, they skip it. They ask questions; lots of them. They ask if the seemingly vegan miso soup at the Japanese restaurant has the traditional solitary chunk of fish floating in the kitchen pot "just for flavor." They shoot off quick e-mails to companies and ask if the "natural flavors" in the potato chips are from animal sources or from plants. They order Sonic's fries, but skip the tater tots, because the fries are deep-fried alone, while the tater tots are often cooked with the chicken. They'll even avoid orange juice that's fortified with D_3 because, well, unlike D_2, which comes from fungus and yeast, D_3 is usually derived from the irradiated wool of sheep.

Whether you're politely picky, or you let it slide, you're helping the world in a very *big* way. No doubt about it. So do *whatever is best for you* as you transition to being vegan. Being vegan isn't about living as a purist, it's about doing the best we can, while keeping an eye on the big picture: what's best for the animals, the environment, and our health. As for me, personally? After decades of being vegan, I'm now politely picky, with no apologies, and here's why:

- ✑ **FOR MY MENTAL WELLNESS**: I can't help it. There's just something vile about swallowing body parts and excretions that were stolen from an animal who was abused and killed. What we consume becomes us—and I don't mean that in a flattering way. Unlike a fur coat, or a pair of leather shoes, we can't change our mind, and "take off" the animal we ate, and that really bothers me. I don't want to be a walking coffin. I want to be a caring, loving human being. I'm OK with politely avoiding even the smallest bit of animal products because quite simply, doing so puts my mind at peace. Some folks say, "Well, at least they're using every bit of the animal. If the cow is already dead, why be wasteful?" I'm not sure the old saying "Waste not, want not" works when we're talking about killing and eating a cow, much less any animal.

- ✑ **BECAUSE FOOD POLITICS DRIVES ME BATTY**: Whether you're a "let it slide" vegan, a "politely picky" vegan, or a "Mr. I'm never ever going vegan" (maybe you're just living "la vida vegan" vicariously by reading this book?), the deception masterfully imbedded in food labels, advertising, and policy should piss you off a bit. The legal loopholes and lack of transparency when it comes to our food just blows my mind. Vegan or not, everyone should become adept at reading food nutrition labels and ingredients lists. Once you understand how they work, not only can you avoid what you don't want to eat, you can also become an advocate for making food labels more helpful, accurate, and truthful and get more of what you do want to eat. Chances are you'll become healthier, too, as you'll realize that the healthiest foods are the simplest ones.

- ✑ **BECAUSE ASKING QUESTIONS ABOUT FOOD HELPS EVERYONE**: Believe it or not, in my experience, by asking lots of questions concerning food, I've actually helped folks realize that being vegan is easier than they think, not more complicated. I asked our local bakery, a beach town "hot spot," if any of their fresh breads were vegan, and the girl at the counter quickly replied, "Oh, no, sorry. All of our bread contains eggs or milk." So I politely asked if I could please see their binder of ingredient lists for the baked goods—many bakeries and eateries have them these days—and she kindly obliged. Sure enough, several breads were 100 percent vegan, with very simple ingredients, one of which is a seeded Francese bread that we buy weekly. Delicious! And now she knows that they carry vegan bread for any other customers who might ask.

The same thing happened to me last week when I was at a grocery store. I noticed they had a nice deli inside, so when I was done shopping I thought to grab a veggie sandwich to go. I asked the deli worker if any of their breads were vegan, and she replied with a definitive "No; none of our breads are vegan." So I asked if she wouldn't mind handing me the loaf of bread she had behind the counter so I could give it a quick look over, and yep, sure enough, it was vegan. I explained to her that the allergen warning at the bottom of the ingredients list did indeed list milk and eggs, but it was only to alert people to the fact that the bread was produced in a facility where they make other food items with animal products. That didn't mean that the bread I was holding was made with animal products, in fact, it even had a big green "VEGAN" printed on the package. It was clear that she didn't have much experience reading food labels, but now she was prepared for anyone else who might request a vegan sandwich in the future. I wasn't offensive; I was informative, and most importantly, *polite*.

People have been making bread for over thirty thousand years, first flat with just grains and water, and then leavened with yeast, and sometimes a little salt and sugar. So why is it that so many people assume there are animal products in bread? Well, let's take a look at a common grocery store bread, found across the nation in many supermarkets. This is the ingredients list for Sara Lee's Classic 100% Whole Wheat Bread, sold across the country at Kroger:

Whole Wheat Flour, Water, High Fructose Corn Syrup, Wheat Gluten, Sugar, Yeast. Contains 2% or Less of Each of the Following: Soybean Oil, Calcium Sulfate, Salt, Dough Conditioners (May Contain One or More of the Following: Mono- and Diglycerides, Ethoxylated Mono- and Diglycerides, Sodium Stearoyl Lactylate, Calcium Peroxide, DATEM, Ascorbic Acid, Azodicarbonamide, Enzymes), Wheat Bran, Guar Gum, Distilled Vinegar, Calcium Propionate (Preservative), Yeast Nutrients (Monocalcium

Phosphate, Calcium Sulfate, Ammonium Sulfate), Corn Starch, Vitamin D₃, Soy Lecithin, Milk, Soy Flour.

The name of the bread sounds rather healthy, doesn't it? But look at that novel-length list of ingredients. Keep in mind; it's just a loaf of bread! Vegan or not, this list should raise a few red flags. Why should something as simple as bread require so many ingredients? Because the quicker a company can produce bread (gotta have accelerators), and the longer time it can sit on that dusty shelf before going stale or moldy (gotta have preservatives), the more dough food companies can make. Give a quick glance to the breads at the supermarket the next time you're there; with the typical everything-but-the-kitchen-sink list of ingredients, it's no wonder folks just *assume* all bread contains eggs and milk. Most people think vegans are the complicated ones, but we just want our sandwich bread to have a little flour, water, yeast, a dash of salt, occasionally some molasses for sweetness, and maybe some seeds for extra flavor and nutrition. Simple! Stay tuned for some delicious vegan bread options in Day 9: Fast, Cheap, and Easy!

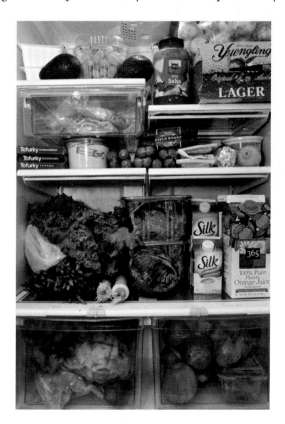

OK, LET'S HOP TO IT!

1. *Empty your refrigerator and pantry.* Sounds horrible, I know, but honestly, even if you didn't want to go vegan, this is a supergood thing to do once in a while. I recently emptied mine, and let me just say, "Eeww!" I think a few things on the far back bottom shelf were about ready to walk out on their own. Once you have everything out, dedicate a couple shelves to the vegan food you already have on hand, and a couple shelves to the non-vegan food. You'll want to do the same for your freezer and your pantry. Since you're already familiar with the biggies like milk, meat, eggs, fish, and cheese, here's a little vocabulary list to help you recognize what's vegan, and what's not, when you're reading the fine print. Some of the crazy ingredients will have you scratching your head, wondering *who on earth* ever thought someone would want to *eat* this stuff?

   - Albumin: Egg whites.
   - Carmine and Cochineal: A bright red pigment from crushed female cochineal insects.
   - Casein, Caseinate, Sodium Caseinate: A protein from dairy milk.
   - Castoreum: Extract from muskrat and beaver genitals.
   - *Cysteine, L-form: An amino acid primarily derived from animal hair, human hair, and chicken feathers.
   - Gelatin: A protein from the boiled tendons, ligaments, hooves, and/or bones of pigs and cows.
   - *Glucose: Usually derived from animal tissues and fluids.
   - *Glycerides (mono-, di-, and triglycerides): An additive in food to help ingredients blend. Usually derived from cows and pigs.
   - Honey: Food that bees make and need for themselves.
   - Isinglass: The internal membranes of fish bladders.
   - Lactose: A sugar from the milk of mammals.
   - Lard: A fat from various areas of a pig.
   - *Natural Flavors: Can contain extracts from animals, fish, eggs, and dairy products i.e.—our lovely castoreum is a "natural flavor." (See Castoreum, above.)
   - Pepsin: An enzyme from the stomach of animals. Usually derived from pigs.
   - Rennet: Enzymes from calves' stomachs.
   - Shellac,* Resinous Glaze, Confectioners' Glaze: Usually extracts from insects. Often from the lac beetle.

- Stearic Acid, Stearate: Fatty substance from the stomach of pigs.
- Tallow: Fat from animals.
- Vitamin D_3: Usually derived from fish or animals.*
- Whey: A serum from dairy milk.

*Can be also derived from a plant source.

This list may look a little long, but trust me; I really narrowed it down for you. There are hundreds of other terms for pesky animal ingredients, but these are the items that I've come across the most; ingredients that have spoiled what could have been a delicious vegan meal or snack. Feel free to learn more if you're up to it. There are animal product apps you can get for your phone, as well as a book called *Veganissimo, A to Z*, by Reuben and Lars Proctor Thomsen, that's filled with three hundred pages of animal ingredients that creep into our food and other products. It makes the mind swirl. But for today, we're keeping things simple.

The good news? I think you'll be pleasantly surprised to discover how many vegan foods and beverages you already have and enjoy. The bad news? You're probably going to feel a bit betrayed by the deceptive practices of food manufacturers and advertisers. After all, most aren't in it for your health; they're in it for the money, and, boy, can they be sneaky. Here are a few pointers on where to look:

- **CARMINE AND COCHINEAL** are often used to color candy and beverages bright red. I've even found them in jam. Until recently, Starbucks used cochineal extract to color their Strawberry Frappuccinos. Starbucks used the excuse that they were just trying to avoid using artificial colors, and therefore smushed bugs were better, but once folks got the word out, Starbucks changed its tune. The bugs are *out*, and a beautiful, all natural, tomato-based extract is in. Where there's a will, there's a way. Thanks, Starbucks!

- **WHEY** likes to lurk in baked goods and dietary supplements. No whey! Yes, whey. It's kind of left over from the "old school" muscle-building crowd that's obsessed with packing protein. Funny thing is, most Americans consume *too much* protein. But if they told you that, they couldn't sell you that jumbo, overpriced tub of cholesterol-filled "get ripped in a jiff!" muscle-building fluff. You don't need whey.

❧ **VITAMIN D₃** is commonly found in fortified orange juice. Unlike protein, many folks are deficient in Vitamin D; however, I'm not sure why anyone would want D3 made from lanolin, aka wool grease, floating in their morning glass of OJ. I know when I'm craving a nice tall glass of orange juice, I just want *exactly that*: the juice of oranges, not an orange-colored mix from the lab. Nor do I want Tropicana's Pure Premium Healthy Heart orange juice; it's anything but pure. It has tilapia, sardines, and anchovies in it, despite being labeled "100% Juice."[1] Blah! Orange juice with squished fish? No, thank you! Check your Worcestershire Sauce for anchovies, too. Oy.

❧ **SHELLAC AND OTHER ANIMAL-BASED GLAZES** are often in candy that's shiny, like those glistening chocolate-covered almonds and colorful jelly beans. It's a real bummer, too. As your vegan adventure unfolds, be prepared to read through candy ingredient lists with a big smile on your face because all of the ingredients seem vegan, only to find that at the *very* end you see . . . dun, dun, DUN: confectioners glaze or shellac. It boggles the mind. There really should be a law against ruining perfectly fine sweets with bugs. If you find fruit in the grocery store that's shiny as hand-polished chrome on a hot rod, it's likely glazed with shellac, too.

❧ **L-CYSTEINE** likes to sneak into bread, especially bagels and pizza dough, as a "conditioner." I've found that when I see this ingredient, it's usually packed into a very unhealthy, overly processed food item that I shouldn't be eating anyway. And besides, who purposely wants hair in their food? This will be an easy one to ditch. Good-bye hairy bread!

This is a good base for you to start with while perusing your cupboards, fridge, and freezer, but if it's too overwhelming, or your eyes start to hurt from squinting at the incredibly small print, just sort your kitchen by looking for those terms you're readily familiar with: milk, eggs, butter, cheese, fish, etc. No need to get frustrated. You can always come back to this list later. We've got 21 days together and we're making things easy. And remember, as I mentioned earlier, no one will *ever* be a *perfect* vegan. Repeat: No one will ever be a perfect vegan. I will never be, you will never be, no one will ever be. It's simply impossible. Even products that are labeled vegan can contain animal ingredients from the equipment they're processed on. A recent study by the Food and Drug Administration found that seven out of eight dark chocolates marked "Vegan" tested positive for dairy.[2] So when it comes to all of these crazy animal ingredients, just *do the best you can*. And remember, I've been vegan for over twenty-eight years. I'm "seasoned," so to speak, so avoiding the smaller animal by-products was just a natural next step for me many moons ago, but you're just starting off. So play it by ear, and do whatever is best for you. I'm your guide, but *you're* steering the ship!

2. *Empower yourself with knowledge.* As you begin to become more aware of what's in your food, you'll likely find that you've been duped into eating a whole heck of a lot of stuff that you didn't really mean to eat. Manufacturers are pretty sneaky when it comes to marketing their food. Vegan or not, it's smart to be aware of the deceitful games they play. They're not just out to get vegans, they're stinkers to *everyone*. For example, if a product is primarily composed of sugar, instead of raising a red flag by listing "sugar" first on the ingredients list, manufacturers simply divide up the sugar by adding different types, and suddenly, high fructose corn syrup, dextrose, glucose solids, and sucrose— all sugars—fall further down the list, bumping something healthier, like a grain, to the top. A quick glance gives your brain the impression that the food is mostly made of whole grains, but if you add up all of those sugars further on, the food is still mostly sugar. Crackers, granola bars, and "energy" bars are notorious for this sneaky masquerade, so arm yourself with facts about sugars and anything else you might eat. Here are a few tidbits you can start with:

- **SUGAR FACTS**: Sometimes sugar isn't vegan. Sounds crazy, right? How in the heck can sugar not be vegan? It's just sugar, for pete's sakes. Oddly enough, to get that pristine white color, some manufacturers use the dried bones of cows as a carbon filter to bleach it. And some brown sugars are a combo of the white sugar with molasses, so you might want to avoid certain brown sugars, too. Because the USDA doesn't allow the use of bones to char sugar from the meat industry here in the U.S., sugar companies use the bones from animals from foreign countries, such as Pakistan and Afghanistan. Like that's safer, right? Far away, where we have no idea what's going on? Go figure. I don't know of many vegans who check every sugary snack when they're eating out, but *I do know* it's getting easier to purchase vegan sugar to have at home. Here's a list of a few brands that don't use animal skeletons to make sugar ghost white: Wholesome Sweeteners, Sugar in the Raw, Florida Crystals, Trader Joe's (Organic Brown Sugar, Organic Evaporated Cane Juice Sugar, and Turbinado Raw Cane Sugar), and Whole Foods 365 Vegan Sugar. One to avoid: C&H Sugar. Thankfully, beet sugar is never made with bones, and don't forget, there are lots of other natural sweeteners beyond cane sugar, such as maple syrup, rice syrup, agave, and stevia. And there's even a delicious "Bee Free Honee" made from apples. Trust me, there's no shortage of vegan sweets; take it from the biggest fan of vegan sweets I know: Me!

✤ **NATURAL FLAVOR FACTS**: I don't know about you, but before I started to research food policy, the term "natural flavors" always conjured up nice thoughts of fresh herbs and fruit extracts. Little did I know it's a common façade for animal bits and pieces, like blood and chicken fat. Making matters worse, if you take the time to call and ask a food company what's in their "natural flavoring" they can say it's "top secret" or "proprietary information" followed by "have a nice day, good-bye!" It's perfectly legal to leave us in the dark about what we're eating. And whether you're vegan or not, that's neither fair nor safe, especially for those with allergies. Food policy advocates have been fighting for years to pass a "Food Ingredient Right to Know" Act, which would require that "flavoring or coloring derived from meat, poultry, or other animal products (including insects) bear labeling stating that fact and their names." But no matter how often it's introduced, it dies in Congress every single time.[3] I'm guessing if they told us, we wouldn't eat it. Unless a company tells me the natural flavors they use are derived from plants, I steer clear of the food. I avoid artificial flavors and colors, too. Knowing they can stick just about anything in, including a vanilla "flavor" from beaver anal glands, you may want to avoid "natural flavors," too. Heck, they've even derived vanilla "flavoring" from cow poop![4] Not kidding. Secret flavors? No thank you. You can keep your secrets, and your food! Here's the *official* definition of "natural flavors" or "natural flavoring": "[T]he essential oil, oleoresin, essence or extractive, protein hydrolysate, distillate, or any product of roasting, heating or enzymolysis, which contains the flavoring constituents derived from a spice, fruit or fruit juice, vegetable or vegetable juice, edible yeast, herb, bark, bud, root, leaf or similar plant material, *meat, seafood, poultry, eggs, dairy products*, or fermentation products thereof, whose significant function in food is flavoring rather than nutritional."

✤ **DAIRY FACTS**: Sometimes the words on food packaging can be very misleading. If a label is marked "non-dairy" you'd think that would mean there's no dairy in the food. Wrong. The FDA says it's A-OK for foods labeled as such to contain multiple forms of dairy disguised by variations of the word "casein." The FDA recently directed manufacturers to clearly note milk derivatives in the ingredients list; strangely, they still allow the food item to be accompanied by a "non-dairy" claim emblazoned on the front of the carton or package. As you can imagine, that's not only misleading for vegans, it's a hazard to those with allergies, too. You'll notice this happens a lot with "non-dairy" creamers. Making matters worse, the FDA doesn't even define the term "dairy-free," so watch out for that claim, too. Bottom line? Be sure to turn the package over and read the ingredients, just to be safe.

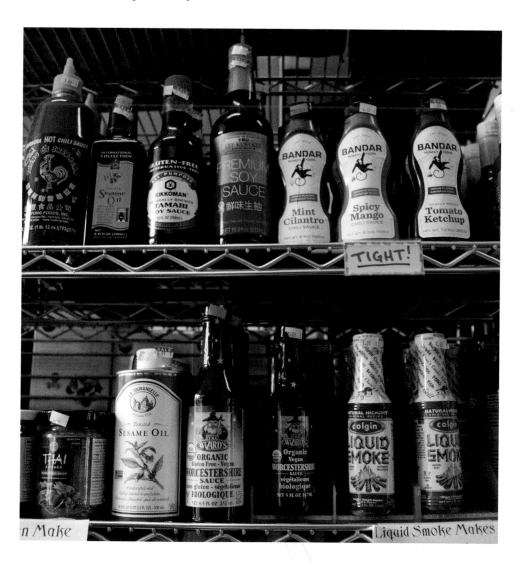

3. *Figure out what you'd like to do with your non-vegan food.* As you sort through your kitchen, continue assigning shelves that will be just for vegan food, and shelves that will be for everything else. Some folks find that it's easier if the non-vegan food is out of their home altogether. If you think that would be helpful to you, consider donating the nonperishables to a local charity, church, or food bank, and the perishables to a neighbor or a friend. Just follow your heart, and do whatever you think will be best for you.

4. *Make a list of vegan pantry essentials.* As you start to eliminate animal products in your pantry, consider replacing them with healthier fare. You probably can't restock your entire kitchen with one visit to the market, but it's good to make a list to peruse so you can slowly add things to your collection of yummies as you progress. Here's what I usually keep in my disorganized but functional vegan pantry:

- Canned Beans (whole, refried, and baked)
- Canned Soups
- Dried Beans and Lentils
- Dried Rice (many varieties)
- Chia Seeds
- Sunflower Seeds
- Sesame Seeds
- Flaxseeds (refrigerate once opened)
- Flour
- Sugar
- Baking Powder
- Baking Soda
- Almonds
- Cashews
- Coconut Milk (canned)
- Coffee
- Tea
- Herbs and Spices
- Hemp Hearts
- Extracts (vanilla, almond, etc.)
- Cereal
- Oatmeal
- Grits
- Chips
- Crackers
- Nutritional Yeast
- Dry Pasta
- Pasta Sauce
- Canned Pumpkin
- Potatoes
- Onions
- Sweet Potatoes
- Garlic
- Tomato Sauce
- Coconut Oil
- Walnuts

5. *Make a list of food you'd like for the refrigerator, too! Here are a few ideas:*

- Fresh Produce (lots!!)
- Fresh Herbs
- Sriracha
- Tofu
- Tamari
- Bragg's Liquid Aminos
- Olives
- Sun-dried Tomatoes
- Crushed Garlic
- Pickles
- Kimchi
- Capers
- Chutney
- Vegan Mayo
- Relish
- Mustard
- Ketchup
- Dressings
- Vegan Butter (Earth Balance, Organic Smart Balance, or Miyoko's Kitchen VeganButter)
- Tahini
- Maple Syrup
- Agave
- BBQ Sauce
- Red Chili Sauce
- Hummus
- Sauerkraut
- Salsa
- Nut Butter
- Hot Sauce
- Vegan Worcestershire Sauce (Annie's)
- A.1. Original Sauce
- Shredded Jackfruit
- Vegan "Meat"
- Vegan "Cheese"
- Vegan Yogurt
- Nut Milks
- Seed Milks
- Coconut Water
- Juice

6. *And while you're at it, here are a few things to consider for your vegan freezer:*

- Frozen Veggies
- Frozen Fruits
- Sorbet
- Vegan Ice Cream
- Veggie, Black Bean, Quinoa, and Tempeh burgers
- Vegan Chick'n Strips
- Beefless Crumbles
- Vegan Mac 'n cheese
- Vegan Meatballs
- Vegan Roasts
- Burritos
- Enchiladas
- Ravioli
- Gnocchi
- Pizza

And don't forget to stock the fruit bowl!

SSHH . . . IT'S A SECRET!

The FDA allows over 10,000 chemical additives to be mixed in with our food. Making matters worse, over 1,000 additives in our food have never been approved, nor even reviewed by the FDA—and according to a law that's been on the books for fifty-eight years, that's A-OK.[5] If a company doesn't want to submit their new "flavor" or "preservative" to the FDA for review, they can declare it "Generally Recognized as Safe" (GRAS) and bypass the entire regulatory agency altogether. Food companies are allowed to select and pay any scientists they want, and with their thumbs up, BOOM—off to the market it goes. As you can imagine, some scientists are called upon over and over again—some of whom worked for Big Tobacco back in the day when cancer sticks were pitched as safe. I'm pretty sure, folks, for the most part, we're familiar with the simple ingredients they ate back in the '50s. Maybe now that we can barely pronounce them, it's time to revisit the law.

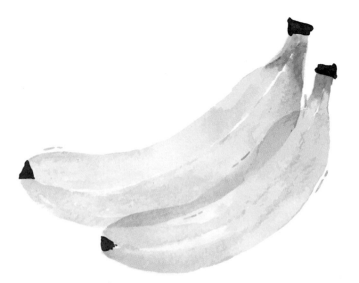

My Sweet Bah Nah Nahs

Here's something simple I love to whip up when I just want a little easy-to-make, sweet-and-warm comfort food. It tastes, and smells, so good!

1 banana

1 to 2 teaspoons vegan butter or coconut oil (if you're using coconut oil, add a pinch of sea salt; vegan butter usually has salt in it)

Sweetener and spices of choice

1. Slice the banana in half horizontally, and then again, lengthwise.

2. Melt the vegan butter or coconut oil in a pan over low heat.

3. Add the banana slices to the pan and cook on low to medium heat until slightly brown, using a spatula to flip now and then to make sure the banana slices don't stick to the pan. If you're using coconut oil, add the sea salt at this point.

4. Once slightly brown, remove the banana slices from the pan and drizzle with the sweetener of your choice. I like using maple syrup, but agave or brown sugar works well, too.

5. Sprinkle the spices you enjoy. I like using a "pumpkin pie" mix blend that's made with cinnamon, ginger, lemon peel, nutmeg, cloves, and cardamom, but any spice you like will do.

Grab a book, a blankie, and your warm bah nah nahs, and you're set for the night!

Checklist

☐ Did you become familiar with a few pesky ingredients that are made from animal products?

☐ Did you organize your refrigerator, freezer, and pantry and create a space for everything that's vegan?

☐ Did you figure out what to do with your non-vegan food?

☐ Did you make a yummy vegan shopping list?

Thought FOR THE Day

In 2012, "Strongest Man of Germany" Patrik Baboumian set a world record by lifting a 331-pound beer keg over his head. In 2015 he broke his own world record for the yoke walk, carrying 1,234 pounds across the floor. Where does he get his protein? The same place elephants and rhinoceroses do: PLANTS!

DAY 3

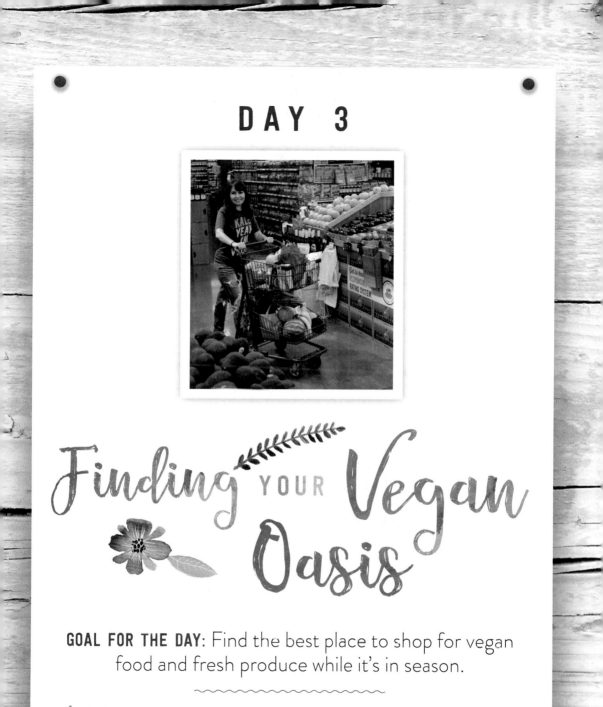

Finding YOUR Vegan Oasis

GOAL FOR THE DAY: Find the best place to shop for vegan food and fresh produce while it's in season.

1. *Evaluate your shopping options.* Now that your pantry, refrigerator, and freezer are well organized, it's time to figure out the best spots to shop for vegan foods. This list is far from comprehensive, but it will get you off to a great start. Let's explore!

FARMERS' MARKETS Farmers' markets are a gold mine for tasty, affordable, healthy food, and with good reason. The produce is generally picked less than twenty-four hours before it's taken to the market (often that very morning!), so it's usually *very* fresh. You'll rarely find a bruise, brown stem, or wilted leaf, commonly found in grocery store produce. Farmers' markets are also a great place to find organic produce at a fair price. What's also "vegantastic" is that farmers' market foods are grown locally, so it doesn't take massive amounts of energy and resources to schlep the produce to us. I live within an hour of Gilroy, California, the "Garlic Capital of the World," but you wouldn't know by the label on the jar of chopped garlic in my local grocery store: "Made in China." I'm not kidding. Even much of the fresh garlic is shipped in from China, nearly seven thousand miles away! Boggles the mind.

Where I live, there's a local farmers' market that's open every Saturday morning *all* year long, and I look forward to it every weekend. If you want to find out where the closest farmers' market is to you, or maybe just explore a new one, the USDA recently set up an awesome search engine so you can find one easily. I rarely complement the USDA, but honestly, this website tool is brilliant. Not only can you search by location, you can find a farmers' market based on the products available and the form of payment accepted; they even note which are open during the winter. With nearly nine thousand farmers' markets listed, chances are good that there's a nice one near you. See Farmers' Market Database: http://search.ams.usda.gov/farmersmarkets

FARMERS' MARKET TIP

Many farmers' markets get their claim to fame because they're incredibly large and attract so many tourists, but just because they're über popular, doesn't mean you'll have the most enjoyable or fruitful (pun intended) time there. Pikes Place in Seattle, Washington, and Farmers' Market in Los Angeles, California, have a large variety of offerings, but they're extremely crowded, parking is a pain in the booty, and they sell a great deal of unhealthy, overly processed food that can tempt even the most seasoned vegan. If your only experience has been a visit to one of the "heavyweights" and it wasn't a particularly fond one, consider exploring a smaller market; you might be pleasantly surprised.

While you're perusing the stands, don't be wary of asking questions; farmers are generally more than happy to chitchat about what to do with those beautiful green tops on beets, how to cook with fresh herbs, or when the first tomatoes of the season are expected to arrive. Try to be open to trying new-to-you fruits and veggies, too. I've found lemon cucumbers, purple potatoes, and the biggest variety of mushrooms and sprouts I've ever seen. Remember, eating a plant-based diet is truly a diet of abundance, not scarcity; I eat a far bigger variety of food than any non-vegan I know. Just grab your bag or basket, give yourself a reasonable budget, meander in the fresh air, mingle with the farmers, and you'll have a great day!

FRESH PRODUCE DELIVERY SERVICES Good news! If you don't have a local farmers' market, no need to fret. Community Supported Agriculture, commonly known as CSAs, provide fresh produce across the country, either straight to your doorstep or at a nearby pickup location. In a nutshell, CSAs consist of a community of individuals who pledge support to a farm operation so that the farmland becomes, either "legally or spiritually," the community's farm, with the growers and consumers providing mutual support and sharing the risks and benefits of food production.[1] Folks pay the farmers in advance, and then upon harvest, they get a nice box of produce in return.

CSAs generally let customers select what category of produce they'd like to receive (i.e. fruit, veggies, a mix of both, etc.), the amount, and how often they'd like it to be delivered. When I lived in Los Angeles, I signed up for a CSA delivery and really enjoyed it. When my biweekly fruit and veggie box arrived on my doorstep, it felt like Christmas morning! I never knew what to expect, but when it arrived, I always found all sorts of unique fruits and veggies that I was eager to try. I'm fortunate enough to live near an abundance of farmers' markets now, and prefer the experience of buying my produce in person, so I no longer use a CSA, but they're out there for those who need one. Local Harvest lists over four thousand CSAs in their database, some of which deliver fresh produce hundreds of miles away, so chances are, there's a CSA near you.

FOOD CO-OPS Another hot spot for vegan goodies are food co-ops, which are sprinkled throughout the country; there are over twenty-nine thousand of them in the U.S. alone! Instead of being owned by investors, co-ops are owned by community members; just average folk like you and me. They're known for offering fair wages to their employees, support for local farmers, as well as having strong environmental standards to minimize the impact of their operation. Many co-ops donate a share of profits to charity, too. Here are a couple of co-op databases to help you find one near you: grocer.coop/index.php?q=coops and www.ncg.coop. And if you don't currently have one nearby, here's a map of all the new co-ops in development: foodcoopinitiative.coop/content/co-op-directories. Cooperation is growing, and that's always a good thing!

GROCERY STORES

WHOLE FOODS MARKET

It's no secret: Whole Foods Market (WFM) is far from perfect. It's been publicly slammed for repeatedly overcharging shoppers, blasted for its brief foray in selling headless, skinned rabbits, and became ensnarled with the Federal Trade Commission during its messy acquisition of Wild Oats Markets.[2] And their so-called "humane meat" is by some reports a complete sham.[3] Sure, I'd fix a few things about WFM if I had my druthers, but the bottom line is: they have over 420 locations scattered throughout the United States, the UK, and Canada, and they are *by far* one of the most accessible markets to shop for vegan food, toiletries, and household items. Many WFM locations have on-site nutrition specialists who are more than willing to help you find what you need and if you visit their website there's an entire section on vegan food, where they list animal ingredients that sneak into supplements, their top plant-based picks for vegan nutrients, and even vegan recipes. Whole Foods Market stocks everything from vegan stuffing to vegan powdered sugar—both of which are clearly marked "Vegan" on the front of the package. Sure makes shopping easy! When it comes to shopping for vegan food, Whole Foods Market rocks! Here's some tips to help:

- Always check out their list of weekly sales items, and pick up a WFM coupon book near the front door on your way in. There's a cell phone app, too!

- If you don't see an item you want, let a team member at the information desk know, and they might be able to order it for you.

- Inquire about store tours and demos, as they often offer free vegan activities and events.

TRADER JOE'S

Ah, where to begin? Baked Onion Rings, Soy Chorizo, Strawberry Coconut Ice Cream, Pad Thai, Cinnamon Rolls, Enchiladas, meatballs, cookies, red wine—all 100 percent vegan! And fresh organic fruits, vegetables, seeds, grains, and nuts at a reasonable price, too; TJ's has got it all! Hard to believe TJ's started out as Pronto Markets, a convenience store in the 1950s, but the founder, Joe Coulombe, was so worried about the competition from 7-Eleven that he completely revamped the stores into what they are today: a vegan treasure trove! Thank heaven for 7-Eleven! As an added bonus, their private label products don't contain any preservatives, artificial flavors or colors, and they're even phasing out BPA (found to be toxic even in low doses) from all of their private label cans and packaging.[4] There are currently over 450 Trader Joe's across the country, with more opening soon, so if you've never been to one, keep your eyes peeled! TJ's is a vegan paradise not to be missed. Here's some tips to help:

- TJ's website has a list of their vegan products—which they update regularly—however, there are many more vegan items not included, so don't think you need to limit yourself to the list. If you ask sweetly, they'll even print out the list for you at the store if you need it.

- Be mindful that you're not filling your cart up only with food that's shipped in from lands far, far away. For most folks, it's close to impossible to *only* buy food that's sourced within a few miles; just try to keep our environment in mind while shopping and make sure your basket isn't a giant heap of international goodies, for which TJ's is known. Remember, it requires a lot of nonrenewable resources to ship food.

- Check out their sampling station, usually located toward the back of the store. TJ's often whips up vegan dishes for customers to try, and provides the recipes, too. And if you need a little extra pep in your step, you can even grab a sample cup of Joe.

KROGER (RALPH'S/FOOD 4 LESS)

If for some reason you don't live near a farmers' market, a Whole Foods Market, or a Trader Joe's, no worries! Kroger, America's largest supermarket chain, has thousands of stores in thirty-one states. They stock tons of vegan items to help you make the transition: vegan ice cream, vegan yogurt, vegan cheese, vegan deli slices, and a beautiful array of healthy organic produce. Thanks to the growing demand for vegan food, they even have a selection of vegan meat without any artificial flavors, colors, or preservatives under their own private label, Simple Truth.

GROCERY OUTLET

This independently operated grocery store, with over two hundred locations throughout California, Idaho, Nevada, Oregon, Pennsylvania, and Washington, just might be one of the best-kept vegan secrets out there. It's just one of those stores that looks like it would be rather ho-hum, but when you venture inside, you suddenly find that there's a ton of yummy vegan food, at a great price, too. The store is very eclectic and there's certainly a fair share of unhealthy food you'll want to avoid, but intermingled is a fantastic array of products that vegans love to eat! I've found everything from flax milk and carrot juice to chia seeds and coconut milk ice cream. I've also bought vegan jerky, granola bars, veggie burgers, barbecue sauce, quinoa, sorbet, organic soups, vegan cheese, vegan yogurt, and delicious seeded bread. And I've scored lots of fresh and frozen fruits and veggies at less than half of what I would have paid in a traditional grocery store. The reason they can sell everything at such a good price is because they buy surplus inventory and products that are undergoing packaging changes. Just be sure to check the "best by" dates as some are close to expiring. And if you see something you like, buy enough to keep you happy since it might not be there the next time you shop. The inventory is constantly changing, but that's kind of nice; you never know what goodies you'll find next!

COSTCO

Costco is the largest membership warehouse chain in the United States and has almost seven hundred stores worldwide, and their stores are huge! Every time I go to one, I'm impressed by the assortment of vegan food they have: grains, organic fruits and veggies, vegan egg rolls, vegan soups and chili, veggie burgers, flaxseeds and chia seeds, nut milks, vegan snack bars, cruelty-free laundry detergent, organic strawberry jam, and my good ole' pantry staple, Kirkland's Organic No Salt Seasoning, a mix of twenty-one organic spices, that I use almost every day. My local Costco even sells the infamous Hodo Soy. Hopefully your Costco will have something especially wonderful, too. All of the stores are a bit different, though, so before purchasing a membership, ask politely if you can just walk around and check it out.

ETHNIC GROCERY STORES Do a quick search to see if you have a local ethnic market in your community. If so, you're in for a real treat! Ethnic grocery stores have all sorts of unique vegan items. For example, you'll find a nice selection of vegan sauces and unique spices in Indian grocery stores, and fresh jackfruit, vegan won ton wrappers, fresh wasabi, and a huge selection of tofu products in Asian markets. One of my favorite finds at a tiny Korean grocery store was a Japanese dessert called Daifuku, which means "great luck." It's mochi, a soft and doughy rice cake, stuffed with a sweet red bean paste made from azuki beans. They are so good! Keep an eye out for Mexican markets, too; they usually have great deals on rice, beans, hot sauce, masa harina, and fresh produce such as cilantro and tomatillos. And if you're lucky enough to live near a Jons International Marketplace, they have amazing weekly deals. When I lived near one in Los Angeles, I'd snag three heads of organic romaine lettuce for ninety-nine cents. Can't beat that!

VEGAN GROCERY STORES Here are a few 100 percent vegan brick-and-mortar grocery stores for the lucky duckies who live close to these locations. If you do, consider me jealous!

Artichoke Red Vegan Market (Orlando, Florida)
Food Fight Grocery Store (Portland, Oregon)
Vegan Haven Grocery Store (Seattle, Washington)
Rabbit Food Grocery Store (Austin, Texas)
Nooch (Denver, Colorado)
Veganz (Portland, Oregon, and multiple locations in Germany, Czech Republic, and Austria (keep tabs on them, as they expand! veganz.de/en/stores/)
Un Monde Vegan (Paris, France)
GreenBay Grocery Store (London, England)

ONLINE VEGAN GROCERY STORES
Pangea veganstore.com
Vegan Essentials veganessentials.com
Vegan Perfection veganperfection.com.au/index.php
Shop Vegan shopvegan.co.uk
Vegan Cuts vegancuts.com

OTHER OPTIONS FOR SHOPPING ONLINE
Amazon (go to the grocery section and select "vegan" on the left-hand side of the page) amazon.com
Vitacost (search "vegan" on the website) vitacost.com
Abe's Market (search "vegan" on the website) abesmarket.com
shopOrganic (search "vegan" on the website) shopOrganic.com

2. *Think about eating seasonally:*[5] Eating a diversity of produce that's in season is good for your health *and* the planet. Here's a list you can copy and post on the fridge so you know what and *when* to buy the best of nature's bounty!

ORGANIC ON A BUDGET?

When the price of organic produce shoots through the roof, you can use these two lists to help guide you. Ideally, it would be great to buy organic 100 percent of the time, but if that's not possible, at least you can make educated shopping choices and prioritize your purchases by knowing which produce contains the *most*, and the *least*, amount of pesticides.

ENVIRONMENTAL WORKING GROUP'S DIRTY DOZEN AND CLEAN 15

The "Dirty Dozen (plus)"

1. Strawberries
2. Apples
3. Nectarines
4. Peaches
5. Celery
6. Grapes
7. Cherries
8. Spinach
9. Tomatoes
10. Sweet bell peppers
11. Cherry tomatoes
12. Cucumbers
13. Hot Peppers
14. Kale/Collard Greens

The "Clean 15"

1. Avocados
2. Sweet Corn
3. Pineapple
4. Cabbage
5. Sweet Peas (frozen)
6. Onions
7. Asparagus
8. Mangoes
9. Papayas
10. Kiwi
11. Eggplant
12. Honeydew Melon
13. Grapefruit
14. Cantaloupe
15. Cauliflower

WHAT'S IN SEASON IN THE USA (Are we lucky, or what?!)

WINTER

Apples

Bananas

Beets

Brussels Sprouts

Cabbage

Carrots

Celery

Grapefruit

Kale

Leeks

Lemons

Onions

Oranges

Parsnips

Pears

Pineapple

Potatoes

Pumpkins

Rutabagas

Sweet Potatoes
and Yams

Turnips

Winter Squash

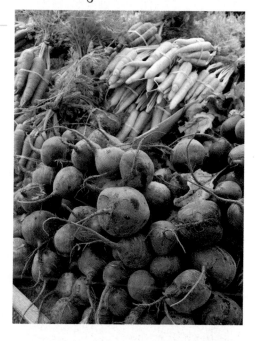

SPRING

Apples

Apricots

Asparagus

Bananas

Broccoli

Cabbage

Carrots

Celery

Collard Greens

Garlic

Greens (cooking)

Lettuce

Mushrooms

Onions

Peas

Pineapple

Radishes

Rhubarb

Spinach

Strawberries

Swiss Chard

Turnips

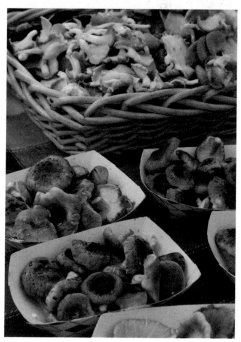

SUMMER

Apples

Apricots

Bananas

Beets

Bell Peppers

Blackberries

Blueberries

Carrots

Cantaloupe/
    Muskmelons

Celery

Cherries

Collard Greens

Corn

Cucumbers

Eggplant

Garlic

Green Beans

Honeydew Melon

Kiwifruit

Lima Beans

Mangos

Nectarines

Okra

Peaches

Plums

Raspberries

Strawberries

Summer Squash
    and Zucchini

Tomatillos

Tomatoes

Watermelon

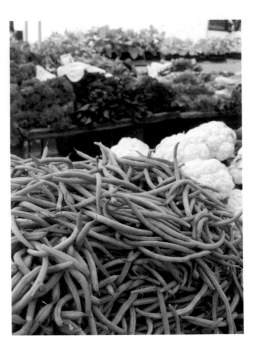

FALL

Apples

Bananas

Beets

Bell Peppers

Broccoli

Brussels Sprouts

Cabbage

Carrots

Cauliflower

Celery

Collard Greens

Cranberries

Garlic

Ginger

Grapes

Greens (cooking)

Green Beans

Kale

Lettuce

Mangos

Mushrooms

Onions

Parsnips

Peas

Pears

Pineapple

Potatoes

Pumpkins

Radishes

Raspberries

Rutabagas

Spinach

Sweet Potatoes and Yams

Swiss Chard

Turnips

Winter Squash

WHAT'S UP, DOC?

I've followed the great work of Dr. Neal Barnard for nearly three decades, but never knew exactly what made the lightbulb come on for him, as far as ditching animal products for healthier, plant-based fare. I had a chance to catch up with him recently and he explained the "aha moment" for him occurred after assisting with an autopsy during medical school. The pathologist he was observing carved open a man who died of a heart attack, and while doing so, Dr. Barnard saw firsthand how the arteries to the heart, and the brain, were clogged up with fat. When the autopsy was completed, the pathologist assigned Dr. Barnard the task of closing the man up. As instructed, Dr. Barnard put each of the man's ribs and skin back in their proper place, and then went to the cafeteria for lunch, where happenstance would have them serving, you guessed it: ribs. From that moment on, he associated meat with dead bodies, and as he aptly points out, when folks eat meat, "that's exactly what they're eating."

DR. NEAL BARNARD'S MEALS ON A TYPICAL DAY:

Breakfast: "I eat oatmeal for breakfast, usually a bigger serving than most people do. Sometimes I flavor it with blueberries, raspberries, or strawberries and sometimes slivered almonds, too. I'll even have a green vegetable for breakfast. I steam up spinach or broccoli. It's really just like an omelet except without the eggs. There's no reason why the time of day matters when it comes to eating vegetables. Occasionally I'll also have tempeh, which has the texture of sausage. I marinate it in soy sauce, and then put it in the pan. It doesn't even need oil."

Lunch: "For lunch I eat lots of different things. If I'm out, I'm not above getting a sub, with lettuce, tomatoes, olives, and red wine vinegar; I just skip the meat and the cheese. Or if there's a Mexican restaurant nearby, I'll get a burrito, with enough jalapeños to make it almost life threatening. I love sweet potatoes, too. I puree them, and then put them in a Pyrex bowl, along with asparagus or other greens on top, and just microwave it."

Dinner: "Yesterday I ate at an Italian Restaurant where I ordered pasta, with a wild mushroom sauce with artichokes. And I had a side of vegetables . . . asparagus and steamed broccoli with garlic. It's very common to find vegan food at Italian restaurants."

—DR. NEAL BARNARD, founder of Physicians Committee for Responsible Medicine and the Barnard Medical Center

Checklist

☐ Did you explore the USDA Farmers' Market Directory and jot down the time and day of a farmers' market near you?

☐ Did you find a brick-and-mortar store in your community that has a nice variety of scrumptious vegan food?

☐ Did you check out an online store or two just to check out their vegan selection?

Thought FOR THE Day

Oprah was fired from her first TV job. Thomas Edison was told he was too stupid to learn. And poor "Dr. Seuss" faced the rejection of his first book by twenty-seven different publishers. So remember, if your vegan voyage at first seems daunting, don't fret; today's setback does not dictate tomorrow's outcome. Stay strong and march on!

DAY 4

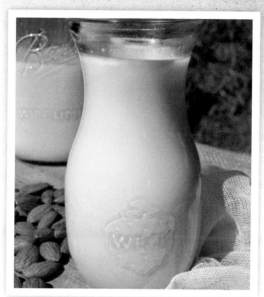

Let's GET Nutty!

GOAL FOR THE DAY: Switch out dairy from your morning beverage or cereal and replace it with a healthy plant-based milk.

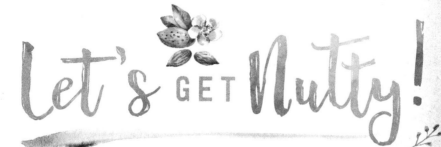

Got *Dairy* Milk? Nope, not me. The folks who launched the "Got Milk?" campaign know others are ditching it, too. Despite a whopping 91 percent of Americans being familiar with "Got Milk?" ads—which is no less than golden in the world of advertising—dairy milk consumption continues to spiral downward. Publicity thirsty celebrities donning goopy mustaches couldn't get adults to drink more dairy milk. Mattel's "Got Milk?" Barbie dolls and Hot Wheels "Got Milk?" delivery trucks couldn't drive in the kids. In fact, according to the USDA, between 1977 and 2007 the number of preadolescents who ditched dairy milk in the U.S. *doubled* and more than half the adults and adolescents in the United States now skip the stuff altogether.[1] So after a run of nearly twenty years, with little fanfare, the national "Got Milk?" campaign got *dumped*, and 50 million bucks was poured into a new campaign urging folks to drink milk for protein, because, you know, rumor has it, everyone is running around deficient in protein. Yawn.

So what could possibly have gone wrong for the dairy milk industry? They had the money. They had the fame. They had the USDA's support, and still do. They even plastered big poster-size ads in classrooms across the nation for decades duping a captive audience of schoolchildren into thinking their bones would break without dairy. How could they have possibly failed? Well, for one, a *huge* secret got out. This will blow your mind. Are you ready? OK, here it is: Cow's milk is for baby . . . *cows*! Yep. It's not for baby hippos, or for baby birds, or for baby gophers, *or for baby people*; it's for baby cows, and only while they're babies. Humans are the only species on the planet that seeks out the nipple of another species and drinks their milk. And incidentally, we're also the only ones to keep drinking a mother's milk past weaning.

Once people learned that cow's milk is truly just meant for baby cows, they began to understand why: it's full of saturated animal fat, which is a risk factor for heart disease.[2] Nature wants babies to be nice and chubby, but few adults want to look like supersize babies, nor tackle the myriad health problems that accompany excess weight. Even if you remove the fat from dairy milk, you're still left with lactose: aka milk sugar. Not only is it difficult, and often impossible, for most folks to digest lactose, researchers analyzed more than 500,000 women and found those with high intakes of lactose had a higher risk of ovarian cancer, compared to women who consumed the least.[3] And men who consumed three or more servings of dairy products per day had a 141 percent higher risk of death due to prostate cancer compared to those who consumed less than one serving.[4]

You don't need to get your protein from milk either. In fact, most Americans already consume *twice* the amount of protein they need.[5] Just take a moment to reflect: when was the last time that a friend or family member told you they were deficient in protein? Any mention of protein deficiency diseases such as marasmus or kwashiorkor? Probably not. I've had my blood tested with full CBC blood panels many times over the course of my twenty-eight plus years of being vegan, as well as routine physicals, and

I've never been told that I need to eat more protein, by any health professional. Ever. But I know of many folks who have been told they consume *too much* cholesterol, *too much* saturated fat, and *too much* sugar. And I bet you know of some, too. The vast majority of today's health problems, particularly in the United States, are spurred by excess fill-in-the-blank, not deficiencies, and judging by the decline in dairy milk sales, the general public is catching on.

As people began to make the important mama cow/baby cow connection over the past few decades, another major development that would shake up the dairy industry like never before was quietly brewing behind the scenes. In the early '70s a down-to-earth vegetarian guy named Steve Demos borrowed five hundred dollars from his upstairs neighbor and started making tofu in his apartment kitchen, selling chunks of the bean curd to his tai chi friends. Demos experimented making other soy products, too, including organic soy milk, and with a two-thousand-dollar loan in 1977 launched WhiteWave Foods[6], maker of Silk. Armed with a savvy ad campaign, coupled with giving away more than 3 million half-pints of free soy milk, Demos galvanized consumers who were looking for an alternative to dairy, and grew the company to a net worth of nearly 20 million bucks. What happened next is nothing short of genius. In 2000, Demos entered into an agreement to sell WhiteWave to Dean Foods, which, at the time, was a 10-*billion* dollar company and the largest distributer of dairy in the United States. This made most vegans shudder; some even boycotted the brand. Fortunately, Demos was, and is, a very smart man.

Demos got Dean Foods to agree to give WhiteWave an initial investment of 5 million dollars, with the understanding that three years later they would purchase WhiteWave for its full market value. During this three-year period, WhiteWave would have complete control over all capital expenditures, all distributions of resources, and all marketing initiatives.[7] With Dean Foods footing the bill, and Demos steering the ship, Silk soy milk was launched in supermarkets across the nation, placed on coveted eye-level shelf space, and landed smack-dab in the middle of all the dairy milk. And the cartons didn't just sit there innocently with a photo of soybeans. Demos is smarter than that. If you've read a Silk soy milk, almond milk, or cashew milk carton lately, you'll see Silk is no friend of the dairy industry. Cartons are emblazoned with nutritional claims showing how much better plant-based products are compared to dairy milk. I wouldn't be surprised if something hit the fan at Dean Foods' headquarters thanks to the sweet deal. Within three short years, WhiteWave grew its 20-million-dollar vegan company into an unstoppable, powerhouse corporation with a market value of 296 million dol-

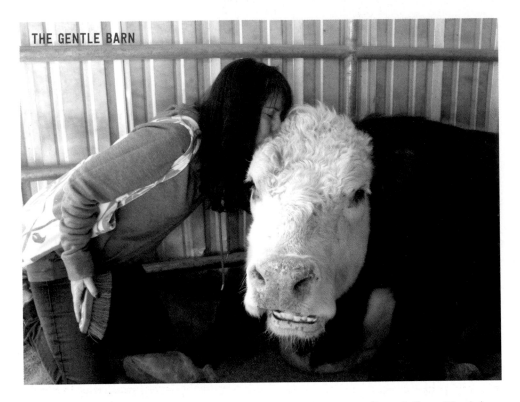

lars, ensuring its permanent spot in the dairy case. Yep, 296 million dollars. That's how many smackers Dean Foods had to fork over to the company that made, and continues to make, folks understand why dairy sucks.

And sucks it does. I don't like watching animal abuse, reading about animal abuse, or writing about animal abuse, but I promised I wouldn't skirt the truth about what *really* happens to the animals. With that in mind, I'll keep this next bit brief, because I think most of you just want to know enough to be inspired into action, but not *so* much that you wind up curled up in a ball in bed with a box of tissue and a closed book. So, here we go.

There are over 9 million dairy cows in the United States alone, and most are raised in very intensive factory farm conditions.[8] Cows have to be pregnant in order to produce milk, so the factory workers force bull semen into their vaginas, which, for an animal, is nothing short of being mechanically raped. Cows who would normally live about twenty years usually die within five due to the horrific conditions in which they live. Their breasts are hooked up to tubes for most of their lives, which causes many to develop mastitis, a bacteria growth in the udder[9]; the impetus for PETA's infamous "Got Pus?" campaign. Because the dairy industry would lose money if the cows die from disease, they pump them full of antibiotics to keep them alive. Thus, the growing concern that the massive, ongoing use of antibiotics in animals is creating a resistance to antibiotics in the humans who eat them. In other words, if you continually consume antibiotics when you eat animal products, the antibiotics you take when you're sick might not work because your body may have already developed a tolerance to them. A recent FDA investigation found that some of the antibiotics used for cows aren't even *approved* by the FDA, nor can the FDA confirm if they're safe for human consumption.[10] As if that wasn't bad enough, the FDA can't investigate the dairy farms in violation because the samples were given anonymously; the government doesn't know which cows are getting the illegal antibiotics, or which unsuspecting people are drinking their drug-infested milk.[11]

And then there's the heartbreak of having your child stolen upon birth. Dairy farmers have no use for most baby male calves—after all, they can't give milk—so within twenty-four to forty-eight hours of birth, most are torn away from their mothers and sold off to the veal industry. In fact, if you take a Sunday drive and see hundreds of tiny boxes in an otherwise barren field, you might just be looking at a veal farm. Here they spend most of their time in small closed crates with tiny holes, all alone in almost complete darkness, unable to even turn around. You see, fancy folks like their veal soft and pink, so if the calves can't move, they can't develop their muscles, and if they live in the dark on a liquid diet, they'll grow pale and anemic, too. Great for the greedy farmer who wants the big bucks; not so great for the baby cow who just wants his mother. Once a mama cow can't produce any more milk, or as is often the case, can't even stand up, her fate is the same as her babies'; they are all slaughtered. This is why some folks call dairy milk "liquid meat," since in the end, it's all the same: misery followed by death. A glass of dairy milk might look pure and white upon first glance, but through my eyes, it's a gruesome bloodred.

Are you still with me? I sure hope so, because I have some great news for you: the abuse of dairy cows will stop when people stop consuming dairy, and today, right now, it couldn't be easier to ditch. Good-bye, dairy milk! Hello refreshing, cholesterol-free plant-based beverages made from nutritious almonds, soy, cashews, oats, rice, hemp, coconuts, flaxseeds, walnuts, and more. So many to choose from! It's really just a matter of preference. For smoothies, some folks prefer lighter ones, such as rice milk or flax milk, but if you're making a delicious curry or whipped cream, I'd jump right over to the thick and creamy coconut milk. I generally use almond milk for smoothies and in my coffee, but our taste buds are all different, so just enjoy whatever you prefer. The cows will be happy no matter which one you pick!

Plant-based milks also offer a wide range of essential nutrients as well. If you think about it, with a little sunshine, soil, and water, a tiny nut or seed can become an entire plant—or even a big tree—so you know there *has* to be a tremendous amount of good stuff packed in those little seeds and nuts to fuel all that growth. Soy milk and cashew milk, for example, are known to be high in protein, while oat milk is a great source of soluble fiber. Hemp milk has omega-3 and omega-6 fatty acids, and walnuts are a powerhouse of goodness, including the gamma-tocopherol form of vitamin E, known for deterring heart problems.[12] As an added bonus, many store-bought plant milks are also fortified with vitamins and minerals such as calcium and B_{12}, which by the way, I get *plenty* of without taking any shots or pills. According to my most recent blood analysis, taken less than a year ago, the normal range for B_{12} is 239-931 pg/ML. If we listen to the naysayers, they'd probably predict I'd have a big fat zero when it comes to B_{12}, having been vegan for over twenty-eight years, but I have over 500 pg/ML of B_{12} in my body, and my calcium intake is normal, too, so they can take *that* to the bank.

When shopping for plant-based milks, just keep in mind that many of them add extra ingredients beyond the nuts, seeds, and water, some of which you may want to avoid. Salt and sugar are a pretty common addition, as well as carrageenan (made from seaweed), which some believe causes stomach ailments. People sometimes prefer carrageenan or gellan gum in their nut milks because it makes them thicker and creamier, more akin to the dairy milk that they're accustomed to. So if you're used to drinking a lot of whole milk, you might want thickening agents in your non-dairy milks as you make the transition, or if you don't mind a thinner nut milk, grab one that's just made with water, seeds, and/or nuts, and whatever else sounds good to you. If you want to save a bit of time, and avoid standing in the middle of the grocery aisle reading every single nut and seed milk label, most companies post their products' nutritional info online so you can check them out in advance. There are also helpful nutritional data websites that post product information as well, such as MyFitnessPal.com. You can plug in the brand name and flavor of what you're interested in, and it should pull up the most recent nutrition information. Just know that manufacturers can change their ingredients at any time, so before you make a purchase, of *any* food or beverage item, always double-check the label in person.

So, what do you enjoy for breakfast? If it involves dairy milk on cereal, in a smoothie, or in your morning hot cup of Joe, simply make a switch-a-roo; just pour in some delicious plant-based milk instead of the yucky moo!

1. *Look at the variety of non-dairy milk out there and decide which one is best for you:* Don't be surprised if you need to try a few before you find the one you like best. It's like dating; it's difficult to know who's really "the one" unless you go out with a few, so live it up and have some fun! Here are a few to consider.

- Soy Milk
- Almond Milk
- Cashew Milk
- Oat Milk
- Rice Milk
- Hemp Milk
- Coconut Milk
- Flax Milk
- Macadamia Nut Milk
- Walnut Milk

2. *Choose foods and activities to keep your bones strong:* Most folks think that if they give up dairy milk, they're opening the door to osteoporosis; after all, we've been told since childhood that consuming dairy products will give us strong bones. But as Harvard's School of Public Health points out, "Calcium is important. But milk isn't the only, or even the best, source. Plus, dairy products can be high in saturated fat as well as retinol (vitamin A), which at high levels can paradoxically weaken bones."[13] In fact, researchers found that in a twelve-year Harvard study of 78,000 women, those who drank milk three times a day actually broke *more* bones than women who seldom drank milk.[14] It turns out that the focus should really be on the big picture: preventing bone loss, rather than just focusing on calcium intake.

How do you prevent bone loss? Exercise! This is particularly important if you're a woman in menopause, since your body is producing less estrogen, which causes a decrease in calcium absorption. I'm not there yet, but at fifty-one years old, I know it's just a matter of time, so I'll be sure to pick up the pace and wiggle around even more. Tennis, anyone? A hike in the wilderness? A bike ride by the sea? Gee, getting old doesn't sound so bad. Bring it!

You should also avoid foods and certain lifestyle habits that have been shown to have a detrimental effect on your calcium levels, too. Sodas with phosphoric acid, typically the colas, can leach calcium from your bones and have been shown to create lower bone density.[15] Diets high in caffeine and sodium can also contribute to the loss of calcium. And diets high in protein can cause you to pee calcium out through your urine. The good news is that plant protein is *less* likely to cause calcium loss than animal protein.[16] Hurray! Yet another great reason to say "so

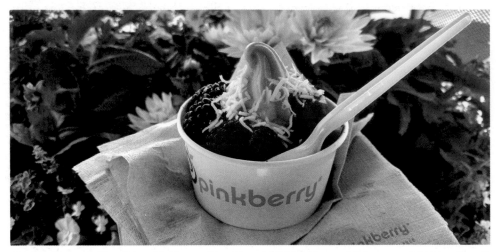

Craving fro-yo? Menchies, Pinkberry, Tutti Frutti, TCBY, Pressed Juicery, and 16 Handles all have vegan options.

long!" to dairy milk! Hello collards, bok choy, fortified nut milks, and baked beans, all of which are recommended by Harvard's School of Public Health as good sources of calcium. You'll also notice that most tofu is made with calcium sulfate, yet another good option if you want to gobble up a little more of the healthy mineral.

3. *Check out your Vitamin D level:* The next time you visit your doctor, you might want to ask for a blood panel just to take a peek at your Vitamin D. It plays a key role in bone health, and many Americans don't get enough. Your body can make vitamin D from sunshine, but sometimes it's hard to get enough, and no one wants skin cancer, so soaking up a ton of sun isn't always the best plan. Other options include consuming foods that are fortified with Vitamin D (like most store-bought nut milks!), or taking supplements. Vitamin D_2 is made from yeast (it's vegan!) but vitamin D_3 is usually derived from fish or sheep (boo!). If you want a vegan source of D_3, Nordic Natural's and Vitashine have supplements that are made from organic lichen—those pretty little fungus-algae growths that look similar to moss on coastal rocks and trees. Nice!

4. *If you start your day with coffee, find a local place that also serves plant-based milk:* Is coffee good for us? Or bad? Who knows; research findings seem to change as often as the weather. Rain or shine, that first cup of java in the morning is an important

ritual for many, so if you normally drink coffee with dairy milk, find a place near you that offers a nut or seed milk as a refreshing alternative. I'll bet there's a barista in your neighborhood who'd love to make you a vegan latte every day. Here are a few options to get you started:

COFFEE SHOPS WITH NUT MILKS FOR YOUR MORNING CUP OF JOE!
- Starbucks (soy milk, coconut milk, and almond milk)
- Dunkin' Donuts (almond milk)
- Peet's Coffee and Tea (soy milk and almond milk)
- Caribou Coffee (soy milk)
- Tully's (soy milk and almond milk)

And here's some vegan-friendly shops that have vegan donuts to go with your coffee for an occasional sweet treat! And yes, vegan custard–filled chocolate glazed donuts really *do* exist. And they're darn tootin' good, too.

- Mighty-O Donut (Seattle, Washington)
- Dottie's Donuts (Philadelphia, Pensylvania)
- Donut Friend (Los Angeles, California)
- Donut Farm (Los Angeles, California)
- Dun-Well Doughnuts (Brooklyn, New York)
- Hypnotic Donuts (Denton and Dallas, Texas)
- Voodoo Doughnut (Portland and Eugene, Oregon, and Denver)
- Le Cave's Bakery (Tucson, Arizona)
- Tandem Doughnuts (Missoula, Montana)
- Pepples Organic Donuts (Berkeley, Oakland, and San Francisco, California)
- Ronald's Donuts (Las Vegas, Nevada)
- Vegan Treats (Bethlehem, Pennsylvania)
- Whole Foods Market (available in selected locations)

BONUS ACTIVITY FOR THE DAY: If you're feeling adventurous, here's a simple recipe to make your own nut milk. It does take a bit of planning, so I don't make it very often, but some folks just can't get enough of homemade nut milks. They're thinner than most store-bought nut milks, which makes them extremely refreshing and thirst-quenching. If you've got the time, go for it! And, when you've made it, you can also use it to create a great breakfast without milk. See My Overnight Oats (page 135).

Easy Almond Milk

1 cup almonds

Water, as needed

Flavoring of choice (optional)

Fine cheesecloth, for draining

1. Soak the almonds overnight in enough water to cover them, plus a few extra inches.

2. The next day, drain and rinse a few times, discarding the water.

3. Add to a blender with 3 to 4 cups of fresh water; the less water you use, the thicker the milk will be.

4. Add additional flavorings, such as maple syrup, cinnamon, pitted dates, or whatever else suits your fancy. Or keep it simple, with just the almonds.

5. Blend at high speed for 1–2 minutes, until the almonds are ground to a fine meal and the water is white and opaque.

6. Transfer to a cheesecloth-lined strainer set over a bowl and drain. Using the cheesecloth, gather the nut mixture into a ball and squeeze out any excess liquid that remains in the bundle of almond meal. Save the almond meal for smoothies, cookie batter, or anything else that sounds good to you. Place the almond milk in the refrigerator where it should keep fresh for several days. Don't worry if it separates a bit; that's normal. Just stir it up before serving.

7. Enjoy your refreshing almond milk! Cheers!

WHERE DID THE "V" WORD COME FROM?

The term *vegan* was coined in 1944 by Englishman Donald Watson at a meeting in London where a few like-minded folks gathered to discuss non-dairy vegetarian lifestyles. They created the word *vegan* by simply combining the beginning and end of the word *vegetarian*.

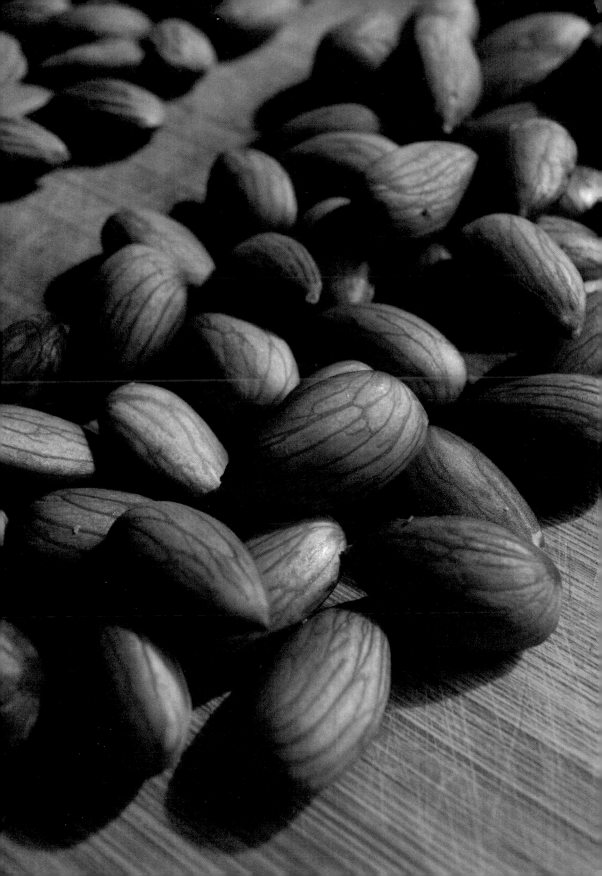

Checklist

- ☐ Did you select a nut or seed milk you'd like to try out?

- ☐ Did you make a plan to limit foods that reduce calcium absorption?

- ☐ Did you make a plan to get some exercise?

- ☐ Did you find a shop that serves a vegan beverage to start your day?

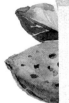

Thought FOR THE Day

It's impossible to look into the eyes of an animal and not see a small reflection of oneself.

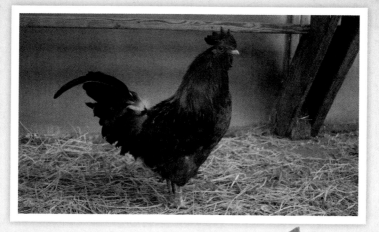

Eggs MAKE BABIES, NOT Breakfast

GOAL FOR THE DAY: Turn an egg-based meal into a scrumptious vegan delight.

I loved Sunday mornings so much as a little girl because that's the day we'd always have my favorite breakfast: French crepes! I wasn't allowed to watch my mom turn them over in the pan, though, because the perfect flip required intense concentration, and if I was watching, my mom would lose her focus and they'd invariably fall apart. So I knew the drill: if crepes were about to be flipped, I had to run out of the kitchen.

I was allowed to watch my mom make the batter, though. She'd whisk together all the basics: eggs, milk, flour, a dash of salt, and her special little addition of juice from a fresh-squeezed orange. One day, however, I noticed something strange about the egg she had just cracked as it sunk into the pile of flour. There were two little odd-shaped white things dangling about the yolk, and they didn't look like something you were supposed to eat. "What's *that?*" I asked. Trying to deflect my inquiry swiftly, my mom, in her British accent, calmly said, "What do you mean, 'What's that?' It's just the egg. Now go on. Set the table, please."

A guest who overheard the conversation wasn't quite as kind, and tried to stir up a little trouble in the kitchen. "It's the head and the legs," she laughed. From that moment on, my mother had to remove those stringy bits from every batter, and every dough, and everything else that she ever made again with eggs, knowing all along that they weren't *really* the head and the legs, but that her little girl wouldn't eat anything with eggs unless she did. Ah, my mom was the best.

As some of you may already know, those little white doodads are called chalazae (pronounced cuh-LAY-zee) and they serve to tether the yolk so it's protected against hitting the inner wall of the egg if it's bumped around. And although there are no pre-formed limbs in a non-fertilized egg, there *are* plenty of both unappetizing and unhealthy parts in an egg, as well as a tremendous impact on chickens and our environment. The more I learned, the more I realized that feeling that something just *wasn't quite right* about eating eggs back when I was a kid was actually spot on. Here are a few things to keep in mind as you toss eggs from your diet:

THE YUCK FACTOR

This isn't the *best* reason, but for some, it's more than enough: if you think about it, eating eggs is kind of, well . . . *gross.* Just as women have their "period," chickens do, too. The eggs in the carton are similar to the eggs women of childbearing age release each month, only much larger and with a hard shell. They hold the hen's DNA and lots of saturated fat for the baby chick, should the egg become fertilized. Can you imagine someone forcing you (or your female friend) to ovulate faster to produce more eggs, and then snatching

> "There is no specific federal humane handling and slaughter statute for poultry."
>
> —Treatment of Live Poultry Before Slaughter, USDA Federal Register

them up to make breakfast? Or for birthday cake batter? Don't fault me for being disgusting; *I'm* not the one eating eggs. I'm just the messenger. Wink.

NO MATTER HOW YOU CRACK 'EM, EGGS ARE FULL OF CHOLESTEROL

Cholesterol: that icky, sticky stuff that clings to our artery walls, making the blood's passageway smaller and smaller, until a little chunk of plaque gets loose, and plugs the whole damn thing up. BOOM: a heart attack. Well, eggs are packed with it. Yes, it's true, cholesterol *is* essential for our bodies to function, but the great news is, if your body is working properly, it makes all the cholesterol you will ever need. You don't need to go out and eat a single bite of dietary cholesterol, *ever*. Isn't that nice?

So what's wrong with a little cholesterol? Well, when it comes to eggs, it turns out it's not very little. Instead of just throwing out a random number, let's put things in perspective. A McDonald's Quarter Pounder with Cheese (blah!) has 93.5 mg of cholesterol.[1] That's a *lot*. Guess how much cholesterol a couple of scrambled eggs have? A whopping 370 mg.[2] Almost four times as much! If you buy extra-large or jumbo eggs, the cholesterol in your scramble is even greater. The greasy combo of excess saturated fat and cholesterol is your straight-to-the-front-of-the-line ticket to myriad health ailments including atherosclerosis, heart disease, and strokes—all of which too often lead to death.

Sadly, too many folks seem willing to take their chances and wind up with an early rendezvous with the reaper. About 2,150 Americans die of cardiovascular disease *every single day*. One out of every 3 people will die of cardiovascular disease at a rate of about 1 every 40 seconds.[3] That's just crazy. Let's put faces to figures. If you have three hundred Facebook friends, about *one hundred* of them, on average, are going to die from cardiovascular disease. Knowing that LDL cholesterol contributes to cardiovascular disease, why on earth would you want to gobble it up if you don't need to? No wonder the Easter bunny drops off those eggs. He doesn't want them!

THE CHICKEN OR THE EGG

Spoiler Alert: It really doesn't matter which came first, the chicken dies in the end either way. And they endure a living hell straight through that last desperate gasp to live—all for some fatty food that none of us need. Just as with the plight of dairy cows, I really loathe writing about how animal products wind up in the fridge and on the table, but I know from experience that for most folks, it's information like this that will *really* help you stay the course; you're going vegan, after all, and you'll need to lean back on the *why*

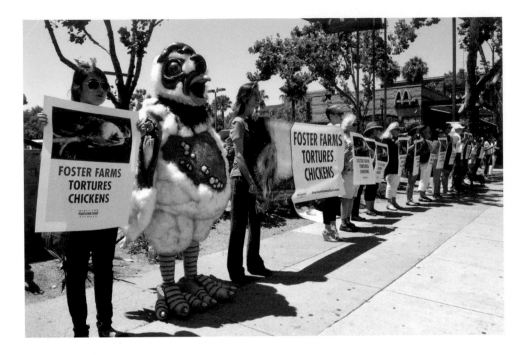

of it all when old habits come knocking. Knowing the facts will help you make an educated, heartfelt decision to say "No thanks!" to food made with eggs. So bear with me here for a few minutes, and then we'll get to the good stuff. Trust me, I won't leave you hanging feeling sad and helpless. This is a book of empowerment, not despair. You and I are changing the world, together, in a very easy and delicious way!

OK, up first, the Humane Methods of Slaughter Act. I know, the words *humane* and *slaughter* go together about as well as "beautiful diarrhea" but that's honestly the name of the Act. Well, guess what? Birds aren't covered under it.[4] Nope. They left them out. Ninety-five percent of *all* the animals who are slaughtered in the United States are birds, and the USDA decided they aren't entitled to even the slightest bit of protection under this law.[5] With so few rules, their death is akin to medieval torture.

Once chickens can no longer lay eggs, they're considered "spent" and they're shackled upside down, paralyzed by electrified water, and dragged over mechanical throat-cutting blades, all while being conscious.[6] The USDA allows this cruel system of slaughter to occur at a rate of 140 birds per minute; that's one bird killed every .43 seconds. Not every 43 seconds, but one every *point* 43 seconds. And it gets worse. Because the machines move *so fast*, many birds miss the blades, and I don't just mean a few dozen or even a few hundred. According to the USDA's own records, nearly 1 million birds are boiled alive each year because they're not killed before they're dumped into the scalding water.[7] Some birds are spared the knife, and instead piled into a small area and poisoned with carbon monoxide. Imagine being trapped in a room with a gasoline-powered leaf blower on full blast until you die from the fumes—all because someone wants scrambled eggs. And here's the kicker: it's all 100 percent legal. It's just business as usual for an industry that profits from snuffing the life out of others on a massive genocide-like scale. The faster they can kill the birds, the more money they can make. It's that simple—and that sad.

As for life before the kill, it's not any better. I'll try to give you a quick tangible example. If you have an iPad handy, please grab it. I have an iPad 2, and you know what? The "guidelines" given by the United Egg Producers state that a chicken doesn't even need to have as much space as the size of my iPad, which is only 9½ x 7¼ inches.[8] Now try to imagine a bunch of chickens being crammed into cages with other birds, each having less space than an iPad; that's less space than an 8 x 10 sheet of paper. That's how 250,000 million birds are living right now, as you're reading this, in the United States alone. They can't spread their wings, they defecate on each other because there's no where else to go, and because the bottom of the cage is made of slanted wires so the eggs roll out, their feet become lacerated and their nails become overgrown and entangled in the metal.[9]

The bodies of the chickens who lay eggs in battery cages are so damaged that by the time they're killed they can usually only be used for chicken soup or "pet" food. The male chicks are useless to the industry—after all, they can't lay eggs—so they're stuffed into garbage bags where they suffocate on top of one another, or are tossed into grinders while alive. Again, all 100 percent legal. I wish there was a nicer way to tell the story of a factory-farmed chicken, but it is what it is: inexcusably sad. It's a madman's house of horrors, far removed from any semblance of the bucolic farm most people imagine.

THE EGG INDUSTRY IS SCRAMBLING

As you'll see on pages 107–110, there's a huge array of scrumptious alternatives to eating eggs or foods made with eggs. So *huge* that it's scaring the bejesus out of the egg industry. Folks want healthier, more compassionate options, and with good reason. It's not the '50s anymore; people, like you (hurray!) are learning the truth and making smart lifestyle changes. As you can imagine, watching a bunch of lightbulbs turn on in our heads isn't going "over easy" with the egg industry. They'd rather we stay in the dark. Selling bird eggs fills their coffers, and they like their fancy things regardless of the consequences to those who consume eggs, or to those who die producing them. They've been worried about consumers learning the facts for a very long time, but no matter how hard the egg industry tries to persuade us, in the end, the truth always prevails.

Frustrated with the outpouring of scientific evidence that shows eating too many eggs makes folks ill, the egg industry whipped up a little official-sounding committee in the '70s called the National Commission on Egg Nutrition (NCEN) to counteract the bad press. NCEN hired an advertising agency, and began to blast the message that there's "no scientific evidence that eating eggs increases the risk of . . . heart (and circulatory) disease," and that eggs are actually harmless and needed for good nutrition.[10] Say what?! People *have* to eat eggs? Thankfully the Federal Trade Commission (FTC) thought that smelled a little rotten, and filed a complaint charging them with having made "false and misleading statements" regarding the relationship between eating eggs and disease.

The result? Not only did the court issue a cease and desist order prohibiting NCEN from making those statements, they removed the deceptive cloak the egg industry was hiding behind. (Hello?! We see you!) The FTC said if they ever use the name "National Commission on Egg Nutrition" again, they must reveal NCEN's *true* identity and disclose that it's really just a bunch of "egg producers and other individuals and organizations of, or relating to, the egg industry."[11] Studies show eating eggs can be *very* unhealthy. Hey NCEN, disagree all you want, but you can't say the evidence doesn't exist. And while you're disagreeing, you can't pretend you're not the egg industry. Save your creepy costume for Halloween.

Flash forward to 2015 and the industry is *still* trying to strong-arm stores and consumers into buying more eggs. Only this time the feud isn't over scientific studies that prove eggs aren't healthy, but a predictable (and possibly *illegal*) reaction to CEO Josh Tetrick's successful start-up, Hampton Creek, a company that for the first time is on the fast track to make the consumption of eggs obsolete. Backed with investments from fiscal heavyweights, Bill Gates, hedge fund billionaire Tom Steyer, and Li Ka-Shing, who at a net worth of $31.7 billion has been crowned Asia's richest man, Hampton Creek has the financial backing to move mountains, and they are. In just a few short years, Hampton Creek, now valued at $500 million, is the fastest-growing food company in the world, with no end in sight. Thanks to the avian flu, and other health concerns, their tasty egg-free products are being snatched up by consumers across the globe.

Enter the American Egg Board (AEB), responsible for boosting sales of eggs with catchy slogans like "The Incredible, Edible Egg" and other promotional campaigns overseen by the United States Department of Agriculture. While Hampton Creek's sales have soared, egg sales have soured, falling 10 percent this past year alone.[12] The egg industry watched on as Hampton Creek's eggless Just Mayo replaced egg-based mayonnaise in every sandwich in every 7-Eleven across the United States. They endured the pain of seeing Compass Group, the largest food service company in the world, give up their egg-based cookies in exchange for Hampton Creek's *eggless* cookies. Thanks to Hampton Creek, products that traditionally contain eggs are being replaced across the planet, from Yale University to the United States Senate; egg-free food is everywhere. Hampton Creek's products are rolling out in Asia, Mexico, and Europe, too.

As you can imagine, this makes the egg industry a wee bit cranky. Actually, more like raging mad. *So* mad that according to e-mail documents provided to The Associated Press, the AEB engaged in a two-year effort to damage Hampton Creek, including a documented e-mail exchange illustrating a plan to get Whole Foods Market to ditch the brand.[13] Thanks to The Freedom of Information Act, the public was able to acquire and read six hundred e-mails sent out by the AEB, some of which showed that they went far above and beyond promoting eggs; they attacked a competitor, which is a big fat no-no for a USDA-run agency. The AEB allegedly sought out Google adds that promoted eggs whenever someone searched for "Hampton Creek" and the AEB advised Unilever, makers of Best Food Mayonnaise, on how to proceed in a false advertising lawsuit against Hampton Creek last year.[14] One AEB member even joked (at least I *hope* it was a joke), that they "put a hit" out on Tetrick.[15] As for the American Egg Board CEO Joanne Ivy, who told a consultant that she'd like to accept an "offer to make that phone call to keep Just Mayo off Whole Foods shelves," well, she just "retired." *Early.* As Upton Sinclair noted, "It is impossible to get a man to understand something when his salary depends on him not understanding it."

All of this craziness should help you realize something supercool: It's a great time to be vegan. The egg industry feels threatened with good reason; the good guys are winning

A PICTURE SPEAKS A THOUSAND WORDS

The Humane Society of the United States recently sent an undercover investigator out to Butterfield Foods Company in Minnesota to document the slaughter of "spent" chickens in the egg industry. If my words aren't enough to help you stop eating eggs, you can watch their video, "Spent Hen Slaughter Exposé: Birds Abused and Scalded Alive" on YouTube. As promised, there are no sad photos in this book, but there's no shortage of visuals if you need them to help drive the message home.[16]

and that means there will be plenty of yummy vegan food for you to eat. Lot's of plant-based options coming down the pipes! Vegan eggs? Heck, when I went vegan, my doctor didn't even know what the word *vegan* meant. If I said "vegan eggs" he probably would have sent me to the loony bin!

OK, let's get crackin'!

1. *Think about all the meals and treats you currently enjoy that contain eggs, select one, and "veganize" it! Easy peasy.*

   PASTA: Believe it or not, most store-bought pasta doesn't contain eggs, so if you love eating pasta like I do, you're in luck! Check out the ingredients on your favorite dried pasta and you'll likely see that it's made from 100 percent flour (wheat, rice, quinoa, etc.) with little, or nothing else, added. Trader Joe's has lots of vegan pasta for about a buck, and mainstream supermarkets have vegan pasta at a good price as well. It gets a bit trickier when you buy "fresh" pasta, which often contains eggs, so be sure to double-check the ingredients.

   MAYONNAISE: Vegan mayo? Not a problem. Check out Follow Your Heart's Vegenaise, Nasoya's Nayonaise, Spectrum Natural's Vegan Mayo, Sir Kensington's Fabanaise, or Hampton Creek's Just Mayo. Heck, even Unilever, who sued Hampton Creek, created its *own* vegan mayo called Hellmann's "Carefully Crafted Dressing & Sandwich Spread." You can find vegan mayos at grocery stores across the country. I've even found vegan mayo at The Dollar Tree for, you guessed it, one dollar! You can find vegan mayo in different flavors, too: chipotle, sriracha, pesto, horseradish, garlic, and more—perfect for dips, creamy salad dressings, and sandwich spreads. Want to make your own instead? Check out Miyoko Schinner's recipe for "Classic Eggless Mayonnaise." It's from Miyoko's book *Homemade Vegan Pantry* and you can find the recipe posted on Yahoo.[17]

   MERINGUE: Well, here's something "egg-citing!" You know that liquid you pour down the drain when you strain a can of garbanzo beans (chickpeas)? Well, it's been coined "aquafaba": aka bean liquid, and is magical! French chef Joël Roessel recently discovered that chickpea brine can be used in recipes to replace egg whites.[18] You can even make fluffy white meringue with it! Check out my recipe for Easy Meringue Bites on page 221.

   EGGNOG: There's lots of vegan eggnog recipes you can get for free online using a wide range of ingredients: everything from combining cashews with coconut milk to silken tofu with soy milk.[19] I usually just wait for the holidays to roll around and buy some from the grocery store as a treat, or simply warm up some almond milk with a little vanilla, cinnamon, and nutmeg. Califia, So Delicious, Silk, and Rice Dream all make holiday nogs, which come in a variety of flavors and thicknesses, so it's just a matter of taste as to which one you'll like best.

CUSTARD: When I was a child, my mother would always make Bird's Traditional Custard, which was developed in Birmingham, England, by Alfred Bird, back in 1837, because his wife was allergic to eggs.[20] My mother made it with whole milk, but it's easy to make with a plant-based milk, too. You can find it in many supermarkets in a bright red and yellow tin can. It won't be quite as thick, but it's still delicious. There's also a variety of recipes online using a combo of ingredients that usually include cornstarch, vanilla, a plant milk of your choice (the thicker the better) and sugar to taste. And heads up: If you enjoy your custard in the form of a crème brûlée, and are ever in Mendocino, California, swing by Raven's Restaurant; ooh la la!

EGG ROLLS: If you're near one of over 450 Trader Joe's stores, check out their tasty Stir-Fried Vegetable Egg Rolls; they're vegan! Or better yet, make your own! Just find an egg roll recipe of your choice online (so many to choose from!) and substitute a little bit of crumbled tofu or shiitake mushrooms for any animal products. Make sure to add the veggies you love! Most store-bought egg roll wrappers contain egg, but it's simple to make your own. Just mix 1 cup flour with ¼ teaspoon salt, then slowly add ¼ cup of warm water, knead, and let sit, covered with a towel, for 20 minutes. Then roll, cut into the shapes of your choice, dust with a bit of cornstarch, pile them up, and store in the fridge until ready to use. So easy!

SCRAMBLED EGGS AND OMELETS: Most vegans I know, myself included, really enjoy a good veggie breakfast scramble every now and then; trust me, we're not missing the eggs. Vegan scrambles are traditionally so flavorful and satisfying, that cracking a slimy ovum into the pan is the last thing our taste buds crave. Yuck. Check out my recipe for a breakfast scramble on the next page and adjust to taste. Or if you just want a side of fluffy scrambled vegan eggs with a texture similar to chicken eggs, consider trying Hampton Creek's recently hatched Just Scramble, soon to be available nationwide. It's made from Canadian yellow peas, along with other non-GMO plants that together mimic an egg emulsion. Or you can grab Follow Your Heart's VeganEgg, which is also GMO-free. Just Scramble and

VeganEgg both work well for whipping up omelets, and making French toast, quiche, and fritattas as well!

Vegan breakfast scrambles are super easy, hearty, and delicious. I like making them colorful and healthy, too. Here's how I make mine:

My Vegan Breakfast Scramble

SERVES 2 AS A SIDE DISH

1 to 2 tablespoons vegetable oil

8 ounces tofu (about half a standard container of tofu), drained

1 cup chopped veggies (bell peppers, mushrooms, onions, etc.)

2 heaping teaspoons nutritional yeast

2 dashes ground turmeric (for color)

1 tablespoon chopped fresh garlic

Salt and freshly ground black pepper

1 small handful fresh parsley or cilantro, chopped

1. Add enough oil to lightly coat the bottom of a skillet and place over low to medium heat.

2. Break up the drained tofu into scrambled egg–sized pieces with your fingers, and place in the pan. Add the veggies, yeast, turmeric, and garlic and sauté until all the ingredients are hot and lightly browned, seasoning with salt and pepper to taste.

3. Just before serving, fold in the chopped parsley or cilantro, and immediately remove the scramble from the heat so it stays vibrant.

YOUR BREAKFAST SCRAMBLE

Cue Frank Sinatra's "I did it my way," please! Seriously, feel free to get creative here; there are *no rules* when it comes to making a delicious breakfast scramble. The two "biggies" for many vegans are the turmeric, which will give the scramble a beautiful yellow hue, and the nutritional yeast, which adds that distinct umami (pronounced oo-MAH-mee) flavor. I'd stick with those two items, and as for the rest? I say, go for whatever your tummy desires! Add an assortment of veggies you have in the fridge, and spices that you enjoy. There's the organic 21 spice mix at Costco that I love to use, or you can find a smaller version of it at Trader Joe's. I often add a squirt or two of sriracha to the tofu in the pan, and a little Bragg's Liquid Amino once plated. If you want to skip the oil, you

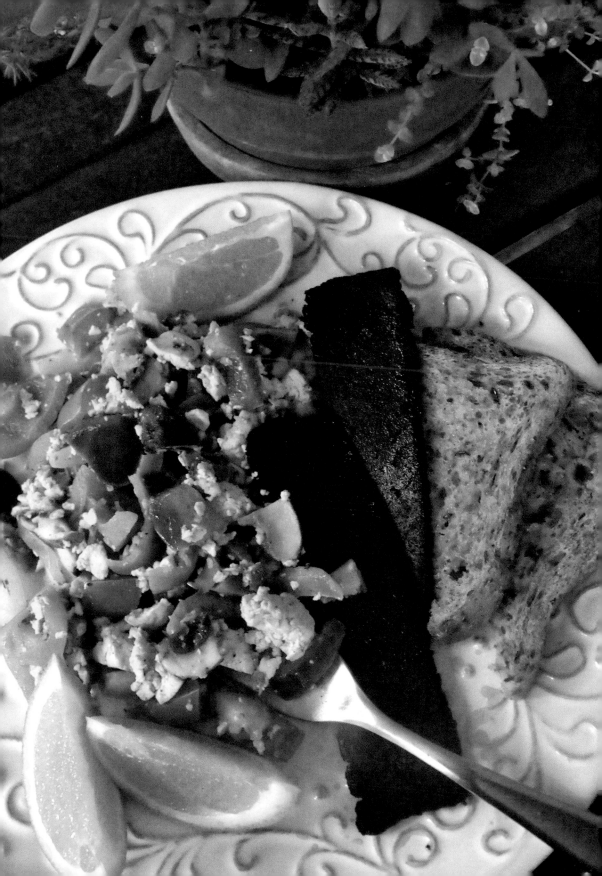

can just sauté your scramble in a little water, and if you'd rather pass on the tofu, you can use potatoes instead. You can bake them in advance, then chop them up for your scramble, or chop into small cubes, and cook them in the pan like "country potatoes" before you add the other veggies. Just remember that some veggies cook a heck of a lot faster than others, and a few, like potatoes, can take a while. I add delicate veggies, like mushrooms and spinach, at the very end so they don't shrivel up and disappear. I like to avoid that "Oh no! Where did they go?" feeling. I add fresh garlic toward the end, too, so it keeps its kick. Some folks even add Kala Namak, a Himalayan black salt (it's actually pink in color when it's ground)—it smells and tastes like eggs. Hopefully your mind is scrambling with ideas; the possibilities are truly endless!

2. *Understand what the terms* free range *and* cage free *really mean.*

So what quality of life do the chickens have while producing these so-called "free-range" eggs?

Your guess is as good as mine. There are *no requirements* for the amount, duration, or quality of outdoor access for animal products labeled as "free range," so who knows? The label "free range" *sounds* like the animals are raised running around happily in a field, but in reality, the USDA only requires that producers must demonstrate to the agency that the chickens have been allowed access to the outside. So, an overcrowded indoor chicken farm could have a small door to a tiny fenced-in concrete parking lot without a single blade of grass, and that would qualify as free range. Gee, thanks, USDA.

But "cage-free" eggs are OK, *right?*

The problem is cage free doesn't mean cruelty-free. Unless you get your eggs from a chicken who was rescued from abuse and lives with someone who you know *personally*, the farm he or she came from likely:

- Still buys their hens from hatcheries that kill the baby male chicks (more than 200 million male chicks are killed each year in the U.S. alone[21]—and over 6 billion annually worldwide.[22])

- Still doesn't allow the hens outdoor access since none is required.[23]

- Still kills the hens at two years old once they're "spent," which is much shorter than their natural lifespan.

- Still doesn't adhere to any regulated method of "humane slaughter" since chickens aren't protected under the Humane Methods of Slaughter Act.

So, although the chickens might get a little extra room, buying cage-free eggs doesn't equal happy chickens. It's like asking someone if they'd rather be punched in the face one hundred times or ninety-five times. Of course they'd pick ninety-five, but heck, who wants to be punched in the face?

Checklist

☐ Did you create a vegan version of a meal or treat that would normally contain eggs?

☐ Did you set to memory what "cage-free" eggs and "free-range" eggs mean so when you're in the store, you won't be tempted to buy them?

☐ Did you exercise today?

Thought FOR THE Day

It's never too late to love. And it's never too late to go vegan. Even folks in their eighties have seen a tremendous improvement in their health, a reduction in chronic pain, and have been able to reduce their medications simply by enjoying a healthy plant-based diet.

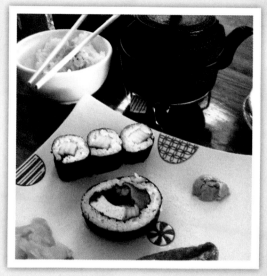

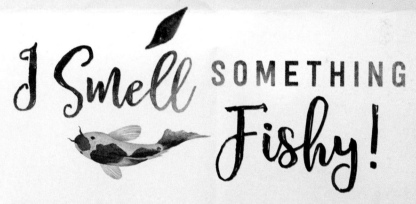

I Smell SOMETHING Fishy!

GOAL FOR THE DAY: Pick a delicious vegan meal that normally contains fish, and "veganize" it.

Surf's up!

People have difficulty relating to fish. Fish don't talk to us. They can't snuggle up to watch TV, sit in our laps for holiday cards, or play fetch. They're always a world away from us, doing their little fishy things, with all their fishy friends, far out of sight under the water. Every now and then, we catch a glimpse of those beautiful eyes, sparkling scales, a few graceful sways and some wide-mouthed "glub glubs." But for the most part, we really don't know fish very well, and that makes them easy to eat. When people feel like they have nothing in common with someone, it enables them to disconnect, landing them in a comfortable, mindless zone of complacent apathy. "Who cares what happens to fish?," folks say, "They're *just fish.*"

If we brush aside our preconceived beliefs, and open our mind and heart a little bit, we'd realize that fish really *do* have a lot in common with us. Fish know how to use tools, perform complex tasks, have excellent long-term memories, recall the location of objects, and cooperate well with each other.[1] They even pass knowledge between one another through social networks, *and* form monogamous relationships.[2] You've got to admit, that's a pretty impressive list for *just a fish.* But that's only "smarts." All animals possess a range of intelligence, and we know brilliance is subjective, so let's set the IQ litmus test on the sidelines for now. After all, whether you're entitled to live or die in this world isn't based on how smart you are, thank goodness.

A far better reason not to eat fish is because, like us, they experience fear and feel pain; there are studies that back this up. When scientists gave fish electric shocks, they not only grunted, but over time they grunted merely at the sight of an electrode.[3] But I don't need science to know fish want to live, and you probably don't either. Anyone who has witnessed a fish squirming on a hook knows firsthand fish don't want to be taken from the water, no matter how enthusiastic good ole' Grandpa may be. Does anyone *really* believe that a fish being hauled onto a ship deck with a sharp gaff piercing his eye isn't in pain? A fish flailing above water is akin to a person struggling for air beneath. Surely it must be a horrible way to die. Drowning is what nightmares are made of. Now we just need to *make the connection,* and extend our compassion to the creatures of the lake, river, and sea, just like cutie-pie Luiz Antonio did when his mother served him a plate of octopus ravioli. Check out his epiphany on YouTube. In less than three minutes, this three-year-old says it all, far more effectively than words on paper ever will.

As for the "but eating fish is so healthy" mantra, you can easily get healthy fats and omegas elsewhere. There's no shortage of healthy fats in plants: avocados, olives, nut butters, hellooo? I love them all. For omega-3 fatty acids, just enjoy some nuts, seeds, beans, or soy.[4] Flaxseeds are another great option; they have both omega-3 and omega-6 essential fatty acids. I toss ground flaxseeds into smoothies almost every time I make them. Delicious! And those chia seeds? They have, by weight, more omega-3s than salmon.[5] A handful of walnuts provides those healthy omegas, too.

And those heart-healthy fish oil claims? Don't be so fast to take the bait. Despite eager Americans spending $1.2 *billion* a year on fish oil supplements (yes, that's billion!), the National Institute for Health notes, "Omega-3s in supplement form have not been shown to protect against heart disease."[6] Say, what? Well, here's the scoop. The craze for this alleged fish oil panacea arose from an expedition to the Arctic Circle led by two Danish researchers in the 1970s. The Danes set out to study the Inuit population and concluded that eating fish, coined the "Eskimo Diet," prevents heart disease. Here's the crazy part: they never studied the Inuits' hearts. Since so many of the Inuits lived in isolation up in the Arctic, they often died without any doctor looking at their body at all. The medical records they studied were often incomplete, and many death records simply didn't exist.[7] Recent studies have found that this population actually had the same, *or more*, heart disease. Fish oil? Sounds more like snake oil to me.

For anyone concerned about food safety—and I'm hoping that's everyone—there's also something mighty fishy about how often fish is contaminated. Fish is by far the most contaminated food people eat, and if you think about it, it's easy to understand why.[8] Here's how it works. Toxins flow through fish gills, settling inside fish muscles until you chow down and gobble them up. That's not good, but making matters worse, fish eat a lot of smaller sea life, and each time a bigger fish eats a smaller one, it's compounding all of those toxins, so by the time you eat "big fish D," you're consuming everything little fish A ate, who was eaten by fish B, who was eaten by fish C, before big fish D ate fish C. You know what I'm sayin'? And what exactly are the smaller fish and other sea life eating before you eat that bigger fish? Sadly, the rain washes all of our toxic air pollution down to the ground where it meets countless poisonous chemicals found on our highways, factory dump sites, parking lots—you name it—and then carries those toxins into lakes, rivers, and the ocean where fish eat. I'm not just talking about dog poop and old chewing gum being washed into the water, we're talking a bazillion chemicals, including the heavy metals: mercury, lead, cadmium, and copper, all of which can cause damage to the brain and nervous systems of people who eat them.[9]

If you're hoping the government is doing their job looking out for your well-being when it comes to consuming fish, think again. Despite the USDA's mandatory Country of Origin Labeling (COOL) law to help folks know where fish came from and how they were raised, *all* processed seafood is exempt. Fish sticks, surimi, mussels in tomato sauce, seafood medleys, coconut shrimp, soups, stews, chowders, sauces, pâtés, smoked salmon, marinated fish fillets, canned tuna, canned sardines, canned salmon, crab salad, shrimp cocktail, gefilte fish, sushi, and breaded shrimp are all processed.[10] Good luck trying to figure out the twists and turns of their long journey before all that fishy stuff got to your plate. I'm a little hesitant to drink Japanese tea after the massive Fukushima Daiichi radiation leak, especially since so many teas have been found to be contaminated; can't imagine someone wanting to consume any fish from Japan.[11] But if you eat processed fish, how would you ever know? Even bluefin tuna caught off the coast of California was found to contain the radiation from that disaster. Not to worry, though. In a moment I'll show you how to make a yummy vegan tuna fish sandwich, without all the toxic crud. And I'll even let you know where the ingredients came from. Vegans like to know these things.

Vegans are also happy to know they don't play a part in contributing to the devastating environmental consequences of factory fish and shrimp farming. Did you know tropical coastal forests are cleared for fish and shrimp farming, often destroying the entire local ecosystem? A wide range of antibiotics are used to treat disease on fish farms because, as with chickens and other animals, when you squish too many living beings into one incredibly small and stressful environment, they understandably get sick.[12] Not only is it unwise to consume all of these extra antibiotics, factory fish farms are laden with pesticides and hormones, too.[13] All of these chemicals, along with feces, uneaten food, and carcasses easily float through the cages and into the ocean, causing dire consequences on the surrounding sea life.[14] As for sustainability, it can take up to 6 pounds of wild fish to feed 1 pound of farmed fish. Not a good investment for people, or for the fish. But hey, Monsanto's got our back, and they're pushing for a heck of a lot more fish farms.[15] Nothing like the prospect of selling a little GMO corn feed to the "growers" of frankenfish. Does the craziness ever end? Yes. Yes, it does. With you, right here, right now.

Let's eat!

1. *Become familiar with the wide range of vegan "fishy" food that tastes so good, and you'll skip that trip to the "fish market."* When I became a vegetarian thirty-eight years ago, I didn't need anything to replace the taste of fish because as I mentioned earlier, I think dead fish stink. I never craved eating them. I don't even eat seaweed because it reminds me of fish. But that's just me. For those of you who have a nose that is less offended, you're in luck. There are *plenty* of vegan options to keep both you and the fish very happy. Today you're going to select something that's traditionally made with fish, or other creatures from the sea, and try out the vegan version. Just take a look, and take your pick!

   FISH STICKS: Gardein makes a breaded Golden Fish Filet, which you can bake or fry up very quickly. You can find them in the frozen section of most mainstream supermarkets, including Target and Whole Foods Market. They're packed with protein (9 grams per 2-piece serving) and they're GMO-free, too. Too fishy for me, but my husband loves them. I always squeeze fresh lemon juice on them, and usually whip up a little vegan tartar sauce. It's super easy: just mix up a little vegan mayo, relish, mustard, and pepper to taste and BAM: vegan fish sticks with dipping sauce! Short on time? Check out Follow Your Heart's Vegenaise Tartar Sauce; it's very tasty. If you'd rather make vegan fish sticks from scratch, there are recipes galore online. Vegans use everything from canned hearts of palm with panko bread crumbs, to tofu and seaweed flakes to make them. Just search "vegan fish sticks" and you'll find all sorts of great ideas.

ANCHOVIES: Some vegans have found that using a mixture of capers, tamari, and seaweed will give meals a hint of anchovy taste.

SUSHI: I know I just said I don't like the taste of fish (*eeww!*), but boy oh boy, do I love vegan sushi! Instead of seaweed, I *politely* (always the operative word) request that it's wrapped in soy paper, or even better, sometimes they're kind enough to wrap it in thinly sliced avocado. If you like the taste of fish, just keep the seaweed, and substitute different veggies for the fish (carrots, cucumbers, shiitake mushrooms, avocado, etc.). Once you're dipping your sushi in a nice mix of wasabi and soy sauce, with a side of fresh ginger, you won't be missing that fish. Vegan sushi restaurants are becoming more widespread. You can find everything from spicy tuna rolls and tempura to crab cakes and caviar, all 100 percent vegan. So awesome!

SCALLOPS, SHRIMP, SMOKED SALMON, AND JAMBALAYA: Using elephant yam root (konjac) as a base, Sophie's Kitchen makes a huge array of vegan seafood products, many of which are soy-free. You can find Sophie's vegan fish in health food stores, or order online. They often have a dollar-off coupon on their website, too.

CRAB: If you're craving crab cakes, check out Match Meats at: www.matchmeats. com. Gardein, which is available throughout the United States and Canada, has mini crabless cakes. Here's their website so you can find their product near you: http://gardein.com/products/crabless-cakes/#where-to-buy. For crab steak, May Wah Vegetarian Market has them at their headquarters in New York City, and online at: www.maywahnyc.com. May Wah's selection of vegan fish (and meat) is huge. Sophie's Kitchen makes nice vegan crab cakes, too. There are also a lot of vegan crab recipes online, most of which use Old Bay Seasoning for a crab cake–like flavor.

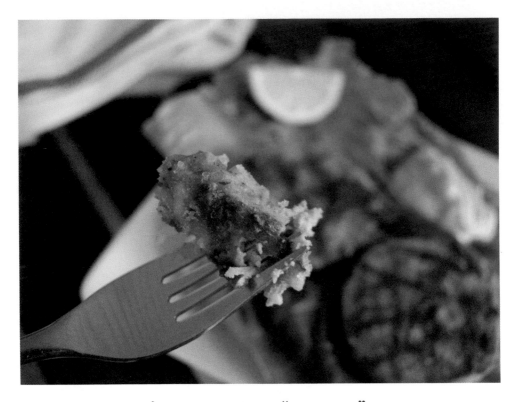

EXTRA TIPS IF YOU'RE STILL MISSING "SEAFOOD"—ONCE BEAUTIFUL SEA *LIFE*:

- Don't forget, you can still enjoy sticky rice, edamame, miso soup, pickled veggies, and other vegan goodies at traditional Asian restaurants that primarily serve fish.

- Seaweed (wakami, nori, kombu, etc.) is the magical ingredient for most vegan fish dishes, so don't be afraid to experiment with it. Seaweed is healthy, too!

- If a recipe calls for fish stock or oyster sauce, there are plenty of easy vegan recipes online that use a combo of ingredients, including dried seaweed, miso, mushrooms, and spices.

2. *Make a scrumptious fishless meal!* Well, I don't miss eating fish, but let me tell you, for my husband, fish was the last thing to go. He craved eating fish more than eating cheese! Here's a simple dish that I created for him and he loves it. I think you'll enjoy it, too. You can select one of the vegan "fishy" foods I mentioned earlier or let the recipe below be your first foray into making a yummy fishless dish that still tastes like it's straight from the sea.

No-Tuna Salad Sandwich

SERVES 3 TO 4

One 15-ounce can garbanzo beans (chickpeas)

⅓ cup vegan mayo

1 to 2 tablespoons kelp granules, to taste

½ teaspoon freshly ground black pepper

1 tablespoon whole grain mustard

1 celery stalk, diced

¼ teaspoon sea salt

2 heaping tablespoons sweet pickle relish

1. In a colander, strain and rinse the garbanzo beans under cold running water, then drain.

2. Transfer the beans to a bowl and smash them up with the back of a fork.

3. Add the rest of the ingredients and mix to incorporate.

4. Serve on bread, open-faced, or as a sandwich filling.

NOTE: As promised, I said I'd let you know where I got my "fishy" flavor for the sandwich: the dried kelp is from Maine Coast Sea Vegetables Inc. It's nutrient dense, sustainably harvested, and organic. Sure beats guessing how a dead fish got to your plate.

3. *Now that fish are your friends, and not food, consider incorporating a little flax into your meals for fiber, lignans, and omegas!* Flaxseeds have been consumed for good nutrition for over seven thousand years.[16] In our current age of fly-by-night food fads, you've got to admit, that's a long time! Hippocrates swore flax helped with ulcers, and Charlemagne was so convinced of its health benefits that he ordered, *by law,* that his royal subjects eat it daily.[17] The steadfast obsession with flax is with good reason: not only are flaxseeds a powerhouse for omegas, they're also packed with protein and fiber, and are believed to help lower the risk for heart disease, stroke, and some cancers, too.[18] But here's the royal dilemma: flaxseeds are best absorbed when ground, not in whole seed form, but when ground they can go rancid quickly, especially if exposed to light. Ground flaxseeds have a very short shelf life. Solution? Buy flaxseeds whole, and grind them yourself, as you need them. I found a little coffee bean grinder online for ten bucks that I only use for seeds, and it works great. Freshly ground flaxseeds in a flash! Done and done. Feel free to zip ahead to Day 9: Fast, Cheap, and Easy!, if you want to see how I make my morning smoothies with flaxseeds in My Vegan Smoothie (page 134).

FISH FACTS

- Surprised by the abundance of wild salmon available during off-season, Marian Burros, a veteran reporter for *The New York Times*, bought "wild fresh salmon" from eight different stores in New York and sent them off to a lab to see if they really were "wild." The lab examined each fish sample using a method of testing that was acceptable to the FDA. The verdict? Only *one* fish was actually from the wild.[19] Speaking of labels, genetically modified salmon doesn't need to be labeled as such. According to a 2015 poll, 93 percent of Americans think the government should mandate the labeling of GMO foods, yet once again, we're left in the dark. GMO—just three letters. Is it really that difficult to print? No matter *what* side of the GMO debate you're on, something stinks here, and it's not just the fish!

- According to a 2003 study by Dr. Lynne Sneddon, director of Bio-veterinary Science at the University of Liverpool, trout have twenty-two pain receptors in their face.[20]

- Watch out for fish in strange places. Anchovies show up in Worcestershire sauce (Annie's makes a good vegan version), and Asian restaurants occasionally add one big chunk of fish "just for flavor" to the giant pot of miso soup in their kitchens.

Checklist

☐ Did you make a yummy meal that tastes like "seafood" without using any sea life?

☐ Did you consider adding flaxseeds to your shopping list?

☐ Are you still using vegan alternatives to eggs and dairy throughout the day?

Thought FOR THE Day

"Think occasionally of the suffering of which you spare yourself the sight."

—ALBERT SCHWEITZER

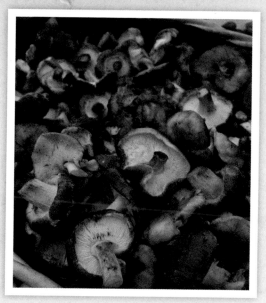

Mystery Meat

GOAL FOR THE DAY: "Veganize" a meat dish!

When I was a little girl, I'd always wait until my mom wasn't looking, stand on my tippy toes, and sneak a piece of raw hamburger meat before the meatloaf made its way to the oven. When caught in the act, my mother would always scold me, "You're going to get sick!" but I didn't care; I thought it was worth the risk. It didn't stop me from scooping out the raw marrow that was tucked in the bone of lamb chops before they'd hit the oven, too. I'd run my finger down the hard crevice, scoop out the gelatinous fat, and lick it up like a finger dipped in cupcake batter. I loved eating animals, especially raw.

The funny thing is, I didn't realize I was eating animals. I thought I was eating meat, and meat was just a type of food. In my young mind, meat had nothing to do with my furry friends. I grew up in the late '60s and '70s, long before PETA or the Internet and social media came to be. Kids like me got their food facts and lore from family, friends, teachers, and commercials sandwiched strategically between Saturday morning cartoons. No one I knew questioned eating meat. No one around me worried about the health effects of chowing down on greasy burgers and hot dogs, or the environmental impact of producing them. No one wondered if children's storybooks depicting happy farm animals relaxing in spacious pastures were actually true. We were blissfully blind and we loved our "meat."

Today's world is far different. Thanks to the relentless advocacy work of those who care, our eyes are now wide open; it's just a matter of opening our hearts. Chances are, for the most part, you already know how cows, pigs, chickens, lambs, turkeys, and other animals wind up on your plate. If you need a refresher, just hop online and watch the short videos "Meet Your Meat" and "From Farm to Fridge," or one of the dozens of undercover investigations. It's not a pretty story, and it's happening at lightning speed. You can visit the United Nation's Food and Agricultural Organization's website at http://www.fao.org/home/en to see exactly how many animals are killed for food each year throughout the world, but the numbers are *so* large that they almost become meaningless. There are so many lists documenting millions and billions of animals that it all becomes a blur of statistics rather than the living, breathing, heart-beating individuals that they really are. A "kill counter" based on United Nations data provides a better sense of what's really going on. ADAPTT, www.adaptt.org/killcounter.html, continually tabulates the number of animals killed for food. The counter moves *so* fast that your eyes can't keep up with the numbers. According to the United Nations' data, 30 dogs are killed for food every minute, 277 cows are slaughtered every 30 seconds, and in *less than 10 seconds*, over 300 rabbits, 425 pigs, and 43,000 chickens meet the same sad fate.[1]

It's true. Americans eat *a lot* of animals: roughly 200 pounds of animals per person, per year.[2] But this wasn't always so. Our primate ancestors ate almost exclusively plants until a change in African climate made plant food scarce, forcing them to scavenge on animal carcasses for survival.[3] As time went on, people resorted to eating animals in order to migrate through colder climates in Europe and Asia, where sometimes weather was so harsh, plant foods simply didn't exist.[4] Throughout our early history, people didn't eat animals because they thought meat was healthy; they ate animals because there was no other option. The intermittent pockets of transition from eating plants to meat were born from necessity, not by choice. Even the hunter-gatherers that Paleo dieters so revere got the majority of their calories from plant foods.[5]

So why is it that with today's abundance of healthy fruits, vegetables, grains, legumes, nuts, and seeds, which we know help us live long, happy, and productive lives, people are eating *billions* of animals and their by-products? MONEY. No surprise there, right? The *amount* of money might come as a shock, though. According to farm receipts, the USDA estimates that the United States meat industry makes over 96 billion dollars a year just from the slaughter and sale of cows and calves alone.[6] The figure jumps to over 186 billion when you account for all the other animals and their by-products sold for food.[7] From the perspective of those who profit, that's an investment worth protecting, no matter what the health, environmental, societal, or ethical consequences are. Be it laws, education, public relations, medical research, or any other aspect of society that affects the profitability of animals sold for food, the meat industry makes sure its voice is heard loud and clear, ensuring its assets are safe. Big money opens doors, and closes minds, each and every day.

Just ask Dr. Luise Light, leader of a group of "top ten" nutritionists assigned with the task of developing the very first food guide pyramid. After lengthy research, the group submitted their final version of the pyramid, recommending a base of 5 to 9 servings of fresh fruits and vegetables every day. Sounds good, right? According to the Union of Concerned Scientists, if Americans ate just one more serving of fruits or vegetables a day, we could prevent thirty thousand premature deaths each year, just from heart disease and strokes, and save 5 billion dollars in medical costs related to those diseases.[8] It makes good sense to eat fresh produce, and lots of it.

As you can imagine, though, Dr. Light's recommendations didn't go over well with Big Ag. They knew eating more fruits and veggies meant eating less meat, dairy, and eggs. Doors flew open and U.S. Secretary of Agriculture John Block listened, changing the official government recommendation to a "paltry 2 to 3 servings" of fruit and vegetables per day.[9] Light's outcry of concern fell on deaf ears. After all, she was *just* a nutritionist, with only one lonely vote like the rest of us come election time. Staying true to *his* twisted vision of good health, Block went on to serve on the Board of Directors for Hormel Foods, makers of SPAM, and currently writes on his personal blog, which is proudly "brought to you by Monsanto."

For those who study food politics, these special interest accommodations come as no surprise. The meat and dairy industries have been in bed with the USDA and other government agencies for many years. Perhaps the most outrageous benefit from this cozy relationship are the federal subsidies and insurance perks imbedded in the Farm Bill, which is tweaked and renewed every five years or so. It was originally created as a temporary program in the 1930s, under President Roosevelt's New Deal, to help folks out during the post-depression era, which makes sense, but today it's taken on an insidious life of its own. If you grow "commodity" items such as corn or soy, which Big Ag uses to produce high-fructose corn syrup and to feed animals in the meat and dairy industries, the government will give you huge subsidies. Just how huge? Between 1995 and 2012, the government gave out $292.5 *billion* dollars in subsidies and the most recent Farm Bill, the Agricultural Act of 2014, signed by President Obama, continues the same gilded favoritism.[10]

Over the next ten years, the United States government will subsidize Big Ag under the Price Loss Coverage (PLC) Program to the tune of over $44 billion dollars.[11] During the same period, they'll also fork over another $89.9 billion in crop insurance to put Big Ag growers at ease. If bad weather destroys crops raised for animal feed, or you lose your hefty profit thanks to a price drop, not to worry: our tax dollars will help cover the tab.[12] It's the law. But if you'd like to know *which* Big Ag farmers receive the insurance dough, don't bother asking. The clause that mandated public disclosure was removed just before the nearly one-thousand-page bill was signed.[13]

So how does all of this political mish-mash affect those, like yourself, who are trying to go vegan? Well, consider this: the USDA only spends a piddly 14.7 percent of total commodity support on fruits and vegetables. The government ensures meat, eggs, and dairy items stay affordable, while those who grow food like organic kale, tomatoes, or berries are comparatively left out in the cold. Fruit and veggie growers fair a little bit better in the most recent Farm Bill, but the bottom line is that this type of politicking keeps the greasy, fatty, cholesterol-laden SAD diet cheap and easier to buy than the *healthier plant-based choices* you, I, and others want and need. And that's not fair.

I learned the effect of this craziness firsthand when I sat down with a high school cafeteria manager in an attempt to have her prepare healthier meals for the students. I showed her my list of delicious vegan food that met government standards for school meals, and in turn, she showed me her long list from which she ordered the food items. Sure enough, the unhealthy items were supercheap compared to the fresh plant-based foods. The manager explained that she was interested in accommodating my requests, but in order to keep within her budget, she had to order the bulk of her food from the government-assigned "commodities" and a nice variety of affordable fresh fruits and vegetables just wasn't part of that deal. Politicians get their votes, the meat and dairy industries get their moolah, and the kids, well, they mostly just get hot, greasy slop.

Speaking of slop, the majority of fast-food isn't much better. Ever wonder what's in a Big Mac? It's a heck of a lot more than the seven ingredients in their jingle, "Two all beef patties, special sauce, lettuce, cheese, pickles, onions, on a sesame seed bun." And if you take into account all of our taxpayer-funded subsides, along with external and hidden expenses, the *true* cost to society for each Big Mac is actually twelve bucks![14] It may seem like a bargain when you're buying one, but trust me, you're paying a heck of a lot on the back end, too—both in your wallet, *and* your pants. Yet another great reason to be vegan: you won't be eating this mess, mistakenly called food. Take a look at the ingredient list for a Big Mac with a side of fries:

BIG MAC INGREDIENTS[15] (SOURCE: MCDONALD'S WEBSITE)

BEEF PATTIES: Beef, Salt, Black Pepper

PICKLES: Cucumbers, Water, Distilled Vinegar, Salt, Calcium Chloride, Alum, Potassium Sorbate (Preservative), Natural Flavors (Plant Source), Polysorbate 80, Extractives of Turmeric (Color)

BIG MAC SAUCE: Soybean Oil, Pickle Relish (Diced Pickles, High Fructose Corn Syrup, Sugar, Vinegar, Corn Syrup, Salt, Calcium Chloride, Xanthan Gum, Potassium Sorbate [Preservative], Spice Extractives, Polysorbate 80), Distilled Vinegar, Water, Egg Yolks, High Fructose Corn Syrup, Onion Powder, Mustard Seed, Salt, Spices, Propylene Glycol Alginate, Sodium Benzoate (Preservative), Mustard Bran, Sugar, Garlic Powder, Vegetable Protein (Hydrolyzed Corn, Soy and Wheat), Caramel Color, Extractives of Paprika, Soy Lecithin, Turmeric (Color), Calcium Disodium EDTA (Protect Flavor).

PASTEURIZED PROCESS AMERICAN CHEESE: Milk, Cream, Water, Cheese Culture, Sodium Citrate, Contains 2% or Less of: Salt, Citric Acid, Sodium Phosphate, Sorbic Acid (Preservative), Lactic Acid, Acetic Acid, Enzymes, Sodium Pyrophosphate, Natural Flavor (Dairy Source), Color Added, Soy Lecithin (Added for Slice Separation).

BIG MAC BUN: Enriched Bleached Flour (Wheat Flour, Malted Barley Flour, Niacin, Reduced Iron, Thiamin Mononitrate, Riboflavin, Folic Acid), Water,

High Fructose Corn Syrup, Yeast, Soybean Oil, Contains 2% or Less: Salt, Wheat Gluten, Sesame Seeds, Leavening (Calcium Sulfate, Ammonium Sulfate), May Contain One or More Dough Conditioners (Sodium Stearoyl Lactylate, DATEM, Ascorbic Acid, Azodicarbonamide, Mono and Diglycerides, Monocalcium Phosphate, Enzymes, Calcium Peroxide), Calcium Propionate (Preservative).

LETTUCE: Lettuce

ONIONS: Onions

AN ORDER OF FRIES

Potatoes, Vegetable Oil (Canola Oil, Soybean Oil, Hydrogenated Soybean Oil, Natural Beef Flavor [Wheat and Milk Derivatives], Citric Acid [Preservative]), Dextrose, Sodium Acid Pyrophosphate (Maintain Color), Salt. Prepared in Vegetable Oil (Canola Oil, Corn Oil, Soybean Oil, Hydrogenated Soybean Oil) with TBHQ and Citric Acid to preserve freshness of the oil and Dimethylpolysiloxane to reduce oil splatter when cooking. (Try singing *that* as a jingle!)

OK, let's talk chow.

1. *Keep these morsels of advice in mind as you continue your transition to a happy, healthy vegan lifestyle:*

   ❧ *The closer you can get to a whole foods plant-based diet, the better.*[16] What does that mean? It means more often than not, the less processed your food, the better it is for you. Instead of eating grains that are smashed and refined, try to eat them whole. In lieu of cookies with sugar stripped from its fibrous source, enjoy sweet whole fruit instead. I always used to tell my students you need to exercise your body, inside and out, and that includes giving your "insides" a workout by letting your stomach break down whole foods. That *generally* means the less ingredients you see on a vegan food label, the healthier it is. Not always, but usually. You should also be familiar with the words on the label, too. It's good to see items like blueberries, celery, and black beans listed (no question what those are) instead of words like potassium bromate and butylated hydroxyanisole (*huh?*). So keep your thinking cap on, and remember being vegan doesn't ensure good health. Being vegan means you're compassionate; being a *healthy* vegan means being smart, so choose wisely.

❧ *It's OK to take baby steps to get from a SAD diet to a healthy one.* If you go straight from eating Big Macs, sodas, and fries to a healthy, whole foods, vegan diet overnight, you'll likely set yourself up for failure. So don't be afraid to enjoy some easy-to-prepare, vegan convenience foods for a little while. Think of them as a stepping stone to get to the other side of a stream. You can even have them as a treat now and then down the road, as do most vegans, myself included. They're tasty! Just don't get stuck here. *Please.* I care about you just as much as I care about the animals. I want us *all* to live happy, healthy, productive lives. We're saving the world together, and I need you, so stay fit!

❧ *If anyone pesters you about eating vegan "fast-food" during the transition, don't let them bring you down.* As my friend and cookbook author Annie Shannon always says, "Fake meat saves real lives," and it's true. If you're vegan, you're saving animals with every bite you take, processed foods or not. You're also being kinder to the environment, and no matter how junky the food may be, there's still *zero* cholesterol in it and your heart is darn tootin' happy about that. So go easy on yourself. If you have to eat a lot of packaged vegan food until you get the hang of things, it's A-OK. No shame, no blame. Just remember to enjoy those healthy whole foods *as often as you can.*

2. *Begin to explore the huge variety of vegan "meat" products available to help you ease into your journey:* The array of vegan burgers, hot dogs, and other yummy options is truly spectacular. Long gone are the days of plain white slabs of tofu, *mon amis.* Peruse the lists and select a few things to help make the transition a savory snap.

VEGAN BURGERS

Gardenburger Veggie Medley
Trader Joe's Thai Sweet Chili Veggie Burger/ Vegetable Masala Burger
Boca Vegan Veggie Burger
Gardein Beefless Burgers
Hilary's World's Best Veggie Burger
Dr. Praeger's California Veggie Burgers
Beyond Meat's Beast Burgers / Beyond Burger
Sol Cuisine Burgers
Tofurkey Veggie Burgers

Sweet Earth Burgers

Field Roast Grain Meat Co. Burgers

Whole Foods Market 365 Everyday Value Meatless Burgers

Amy's All American Veggie Burger

Amy's Sonoma Veggie Burger (Soy-free and Wheat-free)

Engine 2 Tuscan Kale Plant Burgers (Soy-free and Wheat-free)

Sunshine Burger (Soy-free and Wheat-free)

MorningStar Vegan Grillers

MorningStar Spicy Indian Veggie Burgers

MorningStar White Bean Veggie Burger

VEGAN HOT DOGS

Lightlife Smart Dogs

Lightlife Tofu Pups

Loma Linda Big Franks

Tofurky Breakfast Links

Tofurky Hot Dogs

Tofurky Sausages

Yves Tofu Dogs

Yves Meatless Hot Dogs

Field Roast Grain Meat Co. Frankfurters

Field Roast Grain Meat Co. Sausages

Whole Foods Market 365 Everyday Value Veggie Dogs

VEGAN RIBS

MorningStar Hickory BBQ Riblets

VEGAN CRUMBLES FOR SPAGHETTI SAUCE, CHILI, TACOS, BURRITOS, STUFFED PEPPERS, AND CASSEROLES

Lightlife Smart Ground

Beyond Meat Beefy Crumbles

Boca Veggie Ground Crumbles

Trader Joe's Beef-less Ground Beef

Gardein Ultimate Beefless Ground

VEGAN MEATBALLS

Beyond Meat Swedish Meatballs

Beyond Meat Italian Meatballs

Trader Joe's Meatless Meatballs

Gardein Meatless Meatballs

Whole Kitchen Vegan Meatballs

Nate's Vegan Meatballs

IKEA Veggie Balls

VEGAN CHICKEN

Boca Spicy Chik'n Patties

Lightlife Meatless Chick'n Strips

Trader Joe's Chickenless Strips, Chickenless Crispy Tenders, and Chicken-less Mandarin Orange Morsels

Simple Truth Meatless Crispy Tenders (Ralph's/Kroger Brand)

Simply Balanced Korean Barbecue Meatless Chicken (Target Brand)

Gardein (9 different types of vegan chicken. Everything from BBQ wings to scallopini!)

Beyond Meat (7 different types of vegan chicken. Everything from Grilled Strips to Feisty Buffalo Poppers!)

Upton's Naturals Chick Seitan

VEGAN BACON

Lightlife Smart Bacon; Meatless Veggie Bacon Strips

Sweet Earth Hickory and Sage Smoked Seitan Bacon

Betty Crocker's Bac-Os (yep, they're vegan!)

Turtle Island Foods Smoky Maple Tempeh Bacon

Upton's Bacon Seitan

Phoney Baloney Coconut Bacon

Yves' Meatless Canadian Bacon

Vegan Magic (It's vegan bacon grease! Curious as to what's in it? I know I was! Coconut Oil, Non-GMO Soy Protein, Sea Salt, Pure Maple Syrup, Black Pepper, Onion, Garlic, Torula Yeast, and Natural Smoke Flavor.)

VEGAN CHORIZO

Trader Joe's Soy Chorizo (60% less fat than traditional chorizo)

Frieda's Soyrizo (Gluten-free)

Yves Veggie Chorizo (50% less sodium than regular chorizo)

Upton's Naturals Chorizo Seitan

EVERYTHING FROM VEGAN DUCK TO VEGAN MUTTON

Yes, they make it all. Check out May Wah's Vegetarian Market. They're located in New York City, but also sell their huge selection of products online at: www.maywahnyc.com.

3. *If you'd prefer to skip all the prepackaged food, just go ahead and create your own "meaty" vegan meal from scratch. It's easy to do! Here are some ideas to get you started:*

MUSHROOMS: Most vegans I know *love* using mushrooms in lieu of meat for a wide variety of tasty vegan meals. Mushrooms give food an earthy, woodsy flavor and that chewy meaty texture most of us became accustomed to as kids. White button mushrooms work well, but for a special treat, try shiitake, oyster, or cremini (baby portobello) mushrooms grilled alone or added to sauces and stir-fries. Put a giant grilled portobello mushroom in a bun and you've got a scrumptious burger, too. You can even marinade them before grilling if you want an extra juicy kick. Or you can slice a portobello mushroom into strips, marinade overnight, and then bake at 250°F for 1 hour, flip and bake for another, and voilá—you've got mushroom

VEGAN BUTCHERS

They exist! No Evil Foods, based in Asheville, North Carolina, sells "The Pardon" Thanksgiving roast and other various handmade "meats" online and at selected stores: www.NoEvilFoods.com. And check out The Herbivorous Butcher, created by brother and sister team, Aubry and Kale (love the name!), which sells twenty-four types of artisanal "meat" ranging from deli bologna and bangers to Korean ribs and Porterhouse steak. The have vegan cheese and butter, too: Visit www.TheHerbivorousButcher.com. Brilliant! Or visit The Butcher's Son in Berkeley, California. They have everything from roast beef to pulled pork and a sit-down deli where you can grab lunch, too. See thebutchersveganson.com.

"jerky." (The thicker the slices, the higher you'll need the heat.) There are so many types of vegan marinades to choose from! I suggest combining a few of the following and creating your own. It's easy. Just pick a liquid or two, and combine with your favorite seasonings. You can call it: [Your name]'s Vegan Marinade!

SUGGESTED LIQUIDS AND SEASONINGS TO CHOOSE FROM

Lemon Juice	Rice Vinegar	Olive Oil
Chopped Garlic	Smoked Paprika	Thyme
Wine	Apple Cider Vinegar	Soy Sauce
Chopped Onions	Black Pepper	Ginger
Balsamic Vinegar	Sesame Seed Oil	Tamari
Chili Pepper	Sea Salt	Mustard

(Trader Joe's Island Soyaki makes for a nice marinade, too.) The previous suggestions are just to get your mouth salivating. We'll kick it up a notch with more marinade ideas in Day 9, Fast, Cheap, and Easy!

SEITAN: Did you know using seitan (pronounced say-tahn) as a substitute for meat goes clear back to the eleventh century? Proof again that enjoying delicious vegan food is nothing new. Seitan is made from wheat gluten, which is separated from flour. It was discovered by Chinese noodle makers who referred to gluten as "the muscle of flour."[17] Many vegans, myself included, really enjoy the chewy texture, and we love that it can easily absorb so many wonderful flavors. Small pieces of the dough can be fried for tacos, burritos, and stir-fries, or you can toss small pieces into a boiling veggie broth with noodles, chopped celery, and carrots, to make a vegan chick'n noodle soup. Seitan can be shaped into cutlets for grilling or frying, or even made into big roasts that you can stuff with a medley of mushrooms, onions, and garlic, or whatever else you enjoy. Field Roast Grain Meat makes a seitan roast that's filled with cranberries, hazelnuts, and a bread stuffing, and they have another roast accompanied by a pineapple-mustard glaze. No Evil Foods adds sweet potatoes and balsamic vinegar to their seitan roasts. Sweet Earth Foods makes seitan in thin slices, which are perfect for sandwiches, and Tofurky makes seitan strips that can be added to just about anything that's savory. The variety is endless. Truly. Endless. Just don't go to the store and say, "I'm looking for Satan." Unless of course, you'd like a strange look, and a good laugh.

Here's a simple seitan recipe if you'd like to try making your own at home:

Simple Seitan

MAKES 8 BALLS

I use tamari and vegetable stock for the liquid in my homemade seitan, but you can really use any plain or savory liquid that suits your fancy. You can even just use water; you'll just have to season it up a bit after it's done. And feel free to add more yummies to it, look at the list of liquids and seasonings on the previous page. Make this *your* recipe. Get creative and have some fun!

1 cup wheat gluten

½ teaspoon onion powder

½ teaspoon garlic powder

½ teaspoon thyme

½ teaspoon freshly ground black pepper

1 teaspoon nutritional yeast

½ cup vegetable stock

¼ cup tamari

2 or 3 tablespoons olive oil (or oil of your choice)

1. In a bowl, mix together the wheat gluten, onion and garlic powders, thyme, pepper, and nutritional yeast.

2. Add the stock and tamari and stir until incorporated and the mixture forms a doughlike mixture.

3. Using your hands, knead and pound the mixture on a lightly floured surface, as though you were making bread. Continue until you achieve a nice stretchy dough consistency.

4. Shape into a ball. Cut the ball in half, then in fourths, then in eighths, until you get small chunks about the size of a quarter or smaller. (You can also cut the ball into 4 pieces and flatten out to make cutlets.)

5. Add enough oil to coat the bottom of a large sauté pan. Place over low to medium heat, add the seitan chunks, and sauté until browned, using a spatula to turn them now and then so they don't stick to the pan.

6. When browned and slightly crispy, remove them from the pan and set aside on a plate to cool.

7. Add the seitan to your favorite recipe, serve as cutlets, or make Seitan Veggie Kabobs (page 160).

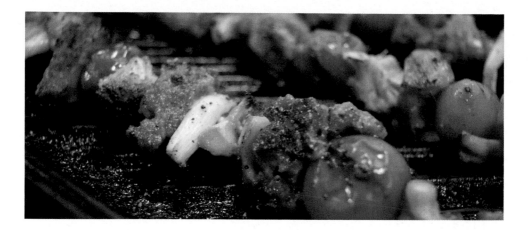

TOFU: Poor little tofu, it sometimes gets a bad rap. Some folks seem to get the willies at just the mention of soybean "curd," despite dairy cheese also being the dreaded "curd" word, too. I once dated a guy who, thanks to all the "tofu is evil" media hype, wouldn't let me cook my tofu in the same pan as he used because he was afraid he'd grow breasts. The fear of tofu-induced "man-boobs" stems from a singular 2008 report of a Texas man who drank three quarts of soy milk a day and complained of "enlarged breasts and decreased libido."[18] When he decreased his consumption of soy milk, he said his breast tenderness disappeared. The authors of the study were quick to point out this case was "very unusual."[19] In fact, no other similar medical cases have been reported.[20] Wow, three quarts? Every *day*? Makes me wonder what else that man consumed. I've seen a lot of men walking around with jiggly breasts, and I'm pretty sure it's not from the tofu. In fact, I bet they'd be very insulted if I ever suggested that it was. "Wow, I see you've been eating a lot of tofu!" Nope, I'm not saying it.

And consider this. It's well documented that people live the longest in Okinawa, Japan, which *also* just happens to be the place where they consume more tofu than anywhere else in the world. Their diet is high in carbohydrates, low in saturated fats, and heart disease, cancer, and Alzheimer's disease are practically unheard of. The residents work and exercise well into old age, all while eating loads of citrus, greens, and tofu.[21] Japan has over sixty-one thousand centenarians, more than anywhere else in the world.[22] For all the naysayers who think tofu is unhealthy: Why are the people of Japan doing so well, and living so long, while eating so *much* of it? I don't think tofu assures anyone will live past one hundred, but there's no doubt that it's great for those in transition to a vegan diet, especially when mixed with other healthy plant foods. Unless you have a soy allergy or a medical condition that warrants avoiding it, I'd suggest tofu over animal products any day.

HOW DO SOYBEANS BECOME TOFU?

Soybeans are soaked in water —> then blended —> then pulp removed —> producing soy milk —> add a coagulant (a natural acid for silken tofu, calcium sulfate for the firmer varieties, or even lemon juice if you're making it at home) —> heat —> strain solids —> press out water (unless it's silken tofu, which isn't pressed) —> and voilà, you have tofu!

I was going to introduce the next section with a witty tofu joke, but decided it was tasteless. Bada Boom! OK, here are the different types of tofu, and once you're done preparing them, you'll find they truly are tasty. Enjoy!

- **SILKEN TOFU**: It's jellylike and silky, just like it sounds, with a high water content. People love to make smoothies, sauces, creams, pies, and puddings with it. If you see a sweet dessert calling for tofu, it often calls for silken tofu. Mori-Nu Silken Tofu is the one you'll likely find the easiest. You'll see it in the refrigerator section, or in small shelf-stable Tetra-Pak boxes that don't need to be refrigerated until opening, making it great for travel, or keeping on hand in the cupboard as a backup. But if you're looking for a sturdy tofu to chop into cubes or throw on the grill, this isn't the one for you.

- **SOFT TOFU**: You'll find this tofu in the refrigerator section, in a package filled with water, and although it's soft, it has a completely different texture than the silken tofu. It's not slippery, just a bit less dense than the medium or firm varieties, so it crumbles very easily for tofu stir-fries or taco filling.

- **MEDIUM, FIRM, AND EXTRA-FIRM TOFU**: The firmer tofu gets, the less water it has, and the sturdier it is to cook with. A firmer tofu will flip better in a pan, and unlike a soft tofu, stands a good chance of staying on that veggie kabob stick without falling through the grill. All of these can be found in the refrigerator section of stores.

- **SPROUTED TOFU**: Sprouted tofu is made from soybeans that have sprouted, making them easier to digest, and increasing the amount of nutrients, such as calcium, protein, and iron. It's my favorite tofu.

TOFU TALK

- If you don't use all the tofu in the package, make sure you fill the container with water and keep the tofu submerged to slow spoilage.
- Most soybeans in the U. S. are doused with pesticides and genetically modified, but all the tofu I've seen in stores lately has been 100 percent organic and non-GMO. Examples of tofu manufacturers that offer non-GMO and organic varieties include: Nasoya, Morinaga, House Foods, SoyBoy, Tree of Life, Wildwood, WestSoy, Hodo Soy, and Trader Joe's.[23] Always double-check the label, just to be sure.
- Ever try Hodo Soy tofu? Hodo Soy Beanery was started by Vietnam refugee, Minh Tsai, who set up shop in Oakland, California, in 1981. What makes Hodo Soy tofu unique is that the soy milk they create and use to make the tofu is almost twice as thick as that used by conventional brands. The texture of the finished product is silky, yet firm. The yield is lower, so the price is a bit higher, but dang, it's good!
- If you want to try something nifty, freeze your pack of tofu overnight. Any type other than the silken tofu will do. Let it thaw the next day, and then gently squeeze out all of the water. The tofu becomes much more porous, with visible holes like a sponge, which will soak up extra flavor when you cook it. Freezing and thawing tofu will make it chewier, too!

AND TEMPEH, TOO!

- Tempeh is fermented whole soybeans. It has antioxidants, all of the essential amino acids, and lots of protein and fiber, too. Steam, bake, marinate, or sauté it with your favorite seasonings. As with tofu, it will take on the flavors you add to it. Just be sure to do something with it, though, because like our little friend tofu, tempeh needs a bit of help to make it taste good.

4. *Get familiar with vegan sources of iron, and which foods help you absorb it:* Lots of folks assume that if they don't eat meat, they'll become deficient in iron, not realizing that there are plenty of plant sources to provide your daily needs. Just as vitamin D helps with the absorption of calcium, vitamin C helps out with iron. So if you want to boost your body's absorption of iron, be sure to eat foods that are rich in vitamin C at the same time. Dark green leafy vegetables, bell peppers, raisins, and oranges are just a few of the smart choices for vitamin C. Some folks like to kick it up an extra notch by cooking in a cast-iron skillet. Just make sure it's not preseasoned with animal fat. (Lodge Cast Iron uses vegetable oil.) I absorb enough iron without giving it any thought, but since you're just starting out on your vegan adventure, it's good to have it on your radar. Check out the list on the next page and see what looks good to you!

THIS LITTLE PIGGY WENT TO THE MARKET

It sounds so sweet when we're counting toes, but in the real world, there's nothing cute about it. Before pigs arrive at the market, most are confined to concrete gestation crates, only two feet wide—an area so narrow they can't even turn around. Ever. Nor scratch an itch. That's where mother pigs lie for most of their lives, without any bedding, in their own waste, biting metal bars, awaiting the birth of their babies.[24] They never get a single breath of fresh air, or a glimpse of earth or sky. When the piglets are born, their teeth and tails are cut without anesthesia. Within ten days the testicles of baby male pigs are torn out without any pain relief.[25] About fifteen days later, all of the babies are torn away from their mothers and sent to stacked cages, where they wallow in the waste of those above.[26] Film footage shows runts of the litter being hung, or having their heads thrown to the floor—or as the industry calls it, being "thumped."[27] That's what *really* happens to the little piggy on her way to the market. She cries all the way there, and never goes home.

Want to skip the packaged burgers and hot dogs, and replace animal products with a simple, non-processed plant protein? Check out page 129 for lots of great protein-packed options!

GOOD SOURCES OF IRON

Pumpkin Seeds	Kidney Beans	Swiss Chard
Quinoa	Black Beans	Tempeh
Blackstrap Molasses	Garbanzo Beans	Tofu
Spinach	(Chickpeas)	Cashews
Lentils	Lima Beans	Dried Apricots

Sweet Potato Split Pea Soup

SERVES 4 TO 6

This is one of my favorite soups—sweet, savory, and hearty! It also feels like you get a lot more for your money when you make a big pot of soup yourself, as opposed to buying it in small cans. And what makes this soup *extra* wonderful is that sweet potatoes are a powerhouse for vitamin C, and split peas have iron! But as I always say: get creative, adjust to taste, and make this recipe your own!

Oil of choice (I like using organic cold-pressed olive oil, but any will do)

1 onion, chopped

1 tablespoon chopped garlic

8 cups water

One 1-pound bag split peas, picked over for debris, rinsed

1 medium, unpeeled, scrubbed sweet potato, chopped into cubes

1 medium unpeeled, scrubbed Russet potato, or two Yukon Gold potatoes chopped into cubes

½ to 1 tablespoon sea salt

Freshly ground black pepper

½ to 1 tablespoon seasoning of choice (I use organic no-salt seasoning blends that you can get at Trader Joe's or Costco)

1. Pour enough oil into a large soup pot to lightly cover the bottom.

2. Add the chopped onion and garlic and cook on low heat until slightly translucent and beginning to turn golden brown, stirring occasionally so they don't burn. This shouldn't take more than 5 minutes.

3. Add the water, peas, and potatoes, and bring to a boil.

4. Reduce to a simmer and cook on low to medium-low heat for 1½ to 2 hours, stirring occasionally. (Trust me, this soup is worth the wait!). When the potatoes start to soften, gently smash them against the side of the pot with a wooden spoon to help the soup develop a thick and creamy texture. Continue to cook, and stir every 7 to 10 minutes.

5. Season to taste with the salt and pepper and any other seasonings you like.

6. When the soup is thick and creamy, give it a taste. Adjust the seasoning if necessary. Enjoy!

NOTE: If you'd like more info on the amount of vitamins and minerals in the food you enjoy, visit http://nutritiondata.self.com and simply search the name of the food and it will provide you with loads of nutrition data.

HUMANE MEAT?

"It is normal to have leg-kicking reflexes in an animal that has been properly stunned with electricity, captive bolt, or gunshot. . . . The person assessing insensibility should concentrate on looking at the head and ignore kicking limbs. Gasping is permissible: it is a sign of a dying brain."[28]

—Guidelines for Humane Handling, Transport and Slaughter of Livestock, Food and Agricultural Organization of the United Nations.

MYSTERY MEAT?

There is no law that requires the USDA to label the country of origin when it comes to "beef" and "pork." You don't have the right to know where the animal was born, raised, or slaughtered, despite the fact that 90 percent of Americans are in favor of such labeling.[29] Good luck trying to figure out if that ground "beef" came from clear-cut land that was once a rainforest, or was schlepped in from an alley in China. Fresh fruits and vegetables, however, are required to be labeled with the country of origin by law. Yet *another* benefit to being vegan.

Checklist

☐ Did you select a meatless meal to make?

☐ Did you think about which ingredients would make a nice marinade?

☐ Did you drink any water today?

Thought FOR THE Day

To discuss the causes of climate change without mentioning factory farming is like discussing the causes of lung cancer without mentioning cigarettes.

DAY 8

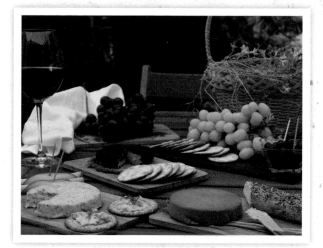

But I love Cheese

(TOO MUCH!)

GOAL FOR THE DAY: Introduce your
taste buds to vegan cheese.

Well, today is the big day! Say vegan *cheeeeese!* Are you smiling? I sure hope so, because there are plenty of reasons to put a big grin above that chin. Let me tell ya, when I went vegan there was no such thing as vegan cheese, not even *gross* vegan cheese. Well, there was one funky creation called Soymage made by Galaxy Nutritional Foods in the '80s, but the reaction from those who dared to taste it was so horrible that I'm not sure if you can even classify it as any type of cheese at all: "I am STILL trying to get the horrible taste out of my mouth! Yuck! I will NEVER eat that stuff EVER again!"[1] and "I would rather eat packing peanuts than the Soymage vegan cheese."[2] Vegan "Sheese" emerged in Scotland in 1988, but most of us didn't have Internet at home back then, so who knew? And even if we did, how many folks could fly to Scotland to pick up a chunk of cheese? "Oh, Brabinger, daaahling, please fetch the jet and fly me to Glasgow. I fancy a piece of vegan cheese." Nope. No one did that.

Oh man, those early days of vegan cheese were bad, bad, bad. I remember the first time I bought vegan cheese. I don't recall the brand, but I remember being so excited about it. I longed for the ooey, gooey, melty, slightly salty, greasy flavor I enjoyed so much during my early college years. I'd always grab a big slice of Blondie's Pizza each afternoon as I walked along Berkeley's Shattuck Avenue, lugging my heavy books back to the dorm. Finally, I thought, *finally*, I'd have cheese good enough for a pizza again. But as anyone who was vegan in the '90s knows all too well, vegan cheese of yesteryear not only didn't taste good, it didn't *melt*. It just sat there in the same shape no matter what you did to it. I tried baking it in the oven, melting it in a saucepan, nuking it in the microwave, grating it, slicing it, chopping it, and heating it over and over again, but to no avail; it *would not melt*. It would just get an ultraglossy sheen, shinier than any top coat of nail polish, and then sit there in full form looking at me like I was a fool for ever thinking there was such a thing as vegan cheese. Vegan cheese?! That tastes good? And melts, *too? Muhahahaaaa.*

Today, it's a whole new world. Vegan cheese is everywhere, and some of it is damn good. During the past ten years, Google searches containing the term "Vegan Cheese" have increased by 833 percent.[3] Why? Because everyone's writing, reading, and talking about making, eating, and enjoying *vegan* cheese. Like I said, it's *that* good. So good that I'm going to skip telling you why it's better than dairy cheese for a moment, and just dive right in and tell you all about it. It's so exciting!

Everyone's taste buds are different, so what I think is super yum, you might think is blah, and vice versa. I don't like anything mint flavored, stevia makes me want to vomit, and I can't stand seaweed (yep, my buds are quite unique!). But I've got to say, I do have some favorites when it comes to vegan cheese. For sandwiches I enjoy Field Roast Grain Meat's Chao Cheese, and I have to admit, I took more than my fair share of allotted samples at this year's Natural Products Expo West . . . *shhh.* And Follow Your Heart's Provolone is tasty, too. When it comes to melting on pizza, Daiya (pronounced day-ah) Shreds are "ah-mAy-zing!" That's what they use on Amy's Kitchen's Vegan Margherita frozen pizza, too. And remember that Galaxy Nutritional Foods'

Soymage that no one liked in the '80s? Well, flash forward a few decades, and they've changed their product name to "Go Veggie!" (smart move!), and also make a super-flavorful, vegan, Chive and Garlic Cream Cheese that pairs perfectly with a warm bagel for breakfast. Kite Hill also makes a delicious Chive Cream Cheese Style Spread. Trader Joe's Vegan Cream Cheese Alternative is pretty darn awesome, too. It's very creamy, doesn't have any artificial flavors, colors, or preservatives, and for under three bucks, I think it's a good deal.

Now, if that wasn't enough to put your fear of losing dairy cheese at ease, hold on to your hats, folks, the next one on the chopping block might just blow you away: Miyoko's Kitchen Cultured Nut Products (They can't be called "cheese" by law. Oy.) I don't even know where to begin. Let me just start by saying if you find Miyoko's cultured nut products, you should try them. I've never, *ever*, tasted anything so close to dairy cheese as these magical, flavorful, wheels of pure heaven. And it's not just me who thinks so. My husband was floored when he tried them, and I drove a few wheels of cheese three hours to my dairy cheese–loving in-laws to sample in gold rush country, and let's just say there wasn't a smidgen of cheese left for the drive back home. They loved it!

When I learned of Miyoko's cheese, I reached out to hear more, and she was kind enough to invite me up to Marin County for a visit. I didn't realize until I set out that day that Miyoko's Kitchen is tucked away behind a little bicycle museum, on the very same street where I went to elementary school over forty-four years ago. The visit was both nostalgic and fun. I put on a hairnet and designated rubber shoes, and was escorted into an aerated room filled with columns of metal shelving, where hundreds of little wheels of cultured nut products were ripening away. Imagine an ancient alchemist laboratory, only impeccably organized, sanitary, and bright, where a wondrous array of flavors, all chosen with fine skill, mingle together until fine perfection. You see, Miyoko isn't just a newbie cook trying to cash in on the unstoppable vegan wave; she's a self-taught chef extraordinaire who is an expert in French, Italian, and Japanese cuisine. Her previous culinary accomplishments are beyond impressive, and yet even so, I don't think *anyone* was expecting vegan "cheese" to ever be *this* good.

Miyoko's cultured nut products range from delicate and creamy to pungent and hard with flavors that can go up, cracker to cracker, against any of the gourmet dairy cheese big boys, if they dare. As you transition from dairy cheese to vegan cheese, consider swapping out your fancy cheese for one of these: Classic Double Cream Chive, Double Cream Sundried Tomato Garlic, High Sierra Rustic Alpine, Fresh Loire Valley in a Fig Leaf, Mt. Vesuvius Black Ash, French Style Winter Truffle, Aged English Sharp

Farmhouse, Aged English Smoked Farmhouse (my favorite!), Country Style Herbes de Provence, or Double Cream Garlic Herb. They're available online and in hundreds of stores. Keep an eye out for the new fresh VeganMozz that melts and browns, too!

Looking for a few more options? Try these:

FANCY CHEESE

Tofutti Milk Free Better Than Ricotta

Tofutti Mascarpone

Kite Hill

Treeline Cheese

Dr. Cow

Miyoko's Kitchen

CREAM CHEESE

Parmela Creamery Creamy Cheese Spread

Go Veggie Cream Cheese

Kite Hill Cream Cheese Style Spread

Nutty Cow Nut Cheese Spread (a variety of flavors)

Tofutti Better Than Cream Cheese

Chia Craft NOT Cream Cheese Spreads

Violife Creamy (dairy-free cream cheese)

PARMESAN CHEESE

Follow Your Heart Parmesan

Go Veggie (Vegan Grated) Parmesan

Parmela Creamery Parmesan

Parma! Vegan Parmesan

Violife Prosociano (with Parmesan Flavour)

Follow Your Heart

Go Veggie!

CHEESE BLOCKS

Daiya

Follow Your Heart

Heidi Ho

Bute Island Foods Sheese

CHEESE SAUCES
Heidi Ho
Nacho Mom's

MAC AND CHEESE
Annie's Vegan Mac & Cheese (box)
Road's End Vegan Mac & Chreese (box)
Earth Balance Vegan Mac and Cheese (box)
Amy's Vegan Mac and Cheese (frozen)

DAIRY CRACK

If you can't find a vegan cheese that you like, it might not be that you're just too picky, but more likely that you're hooked. Cheese really isn't that attractive, at least not compared to a frosted cupcake or even a fresh ripe peach. Sometimes cheese is filled with holes, or even mold, and people *still* gobble it up. Can you imagine people feeling the same way about a moldy bowl of gumbo or a moldy jar of spaghetti sauce? *Eeww!* As for smell, well, "OK, who cut the cheese?" didn't come about because it smells like fresh-baked cookies. The incredibly pungent scent probably explains why I've never come across a cheese-scented candle or any eau de fromage perfume. And yet most people just can't seem to get enough of the cholesterol-laden, saturated fat–filled, antibiotic-infested, chunk of stinky, coagulated cow excretion: aka, good ole' dairy "cheese."

So what gives? Why is *cheese* the most difficult thing to kick for so many folks who are transitioning to becoming vegan? Well, thanks to science, we have a pretty good idea why. It involves a group of proteins called *casein*, that's commonly found in the milk from mammals. In 1981, scientists in North Carolina discovered that when your body digests casein, it breaks up into fragments, which release casomorphines.[4] It doesn't take a PhD in linguistics to see a word embedded in "casomorphines" that sounds an awful lot like a highly addictive drug. At first it sounds crazy; what the heck is *morphine*-like doing in cheese? Well, there's actually a good reason for it, and it all goes back to the mama cow and baby cow bond that we talked about during the chapter on milk. A mother's milk is made for her babies, and it's believed that milk has the addictive properties of opiates to make extra sure that babies crave their mother's milk; it's a product of evolution and the need to survive. Now kick it up a notch, and imagine how concentrated those casomorphines must get in a wheel of Brie or Camembert knowing that it can take ten gallons of milk to produce one pound of cheese.[5] Yep, you're pretty much high as a kite after eating the blasted cheese, without even knowing it. OK, well, maybe just buzzed, but you get the point: it makes you feel groovy, and you want more, more, more!

OK! Are you ready? Here's how you can ditch dairy cheese with ease:

MAKE YOUR OWN VEGAN "CHEESY" STUFF AT HOME

NUTRITIONAL YEAST: I don't know of any vegan who doesn't have a jar, or more likely a giant *tub*, of nutritional yeast in their pantry. The name "nutritional yeast" sounds too healthy to be tasty, and its biological name, *saccharomyces cerevisiae*, sounds even worse, but let me tell you, this stuff can make a lackluster meal into scrumptious chow in a jiff. It has a *je ne sais quoi* about it that satiates even the most picky of vegans when they crave the taste of cheese, and coaxes even non-vegans into a second helping. So what *is* this stuff? It's a bacteria that's usually grown on sugar cane or beet molasses, and unlike the yeast that grows in bread as it rises, or beer as it ferments, nutritional yeast is washed, dried, and deactivated before being sold. And yes, in case you're wondering, vegans are a-OK with killing single-cell bacteria; we're compassionate, not crazy.

In addition to being "cheesy" it's been described as nutty with a pleasant savory taste, similar to umami. I use nutritional yeast almost every day. You can find it in grocery stores worldwide, either on the shelves, or in the bulk section. And if you can't find it locally, you can always order it online, often at a better price. I usually wait for it to go on sale at Vitacost.com, then buy a big 22-ounce tub of it, which lasts for months. It's great on stir-fries, soups, stews, pasta, for mac and cheese, and in sauces to complement veggies, like asparagus and cauliflower. It also works wonders in mashed potatoes, too, either combined or as part of an easy-to-make gravy on top. Spoiler Alert: Gravy Recipe coming up on page 214! You can even sprinkle it on popcorn for a cheese-flavored snack. Love this stuff!

What's extra cool about nutritional yeast is not only is it tasty, it's also really healthy, especially if you use one that's fortified with vegan B_{12}. All brands differ a bit, but here's an example of just *some* of the nutrients in the one that's currently in my kitchen. We sprinkle it on just about everything that's not sweet.

HOMEMADE NUT CHEESE: A second option for those who prefer to make their own

BOB'S RED MILL LARGE FLAKE NUTRITIONAL YEAST

Serving Size: ¼ cup (15g)

Protein: 8g; Thiamin; 790% RDV;

Riboflavin: 570% RDV; Niacin: 230% RDV;

Folate: 270% RDV; Vitamin B_6: 300% RDV; Vitamin B_{12}: 290% RDV cheese-flavored snack is to experiment with nuts. There are a bazillion nut cheese recipes online and they're very easy to make. They don't taste exactly like dairy cheese, but in my opinion, they taste much better. They still give you that fatty, salty taste you crave, only this time, it's from healthy plant fats instead of unhealthy fat shed from animals; and of course, zero cholesterol. Here's an easy recipe to try. It's not only delicious, but also makes a beautiful presentation!

Soft-Crusted Cashew Cheese

SERVES 2

½ cup cashews, soaked

3 tablespoons nutritional yeast

1 tablespoon lemon kombucha or fresh lemon juice

1 garlic clove

1 tablespoon capers (optional)

4 Kalamata olives, pitted

¼ teaspoon sea salt

2 sprigs fresh rosemary, stems removed, needles chopped (or any dried herb you enjoy)

1. In a nonreactive bowl, soak the cashews overnight in the water.

2. The next morning, rinse and drain the cashews and transfer to the bowl of a food processor.

3. Add all the remaining ingredients, except for the rosemary, to the bowl of the food processor with the cashews and blend to the desired consistency, enough that it will stick together when shaped. Add a little more lemon juice if needed.

4. Using a melon baller, scoop out the cheese in balls and place on a plate.

5. Gently press the chopped rosemary on top of the cheese balls. Serve with crudités or crackers.

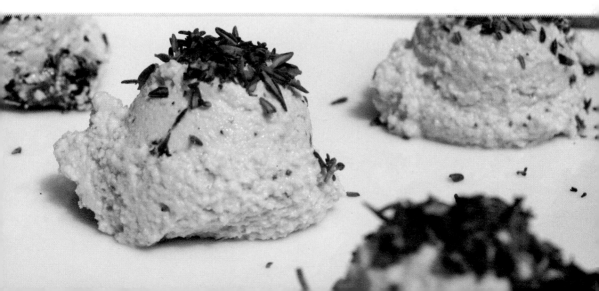

Checklist

- ☐ Did you find a vegan cheese you enjoy, or make your own nut "cheese"?
- ☐ Did you experiment making a meal or snack with nutritional yeast?
- ☐ Are you still avoiding dairy milk, eggs, and other animal products?
- ☐ Did you exercise today?

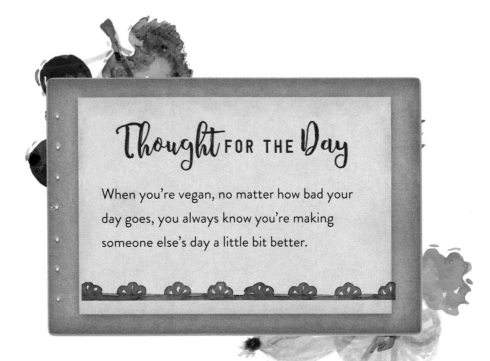

Thought FOR THE Day

When you're vegan, no matter how bad your day goes, you always know you're making someone else's day a little bit better.

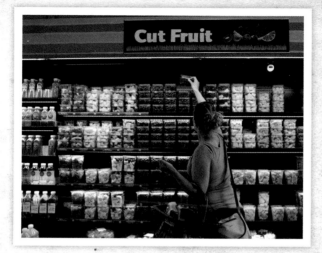

Cut Fruit

Fast, Cheap, AND Easy!

GOAL FOR THE DAY: Make a vegan meal that's fast, cheap, and easy (and delicious, too!)

I'm not sure if fast, cheap, and easy sounds good or bad, but the reality is, sometimes, that's just how we need it. And, honestly, most vegans cook this way, at least the ones I know. Sure, we buy those fancy cookbooks from time to time, and even scroll through the vegan food blogs ogling the screen-lick worthy photos, and drool a bit—OK, drool *a lot*. But hey, when it's time to get in the kitchen, and get cookin', most of us want it stat!

None of this agar-agar or xanthan gum stuff; twenty-eight years of being vegan, and I haven't used them once. No pricey pine nuts in every sauce, and if goji berries are the main ingredient, at a whopping twenty-five bucks a pound, it's just not happening. No spending hours injecting an oblong slab of tofu with yellow goo to recreate a poached egg. Put that idea in your sixth-grade "How to Build a Volcano" box, and head on down to easy street. Vegans, more often than not, just want fresh, delicious, affordable food that we can make in a jiff, and today, you're going to see just how easy it is.

OK, let's hop to it!

1. *First, know that you likely won't have to waste a lot of time thinking about protein.* Ah, good ole' protein. We've got to have it so our cells can build and repair our skin, bones, and muscles, as well as keep our immune system working well. If we were to look into a high-powered microscope, we'd see that protein is composed of beautifully structured amino acids, *so* beautiful that they even make T-shirts and posters of the stained images. Our body makes some amino acids on its own, but others, called *essential* amino acids, we have to go out and get. Here's the great news, though: there's a heck of a lot of protein in plants and you can get *all* of your amino acids from them, even the essential ones. I don't know who started the rumor that you could only get protein from animal products, but sheesh, it's one of those old wives' tales that really needs to be put to rest. Heck, even *watermelon* has protein. The next time you're driving around in the countryside and see a big, strong, and muscular bull, just put your index finger to the side of your chin and ask yourself, "Where does he get his protein?" Yep—from plants. Today you're going to figure out how much protein you need, and then we'll take a look at where you can find it.

Adults need about .36 grams of protein per pound that they weigh.[1] I'm very petite and weigh about 98 pounds so I need approximately 35.28 grams of protein per day (.36 g x 98 lbs = 35.28). That being said, I've never counted out my daily protein intake, other than for one nutrition class assignment. Why? Because I eat enough protein without giving it any thought. You likely will, too, but just to make things easy, I'm listing a bunch of protein-packed plants for you. Peruse the list and jot down what you like in your journal so that when you go to the market, you can pick up a few of them. But rest assured, you really don't need to worry about getting enough protein if you're eating a nice variety of plant foods; as I mentioned earlier, most Americans eat almost *twice* the amount of protein they need.[2] Protein that your body doesn't use turns into sugar, then fat, not to mention it can be hard on the kidneys. Your kidneys are stuck with the task of ridding your body of all of the protein waste by passing nitrogen out through your urine. That's why veterinarians often switch older kitties with kidney problems to a low-protein diet, and doctors encourage those with failing kidneys to eat food low in protein, too.[3] We need protein, but getting enough of it shouldn't be a concern. Leave the obsessive worrying to others. It gives them something to do. We're here to relax, eat good food, and have fun! Here's a list of a few good plant-based proteins you might want to copy and keep handy when you go to the market, though, just to set your mind at ease:

GRAINS
- Quinoa (1 cup cooked) = 8 grams
- Brown Rice (1 cup cooked) = 5 grams
- Oats (1 cup dry) = 6 grams

BEANS
- Black Beans (1 cup cooked) = 15 grams
- Kidney Beans (1 cup cooked) = 16 grams
- Lentils (1 cup cooked) = 18 grams

NUTS
- Almond Butter (2 tablespoons) = 8 grams
- Peanut Butter (2 tablespoons) = 8 grams
- Cashews (1 ounce) = 5 grams

SEEDS
- Flaxseeds (2 tablespoons) = 4 grams
- Sesame Seeds (2 tablespoons) = 3 grams
- Hemp Seeds (2 tablespoons) = 7 grams

VEGETABLES
- Spinach (1 cup cooked) = 5 grams
- Peas (1 cup frozen, boiled, and drained) = 8 grams
- Portobello Mushrooms (1 cup grilled) = 5 grams

2. Adopt some smart vegan shopping strategies that are healthy and will save you money.

⬏ Healthy vegan food begins with your shopping cart, so don't put the junk in your trunk. Once it's home, it's a million times more difficult to avoid eating. Trust me, I know. Yesterday my husband asked if I wanted him to bring home a box of vegan cookies from the store, and I said "No, thank you. If you buy them, I'll eat them." And today, I'm sitting here gobbling up a bag of raw almonds, bananas, and dates. Mission accomplished. For today, at least.

⬏ Shop when you're full to avoid impulse buys, and be especially wary of snacks at the checkout stand.

⬏ Try to shop around the perimeter of the store, or at least go there first. Most of the unhealthy, overly processed products are in the middle of the grocery store.

⬏ Look high and low on the shelves for healthier fare as most of the unhealthy products are strategically positioned at eye level. You'll be surprised at what you'll find, especially in the cereal section. There's actually a lot of healthy whole grain cereals in mainstream supermarkets, they just get swallowed up by all of the psychedelic boxes of "Cholesterol Crunch" and "Obesity O's."

⬏ Bring a healthy, well-thought-out shopping list and try to stick to it. If you add more food to the list once you're at the store, just make sure it's healthy.

⬏ If you're really craving sweets, buy fresh or dried fruit instead. When I want a vegan donut, I pout around the house for about ten minutes (because we don't have them in the house anymore) and then I eat a sweet banana or crisp apple and I'm completely satiated. A handful of cashews or a spoonful of nut butter with a few vegan dark chocolate chips on top works well, too! In the summertime, try frozen grapes. Yum!

⬏ Don't get discouraged if the produce seems to be expensive. I'm lucky to live in California where fresh fruits and veggies are abundant all year. But if you can't find fresh produce at a good price, head over to the freezer section. The fruits and veggies will likely be cheaper, and just as healthy, or healthier. Produce begins to lose its nutrients as soon as it's harvested, but frozen fruits and veggies are usually flash-frozen upon picking, sealing in all of their vitamins, minerals, and antioxidants. Whereas the fresh produce may have traveled over a thousand miles to get to you, and who knows how many moons it has been on the road. Frozen produce often gets a bad rap, but it's actually healthy, and generally less expensive.

⬏ If you get the urge to buy a bunch of highly processed vegan foods like cupcakes and cookies, instead of buying them, or any prepackaged mixes, buy all of the individual ingredients you need to make them. That way you can still have treats once in a while, but because you'll have to work for them, you'll eat them far less, and your homemade treats will likely be healthier, too.

- ᕀ Use coupons! I've seen—and used—online coupons for free Beyond Meat Strips and Crumbles, free Sweet Earth Benevolent Bacon, and free Dave's Killer Bread. Yes, absolutely free! Consider creating an e-mail account just for vegan food, and then sign up for newsletters and promotions from as many vegan food companies as you like. This way you'll always know when there's a good deal for an item, but you won't flood your primary e-mail account. Other food and beverage companies that often have great coupons and promotions for vegan products include Gardein, Earthbound Farms, Jamba Juice, Silk, Lightlife, Amy's Organic, Follow Your Heart, So Delicious Dairy Free, Nasoya Tofu, Go Veggie, Field Roast, and Bob's Red Mill. Just google the company name and the word *coupons* and you'll find them. You might be able to print out the coupon immediately, or you may need to subscribe to a newsletter, but that's OK; you've got your dedicated vegan food e-mail account for it!

- ᕀ Stack Coupons! Most stores accept both the manufacturers' coupon as well as the store's coupon. For example, Whole Foods Market has their own monthly coupon booklet that you can pick up at the customer service counter, as well as a coupon app. They always have at least a few coupons for vegan food and you can stack those discounts on top of the manufacturers' coupons you bring from home. Target often has vegan food and beverage coupons on their website, too. You'll really feel like you've hit the jackpot if you find an item that's on sale, and then use two stacked coupons. It happens!

- ᕀ Check to see if your grocery store has any unique promotions. Sprouts Markets, for example, always has great sales, but on Wednesdays they honor the sale prices from the past week, as well as the current week. You won't get a "double" discount on anything, but you'll have twice as many sale items to choose from, and that rocks!

- ᕀ Check out the Dollar Store and Dollar Tree. There are thousands of locations across the country! I've found so many vegan items at these stores. Peanut butter, oats, vegan mayo, canned coconut milk, soy milk, almond milk, pasta, pasta sauce, dried beans, vegetable samosas, veggie burgers, frozen berries, and at only one buck each. Can't beat that!

- ᕀ Big Lots often has great deals on Bob's Red Mill items, such as a 24-ounce bag of whole flaxseeds for three bucks, or the 13 Bean Soup Mix for four dollars. Big

Lots is also where we usually score our bargain Bob's Red Mill Organic 7 Grain Pancake and Waffle Mix. It's currently $8.37 on Amazon, $4.69 online at Bob's Red Mill, and only $3.70 at Big Lots. Did someone say pancakes? (Spoiler Alert: There's a pancake recipe coming up on page 158!)

3. *Know that if you must have vegan junk food during your transition, it exists. Oh boy, does it exist.*

I don't eat the products in the list that follows, and I don't think you should either. Ever. And that's an "ever" with fifty r's at the end. My brain doesn't even register them as "food" anymore. There are so many reasons to avoid them that I could fill up an entire book telling you why, but today I'm not here to pester you about junk food. Just remember, a whole foods plant-based diet is the way to go, and there are many delicious and healthy options to choose from. But the reality is, if you're used to eating a lot of junk food, as most Americans are, it can be difficult to transition to a *healthy* plant-based diet overnight. I don't think anyone would disagree with that. So if you're about to lose your willpower and grab some crappy "junk food," it's better to munch on Spicy Sweet Chili Doritos (vegan) instead of the Flamin' Hot Cheetos (dairy), or pick up a box of Swedish Fish (vegan) over those colorful Gummy Bears (gelatin). But *please*, just use these as a temporary crutch in the case of a dire emergency. They're *not* healthy. We're making the world a happier, healthier place, and that includes you, too. As I've said before, don't get sick on me, chickadee. I need you!

I CAN'T BELIEVE IT'S VEGAN
Brach's Mandarin Orange Slices
Cap'n Crunch Original Flavor
Cracker Jack
Dum Dums Lollypops
Duncan Hines Cake Mixes (Classic Carrot, Moist Deluxe Butter Golden,
    Classic Yellow, Dark Chocolate Fudge, Devil's Food, Fudge Marble,
    German Chocolate, Red Velvet, Swiss chocolate, Coconut Supreme,
    Lemon Supreme, Pineapple Supreme, and Strawberry Supreme—just
    swap out the eggs when you're making the batter)
Duncan Hines Creamy Home-Style Frosting (classic vanilla and chocolate)

Famous Amos Chocolate Sandwich Cookies (Chocolate, Oatmeal Macaroon, Peanut Butter, and Vanilla)

Fritos (Original and BBQ)

Hubba Bubba Bubble Gum

Jell-O Cook & Serve Pudding & Pie Filling (lemon, chocolate, vanilla, pistachio, banana cream—just use a plant milk in place of dairy milk)

Jolly Ranchers Hard Candy

Keebler Vienna Fingers

Kellogg's Pop-Tarts (unfrosted strawberry, unfrosted blueberry, unfrosted brown sugar—the frosted ones contain gelatin)

Nabisco Lorna Doone Shortbread

Nabisco Teddy Grahams (Chocolate and Cinnamon)

Nutter Butter Cookies

Oreos (original)

Pillsbury Crescent Rolls

Red Vines

Ritz crackers

Sara Lee Oven Fresh Apple Pie (watch out, the Oven Fresh Dutch Apple Pie contains dairy and eggs)

Smarties (USA only)

Sour Patch Kids

Spicy Sweet Chili Doritos

Swedish Fish

Twizzlers

Zotz

I am putting my "health advocate" hat back on now. Whew! Compiling that list for you was painful, but I know for some of you, it will help keep you on track to "Veganville." Some folks need baby steps, and I get that. You're not just going vegan, you're *staying* vegan, so have faith in the process, folks. If you need a box of Cracker Jack as you're starting off, have at it. And you can have the toy surprise, too!

4. *Now, it's time to get cooking!* Here are a few fast and delicious meal ideas to get you started. If you've already made one during an earlier section, pick another one you like, or create your own!

MY VEGAN SMOOTHIE

I *love* breakfast smoothies, and enjoy them three or four times a week. I use a blender that also serves as the cup, so cleanup is a snap. There are a ton of recipes online, as well as in many cookbooks dedicated to the art of smoothies, but the gist of making one just involves three things: the liquid, the produce, and the optional extra nutrients. Here's what I usually put in mine:

Liquid —> 1 to 1½ cups almond milk (any plant-based milk will do)

Produce —> 1 large ripe banana

Produce —> 1 handful frozen blueberries

Extra Nutrient —> 1 heaping tablespoon peanut butter (any nut butter will do)

Extra Nutrient —> 1 tablespoon freshly ground flaxseeds

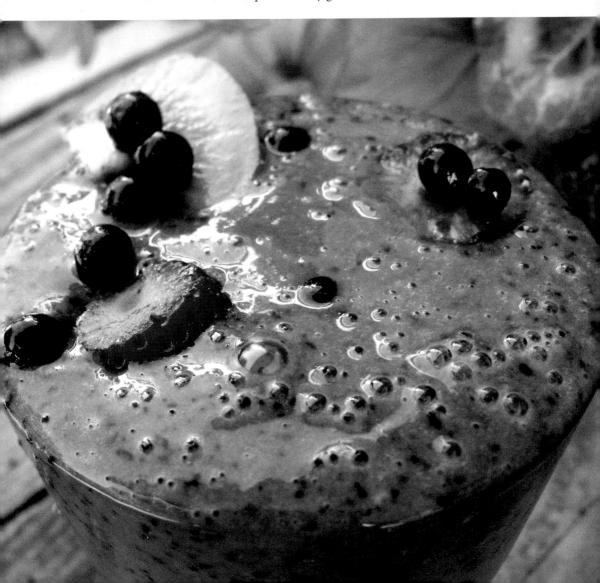

YOUR VEGAN SMOOTHIE

Don't feel like you have to stick with almond milk, there's all of those delicious plant milks we talked about in Day 4: Let's Get Nutty! You can also use any juice you like, or even coconut water. As for the produce, just toss in what's handy. I often add additional fruit, based on whatever I picked up at the farmers' market that week, or whatever was on sale at the grocery store. It's easy to toss in greens, too—just remember to remove the chunky stalks if you don't have a high-speed blender (I nibble on the stalks while I'm making my smoothie). If you're new to adding greens, consider starting slow with a few fresh baby spinach leaves, then you can work your way up toward the heartier greens like collards or kale. Vegan NFL player David Carter adds cannellini beans to his smoothies; now *that* sounds . . . interesting! If you prefer a tropical smoothie, think of the produce you'd find on an island: pineapples, bananas, coconuts, mangos, etc., and give those a whirl. Occasionally, I just want pure sweetness, so I skip the citrus and greens altogether and just blend up bananas, chocolate almond milk, and peanut butter—decadent and satisfying. And there's always cha cha cha chia seeds, or pitted dates if you want a natural sugar boost!

My Overnight Oats

SERVES 1

If you can spare five minutes the night before, this breakfast is ready upon waking up in the morning. You might already be familiar with this as "muesli," a popular breakfast in Germany and Switzerland. Muesli isn't a trendy new vegan dish, but a meal that was created over one hundred years ago by Swiss doctor Maximilian Bircher-Benner, who believed that his patients would heal better if they enjoyed a diet rich in raw fruit, vegetables, and nuts. What? No bacon and eggs? Smart man.

1 cup uncooked rolled oats

¾ cup vanilla almond milk

Fresh blueberries

1. Put 1 cup of uncooked oats in a sealable jar or bowl and mix in the almond milk. Refrigerate overnight.

2. In the morning add the blueberries, and enjoy!

YOUR OVERNIGHT OATS: Blueberries are my favorite, but you can add bananas or strawberries, depending on what's in season. Nuts and seeds make for a nice addition, too. You can even drizzle a little bit of maple or agave syrup on top, if you need a little extra sweetness.

My Breakfast Toast

Most of us vegans aren't sitting at home flipping through cookbooks looking for something to create for breakfast. We have places to go, people to meet, and animals to cuddle. Or we oversleep and just don't have the time. OK fine, a lot of us are simply lazy when it comes to breakfast. There, I said it. Enter, toast! I love lightly toasted bread with avocado, freshly ground black pepper, and a dash of sea salt. If I'm in the mood for something sweeter, I pile on the almond butter or peanut butter, with organic strawberry jam instead. I buy jumbo jars of it at Costco for a great price.

YOUR BREAKFAST TOAST: You can top off your toast with vegan butter, vegan cream cheese, fruit preserves, or even hummus. Sliced bananas with your favorite nut butter on toast is a great on-the-go breakfast, too. Or, as I mentioned, *my* favorite, the "wait until I'm ripe, wait, wait, wait, wait, ready, TOO LATE!" fruit: the avocado.

My Sandwich

My favorite? Avocado sandwiches! I add vegan mayonnaise, whole grain mustard, a slice of red onion and lettuce. I use one of the three breads on the next page, or make an open-faced sandwich with fresh vegan bread. I used to leave the crust behind, but now I eat about 80 percent of it, and give what's left to my husband. I'm improving.

YOUR SANDWICH: Everything that you considered for your toast at breakfast is an option for a yummy vegan sandwich, too. There's also lots of vegan deli meat substitutes and cheeses. And if you have a George Foreman grill, or something similar, it's easy to whip up a vegan grilled cheese or panini, or make a BLT using one of the vegan bacons we talked about on page 109. You don't need much guidance here. Just take 5 minutes and whip one up!

BREAD

If you're thinking it's not the topping, but the bread itself that's hard to find, think again. Here are a few of my favorite vegan breads:

- ⚘ Eureka! Seeds the Day Organic Bread: This bread is packed with lots of seeds—pumpkin, sunflower, flax, sesame, and poppy. And it has a hint of sweetness from a little bit of organic cane sugar and molasses. I've found it at Target, Nob Hill Foods, Grocery Outlet, Save Mart, and a local health food store. Visit eurekabread.com, click on Find a Store, enter your zip code, and it will pull up all the stores where Eureka bread was delivered within the past three days.[4] That's nifty! Eureka makes six varieties of vegan bread, and they're all made without artificial flavors, colors, preservatives, or high-fructose corn syrup.

- ⚘ Alvarado Street Bakery's organic Sprouted Wheat Bread: What's cool about Alvarado's is that it's not only tasty, its creation is rather unique. Instead of using flour, Alvarado Street Bakery soaks whole, organic wheat berries in filtered water, waits for them to sprout, then drains the water, and grinds up the sprouts into dough. The sprouted wheat bread is made with dates and raisins, too. There are several vegan options from Alvarado Street Bakery, including flaxseed bread and sprouted barley, all of which are certified non-GMO and produced in a solar-powered facility. Cool!

- ⚘ Dave's Killer Bread: There's quite a background story here: One in three of the company's employees is a convicted felon, and that's intentional. Even Dave Dahl, the creator of the bread himself, spent fifteen "long and lonely" years behind bars.[4] The company believes in second chances for folks who have been on the wrong side of the law, and wants to prevent recidivism and change the way society looks at folks once they're released.[5] Dave's Killer Bread catapulted from selling one hundred loaves of bread at a Portland farmers' market ten years ago to being sold to Flower Foods, Inc. in 2015 for $275 million, *cash*. Now that's a big pile of dough! I was worried that Flower Foods, maker of the infamous über-processed white Wonder Bread, would change Dave's recipe, but they reassured me with their reply, "We love what you love! DKB will keep using the same recipes for loaves with organic, non-GMO grains and seeds," so fingers crossed! Dave's Killer Bread is expanding throughout the country, and in Canada, too. There are lots of vegan, GMO-free varieties, packed with healthy seeds, whole grains, and sweetened with organic fruit juice and molasses. And if you're missing the super soft texture of good ole' Wonder Bread, check out their White Bread Done Right. You can find loaves of Dave's Killer Bread in mainstream supermarkets and double packs at Costco.

My Salad

I usually like baby spinach leaf salads the best, but I'm on an organic romaine kick at the moment. I chop up the leaves and usually add organic tomatoes, avocado, onions, and mushrooms, and whatever else looks good from my farmers' market haul. If I'm extra hungry, I open a can of black beans, rinse, and toss a few spoonfuls on top. I drizzle it with dressing that I make myself, or a few splashes of balsamic vinegar with freshly ground black pepper. A few of my favorite store-bought vegan dressings are Trader Joe's Asian Style Spicy Vinaigrette and Trader Joe's Goddess Dressing, and several from Follow Your Heart, including High Omega Vegan Ranch and Vegan Thousand Island.

YOUR SALAD: Toss in all the fresh fruits, veggies, grains, seeds, and beans that you enjoy. Everything from olives and artichoke hearts to oranges and strawberries taste good in a salad. Dried cranberries, dates, and raisins also taste good. The more colorful, the better! Then add the dressing of your choice. Easy peasy.

My Dressing

MAKES ABOUT ⅓ CUP

1 heaping tablespoon whole grain mustard (I like the mustard with seeds and sea salt, but you can use any you like)

1 tablespoon brown sugar (agave or maple syrup works well, too, if you prefer)

3 tablespoons olive oil (any oil you enjoy will do)

3 tablespoons balsamic vinegar (rice vinegar also tastes good)

3 pinches dried basil (squish it up between your fingers as you add it to release the oils)

Freshly ground black pepper

1. Mix all the ingredient together in a bowl until the sugar has dissolved and everything is well blended.

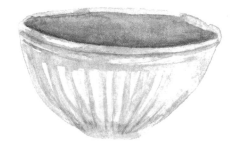

YOUR DRESSING

You can buy dressings or you can use recipes, but there's a certain satisfaction that comes along with creating one yourself. When someone tells you how yummy your food is (and they will!) you can tell them, "It's just a little something I whipped up myself," which feels pretty darn good. Also, you never know when you'll be short on supplies, so by learning how to work with what's on hand, you'll be ready in a pinch.

If you want to keep things simple, just squeeze half of a fresh lemon on your salad, or drizzle a bit of balsamic vinegar. Want more flavor? No problem! It's easy to make your own dressings to tantalize your newbie vegan taste buds. The key is to *combine flavors that excite four key palate areas of your mouth, plus seasoning,* which is exactly what I did when I made my salad dressing. I couldn't figure out why it was so well received until I took apart the elements, and sure enough, there they were: Tart (vinegar and mustard), Creamy/Fatty (Olive Oil), Salty (the sea salt in the mustard), Sweet (brown sugar), plus basil and freshly ground black pepper for spiciness.

Here are some suggestions for making your own salad dressings. Enjoy the freedom to experiment with amounts, and taste as you go. The flavor combinations are endless!

And remember, you can drizzle your delectable creation on a heck of a lot more than salads. Once you find a few combos you like, try topping your potatoes, stir-fries, rice, and whatever else your heart desires with the dressings you like best. You can use them for marinades, too! What you make in the kitchen will likely be tastier and *healthier,* than anything you can buy in the store. Besides, cooking is fun!

Tart + Creamy/Fatty + Salty + Sweet + herbs and spices = Your Yummy Dressing!

Pick at least one from each section:

TART

VINEGAR: Vinegar is simply the next step, after wine. With a little bit of oxygen and bacteria, wine becomes very acidic, thus the name *vin* (French for "wine") *aigre* (French for "sour"). Anything that can be made into wine can be made into vinegar—that's why there are hundreds of varieties, going all the way back to the Babylonians in 4000 BCE who made vinegar from date wine, raisin wine, and even beer.[6] I enjoy making marinades and dressings with balsamic vinegar or rice vinegar, but apple cider vinegar and sherry vinegar are great options, too. There's even pineapple, cherry, and coconut vinegars!

FRESH CITRUS: Just squeeze the juice of a fresh lemon, lime, grapefruit, kumquat, orange, tangerine, or pomelo into your dressing or marinade and you'll get a nice tart kick.

MUSTARD: I love seeded mustard aka whole grain mustard, but no need to limit yourself to what makes *me* happy. There's so many to choose from, including yellow mustard, spicy brown mustard, German mustard, Chinese hot mustard, and the one we always had in the kitchen growing up (and I still do), good old English dry mustard. You can find Colman's English Mustard in a little yellow tin with red writing. One of my favorites! Beware, though; it's *strong.*

WINE: I'm not a big fan of drinking wine, although I do love vineyards and grapes, so count me in for any wine tours! Wine does make for a nice tart addition to a salad dressing or marinade, though. Check out Day 14: Excuse Me, Waiter . . . for a few vegan wine options, one of which is Charles Shaw Red Wine, fondly known as Trader Joe's Two Buck (and a half) Chuck. If you want a slightly sweeter taste, you can "reduce" wine by slowly simmering it with a little bit of sugar, which will make it thick like a syrup. This reduces the water and acidity while increasing the flavor, color, and sweetness—perfect for marinades. Sounds fancy, but it's easy.

CREAMY/FATTY

AVOCADO: I just can't get enough of avocados, which you've probably gathered by now. They make any meal better, in my opinion. If you want creamy, go for the bumpy Haas variety if possible, as the smooth Florida avocados can sometimes be watery.

TOFU: Some folks like to blend up silken tofu to make a creamy dressing. Just toss it into your food processor or blender with the other ingredients. Done.

NUTS AND SEEDS: You can either soak a few nuts overnight, drain, and toss into the blender, or go straight for a nut or seed butter. Tahini, which is made from sesame seeds, and peanut butter are two of my favorites when it comes to dressings and marinades.

OILS: So many to choose from! Some of my favorites include olive oil, and sesame seed oil. I usually go *easy* on the oils, though, and try to add a little more of everything else. And when I do use them, I try to use unrefined, non-GMO oils. As cooking oil expert and author, Lisa Howard, points out, the ingredients in refined cooking oils have been "cleaned, crushed, steamed, pressed with high friction heat, extracted with solvent, distilled, bleached, deodorized, and steamed again."[7] Although they can be more pricey, I think you'll like the taste of unrefined oils better, too. They're pressed and bottled quickly, which seals in the flavor. *Any* vegetable oil is better than a tub of lard, though, even a bottle of canola or corn oil, so just use whatever you have on hand. We're keeping things real, folks; trust in the process.

SALTY

OLIVES AND CAPERS: Olive trees can live for over one thousand years, and have been harvested for over eight thousand. I always keep a jar of their yummy fruit in my refrigerator. The color of olives is indicative of their ripeness. Green olives are picked at the start of the season, and black ones at the end. Kalamata olives are by far my favorite, and when I'm in the mood for a bag of chips, I just nibble on a few olives, and it usually squashes my need for salty junk food. I think they're perfect for seasoning dressings and marinades, too. If you're not sure which variety you like, consider getting a few of each at an olive bar, which you can often find at supermarkets, including many Whole Foods Market locations. Capers, which are simply the little green, unopened flower buds of the caper bush, are a great addition, too.

SEAWEED: As you know, I don't like seaweed (it smells and tastes so fishy!), but if you do, sprinkle a few flakes of kelp or nori into that dressing or marinade.

MISO: This Japanese fermented soybean paste is one of those unsung heroes that usually goes unnoticed tucked away in the refrigerator section at the grocery store. You'll find several varieties ranging from light (sweeter) to dark (saltier), but in Japan they have as many varieties as we have cheese![8] Added bonus: If you're trying to ditch chicken noodle soup, just put a little spoonful of miso in a mug of hot water and you'll have a tasty soothing broth without hurting any birds.

SWEET

FRUIT: Everything from dried apricots and dates to raspberries and raisins can be used to give your dressings and marinades a little sweetness. My friend Amy saves the tops of her strawberries when she makes her morning smoothie, then tosses them into white vinegar and lets them sit for a couple of days to make her strawberry vinaigrette; resourceful and delicious!

MAPLE SYRUP, COCONUT PALM SUGAR, DATE SUGAR, BROWN SUGAR, MOLASSES, ETC.: There are so many types of sugars to choose from these days! I prefer sugars that are less refined, such as organic brown sugar and maple syrup, because they have more flavor than white sugar, and since they're less processed, they have slightly more minerals. Whichever sugar you choose, just try not to eat too much of it. Easier said than done, I know. I love sweets.

SEASONINGS

I usually like basil, sea salt, and freshly ground pepper in most of my salad dressings. But the variety of spices you can use are too numerous to list, so toss in what you love, and enjoy!

Tofu and Grits

I asked the Physicians Committee for Responsible Medicine's in-house registered dietician, Susan Levin, what she likes to eat that can be prepared in 5 minutes or less. Susan's response? Tofu and Grits! I *love* grits, although I make them sweet (with almond milk and maple syrup), which I've heard is a big no-no in the South. Whoops. Here's how Susan makes grits, the *savory* way:

1 cup polenta (yellow grits)

3 cups water

1 block prebaked tofu

"If you grew up where I did, polenta is a fancy way of saying grits. But no matter what you call it, it's easy to prepare and delicious. Boil 3 cups of water, add the polenta, turn down to low, and stir regularly. Within a minute or so, you'll have a nice consistency. Chop your baked tofu and plop it on top (bake or sauté your own if you have more time). Spice as you desire! Add some Tabasco or sriracha sauce if you like some kick."

—SUSAN LEVIN, MS, RD

If times are tough and you need help maintaining your vegan lifestyle, here are a few places and programs that can lend a helping hand:

Vegan Food and Public Assistance Programs
I'll never forget the time a disheartened *My Vegan Journal* reader wrote to me that she was doing her very best to transition to becoming vegan, but was down on her luck, and out of money. It was during the holiday season, and she went to her local food bank where they gave her a big, heavy box of food. When she got home she opened the box and found a dead turkey inside. She wrote to tell me that although she had no money, and barely any food, instead of eating the bird, she buried the turkey in her backyard, and gave him a respectful and loving funeral service. Her pocketbook was empty, but her heart was warm and full.

For most, myself included, life is a roller coaster of ups and downs and there's no telling what tomorrow brings. The "Great Recession" of 2008 was a chilly reminder of this, as so many saw a lifetime of savings and steady career advances vanish overnight. Thankfully, there are several public services and non-profit organizations that can help those in need when it comes to eating healthy vegan food. If you, or a friend, are ever in need, check out the services on the following pages. Remember, you don't need money to be vegan; you just need the will to be kind. How awesome is *that?*

WIC (Women, Infants, and Children)
The WIC program is designed to help pregnant women and infants who are low income and nutritionally at risk. The program also covers women who are breast-feeding (up to the infant's first birthday), non-breast-feeding postpartum women (up to 6 months), and children up to their fifth birthday. WIC serves 53 percent of all infants born in the United States, so it's good to know that there's an array of vegan food that qualifies

under the federal guidelines.[9] The availability can vary from state to state, and from year to year, so be sure to check your local WIC office to see what's available in your area.

CONTACT: http://www.fns.usda.gov/wic/contacts

SNAP Supplemental Nutrition Assistance Program (formerly the "Food Stamp Program") SNAP is a federal aid program that provides food-purchasing assistance to over 46 million Americans who are low income or who have no income. If you qualify for SNAP, you'll be provided with an EBT card that you can use to buy a huge variety of vegan foods, including fruits, vegetables, cereals, grains, seeds, nuts, legumes, and bread, as well as food-producing seeds and plants for your garden. SNAP even has a section on the list of federally approved items entitled "vegan food," the specifics of which can be clarified with your local SNAP office. Be sure to ask about their Farmers' Market Nutrition Program (FMNP), too, so you can enjoy free locally grown fresh fruits, veggies, and herbs.

CONTACT:
State SNAP phone numbers: www.fns.usda.gov/snap/state-informationhotline-numbers
To find out if you're eligible for SNAP: www.snap-step1.usda.gov

VEGAN FOOD AVAILABLE THROUGH WIC:

- Tofu
- Soy-based beverage (flavored and unflavored)
- Any fruit and/or vegetable juice or juice blends
- Peanut butter (creamy or chunky, regular or reduced fat, salted or unsalted)
- Any type of mature dry beans, peas, or lentils, such as black beans, black-eyed peas, garbanzo beans (chickpeas), Great Northern beans, white beans (navy and pea beans), kidney beans, mature lima beans ("butter beans"), fava and mung beans, pinto beans, soybeans, split peas, lentils, and refried beans. Those with limited cooking facilities are eligible for baked beans.
- Fresh fruits and vegetables (states must offer WIC-eligible fresh fruits and vegetables and must allow organic forms of these items; canned, frozen, and/or dried fruits and vegetables are offered at the state agency's option)
- Any plain, dry infant cereal (e.g., rice, barley, mixed grain)
- Infant food fruits and vegetables

NON-PROFIT ORGANIZATIONS THAT PROVIDE VEGAN FOOD

Food Not Bombs

Food Not Bombs is a volunteer-run organization on a mission to end world hunger by providing free vegetarian and vegan food to everyone, without restriction, including those who are "rich or poor, stoned or sober." They promote the benefits of a vegan diet, and never cook with animal products, but occasionally distribute donated food that has dairy in it, so always be sure to ask. Food Not Bombs was the first to provide food to the 9/11 responders in New York, and among the first to offer food to the survivors of Hurricane Katrina.[10] I remember seeing their friendly volunteers dish up a big pot of hearty vegan stew in Berkeley, California, in the late '80s, and most recently, in front of a post office in Santa Cruz. Food Not Bombs has thousands of chapters located throughout the world. Good folks doing good work. I like that.

CONTACT:

To see if there's a Food Not Bombs near you, visit: foodnotbombs.net/new_site/ or call the Hunger Hotline: 1-800-844-1136.

Toronto Vegetarian Food Bank

The Toronto Vegetarian Food Bank was created by fellow vegan Matt Noble in January 2015. Though the name says "vegetarian" they're "committed to providing all vegan-friendly food" of which at least 50 percent is fresh, whole foods. Past offerings have included rice, oatmeal, whole wheat spaghetti, tomato sauce, tofu, dried chickpeas, lentils, soy milk, granola bars, and a vast selection of fresh produce. Sounds good! The volunteer-run organization distributes food once a month at 270 Gerarrd Street East.

CONTACT:

For more information, visit the Toronto Vegetarian Food Bank website: http://tvfb.ca/about/

Additional Options

Many community colleges and churches have free food banks or pantries, some of which offer a nice selection of organic produce, so do a little search on the Internet and make a few calls and see what's available in your community. You can also visit the Feeding America website to see if there's a food bank near you—hopefully they'll have lots of plant-based food to help you make your transition to a vegan diet a healthy one! http://www.feedingamerica.org/find-your-local-foodbank

Checklist

- ☐ Did you find coupons for yummy vegan food?

- ☐ Did you select a tasty vegan bread?

- ☐ Did you create your own recipe for a marinade or dressing combining tart, sweet, creamy/fatty, and salty, with herbs and spices?

- ☐ Did you try making overnight oats, a smoothie, or another quick breakfast?

Thought FOR THE Day

Ralph Horner was an employee at a meatpacking plant in Colorado. One night while at work, his hair and sleeve got caught on a piece of machinery. The fabric twisted around his neck and mouth, strangling him under the conveyor belt. He never made it home to his wife and kids. Sadly, it's no surprise; meatpacking is 2½ times more dangerous than any other industry in the United States. Rapid moving saws, blenders, pumps, knives, chains, and toxic chemicals cause everything from lacerations and lung cancer to muscular disorders and meningitis. When you're vegan, you're not only helping animals, you're decreasing the demand for factory farmworkers, which helps keep people safe, too.

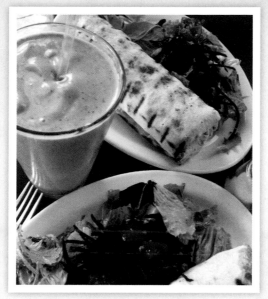

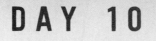

Culinary "Arts"

GOAL FOR THE DAY: Make a tasty vegan meal
that looks beautiful!

I know we shouldn't judge a book by its cover, but truth be told, we do, and the same can be said for food. Now that you've learned to cook fast, cheap, and easy, let's slow things down a bit and make a beautiful meal because presentation means a lot. When we're offered a gorgeous, colorful plate of plant-based foods, our senses become excited. But a hospital tray of amorphous mushed veggies and mashed potatoes? Not so much. In this chapter we'll learn how to make vegan meals pretty, and chances are, the more col-orful the dish, the healthier it will be, too! Consider this the "dress to impress" chapter. Although as kids we're told, "don't play with your food!" we're going to do just that, and it will be fun! It really is amazing how much a few simple culinary techniques—such as slicing veggies creatively, sprinkling dark seeds on light dishes, a few sprigs of an herb on soups and smoothies, or creating rich, deep colors with beets and blueberries—can transform a ho-hum "what *is* this?" dish into a "looks too pretty to eat!" meal. After this chapter's mini culinary "arts" lessons, you will be all set to prepare a feast for your eyes by yourself!

OK, tie on that apron and let's go!

1. *Create a beautiful meal using simple and fun culinary techniques!*

THE PLATE I love pretty, colorful plates, but when it comes to "plating" food for a fancy-pants affair, it's actually best to have a simple, plain white plate. Just think of it as the canvas for your creation; you want it to be clean and white, or very close to it—this is why so many food photographers use simple, clean settings. If the plate itself is already colorful, it will likely detract from your painting: the food. Round plates are the most popular, but square and rectangular plates can be fun, too.

When you're looking at your plate, consider the outer area as the "frame" of your masterpiece. You don't want any food or drips on the frame, so keep it clean, and wipe it before you serve, if necessary. As you focus on the inside of the plate, think of it as a clock, with three main sections: Noon to 4 pm, 4 pm to 8 pm, and 8 pm to midnight. When you put your food on the plate, consider placing at least one item into each section, with the food you want to highlight the most placed in the area from 4 pm to 8 pm, facing the guest. I'm more of a pile-it-on-whatever-dish-is-clean kind of cook and my cupboard is full of colorful mismatched plates. This is just for *very* special occasions, when you get a bit of the Martha Stewart itch and feel like a little "foo foo shoo shoo" fun.

Back to the plate. Make sure your foods are touching, without leaving a big gap in the middle of the plate or between the food, as people will be drawn to the white open spots, rather than the meal itself. If you have a sauce to add, don't smother the whole meal with it, just spoon enough on it to embellish it, rather than drown it, so the lovely details of your masterpiece can show through.

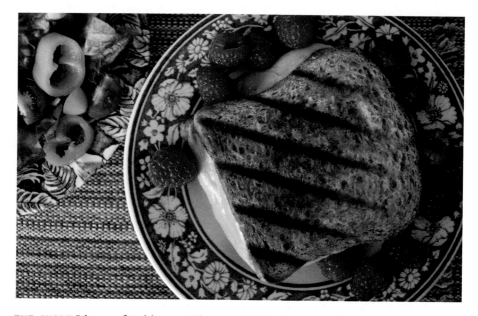

THE SHAPE I love refried beans. I love mashed potatoes. I love jasmine rice. But a round scoop of all three of those on a plate wouldn't win over any artists' hearts. The same could be said of a plate full of Brussels sprouts, baby potatoes, and falafel balls—all delicious, but all the same shape. It's not very exciting, and good luck making it to the table without one rolling off the plate. So just give a little thought as you plan out your meal, as to what it will look like once it's on the plate. If you're having sautéed string beans, you might not want to serve it beside seared asparagus spears, or if you're making couscous, you might not want to serve it with a pile of polenta. It's all pretty much common sense, but still worth thinking about, especially if you're just starting off, or making a meal to impress. Master chefs actually sketch out their plating before they start to cook. Now there's a doodle to keep you busy the next time you're bored at work.

When it comes to slicing fruits and vegetables, there are lots of fancy techniques, from julienne and jardinière to chiffonade and mirepoix, but since this is a guide to going vegan and not French 101, we're going to keep things simple and stick with English here. Just know that you can really liven up a dish by carefully slicing your produce into unique shapes. And if you're trying to get your kids to eat more fruits and veggies as you, or your entire family, transitions to becoming vegan, sometimes just making the food's presentation a bit more interesting will do the trick. If you usually just chop your carrots across, making a round circle, try slicing

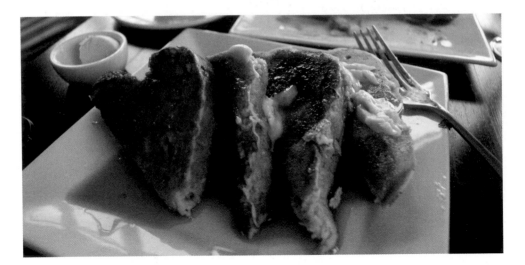

them at an angle. If you normally cut your bell peppers into squares, try a few long strips. Tired of rectangular chunks of tofu? Make them into little triangles. You can even buy a set of stainless steel fruit and veggie cutters—just like cookie cutters, but smaller—to create hearts, stars, flowers, and animals, too. Create a few new shapes, and have some fun!

THE CONTRAST I love to contrast colors as much as possible, and you should give it a go, too. When you're making a dish with light fruits or veggies, add a seasoning or garnish that's dark, and if you're creating a dark dish, top it off with something light. For example, when I'm making a stir-fry that has tofu and light veggies in it, I'll toss in black sesame seeds, but if I'm sautéing veggies that are darker, such as unpeeled eggplant, or asparagus, I'll use white sesame seeds. Around the holidays, I love to make dishes festive by sprinkling pomegranate seeds onto roasted Brussels sprouts or a spinach salad, and I garnish baked beets with chopped fresh dill. I also like to pick a sprig of wild rosemary from the garden, and pierce it through a few fresh cranberries to garnish holiday beverages. Even a simple glass of sparkling water comes alive with this little red-green addition. You can experiment with nuts, dried fruits, and herbs, too. Remember, it's not just the taste that helps folks go vegan, it's how the food looks as well, so get creative and make it as pretty as can be.

THE COLORS I can't emphasize this point enough: the more colors the better! Not just for beauty, but for good health. Many of the most colorful fruits and veggies are packed with antioxidants, with each color providing its own type. You see, our bodies have pesky "free radicals"—sounds more like a rock band or protesters, I know—but they're actually rampaging oxygen molecules that are missing at least one electron, and they zip around trying to find electrons to fill the empty spots. These free radicals are created by all sorts of things: cigarette smoke, environmental pollutants, radiation, pesticides, and industrial solvents, to name a few. In their mad quest to grab another electron, these "hungry" oxygen molecules bump into our healthy cells, screwing up their DNA, proteins, and cell membranes, all of which can increase the likelihood of loads of health ailments, from coronary heart disease to prostate cancer.[1] Enter the amazing *antioxidants* to save the day! They safely interact with free radicals, and end the chain reaction before vital molecules are damaged.[2] Here are some scrumptious options if you're looking for good sources of antioxidants.

- **VEGGIES**: Kale, spinach, artichokes, russet potatoes (with skin), sweet potatoes (with skin), bell peppers, red cabbage, eggplant, and Brussels sprouts
- **FRUITS**: Pomegranate, cranberries, blueberries, blackberries, raspberries, grapes, pears, olives, and citrus
- **GRAINS**: Millet, oats, and barley
- **LEGUMES**: Pinto beans, red beans, black beans, and kidney beans
- **NUTS**: Walnuts, hazelnuts, and pecans
- **GREEN TEA**
- **DARK CHOCOLATE**

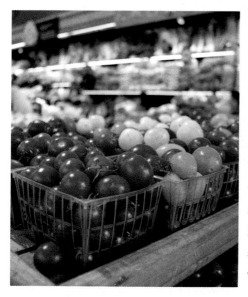

You should eat a variety of as many fruits, veggies, beans, nuts, legumes, and seeds as you possibly can to get the most nutrition possible.[3] Our bodies need a lot more than just antioxidants. Let your plate be a rainbow of beautiful fresh food; it will help ensure you reach the *real* pot of gold: good health! Select at least two or three fruits and veggies you enjoy from each section below, and jot them down in your journal so they're handy the next time you shop. Boring brown and white meals, be gone! Healthy, vibrant, vegan food, get inside that belly!

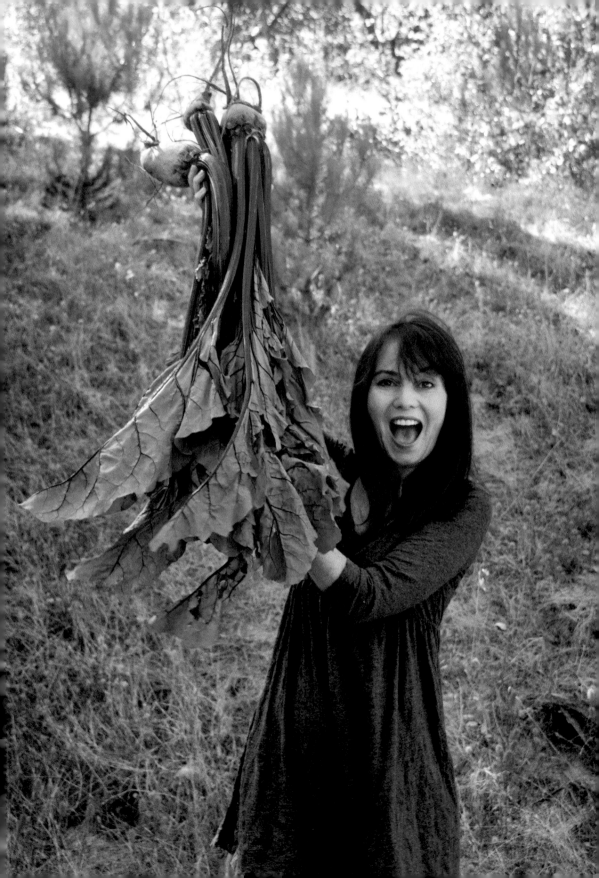

GREEN VEGGIES

Kale	Arugula	Zucchini
Swiss Chard	Sprouts	Broccoli
Collard Greens	Brussels Sprouts	Snow Peas
Lettuce	Green Beans	Sugar Snap Peas
Spinach	Asparagus	Celery
Mustard Greens	Artichokes	
Dandelion Greens	Green Cabbage	

GREEN FRUIT

| Avocados | Green Grapes | Green Pears |
| Green Apples | Kiwi | Limes |

RED VEGGIES

| Beets | Hot Peppers | Rhubarb |
| Red Bell Peppers | Radishes | Red Potatoes |

RED FRUIT

Tomatoes	Strawberries	Red Grapes
Pomegranate	Raspberries	Watermelon
Cherries	Cranberries	

ORANGE VEGGIES

| Orange Bell Peppers | Sweet Potatoes | Pumpkin |
| Carrots | Yams | |

ORANGE FRUIT

| Oranges | Nectarines | Apricots |
| Persimmons | Tangerines | |

YELLOW VEGGIES

Golden Beets	Yellow Winter Squash	Acorn Squash
Yellow Squash	Spaghetti Squash	Delicata Squash
Corn	Butternut Squash	Yellow Carrots

YELLOW FRUIT

| Mangoes | Yellow Peaches | Grapefruit |
| Pineapple | Yellow Tomatoes | |

PURPLE VEGGIES

Red Cabbage	Purple Carrots	Purple Asparagus
Purple Potatoes	Eggplant	Purple Peppers

PURPLE FRUIT

Blueberries	Concord Grapes	Purple Figs
Blackberries	Plums	

WHITE/TAN/BROWN VEGGIES

Turnips	Parsnips	White Carrots
Cauliflower	Mushrooms	
White Potatoes	Jicama	

WHITE/TAN/BROWN FRUITS

Dates	Bosc Pears
Bananas	White Peaches

Speaking of colors, here's a few nifty ideas if you'd like to create them naturally. Nature provides all the hues you'll ever need.

RED

◦ **BEETS**: Beets are one of my favorite ingredients to add to soups and stews. I buy them at the farmers' market, chop them into cubes and toss them into the pot along with the other veggies and liquid. By the time the soup is done, it is rich with color, ranging from an orange red to a deep magenta, depending on the other ingredients added. And they taste good, too! You can also save the beet juice that's left after baking them if you have a sweet treat that you'd like to color pink.

◦ **BERRIES AND CHERRIES**: If you're making something sweet, you can easily color your food with the juice of smashed berries or Bing cherries, too.

YELLOW

◦ **TURMERIC**: As I mentioned with the scrambles, turmeric adds a beautiful yellow color to food. It's so healthy, too! I use it a lot! Just a shake or two produces a nice hue, without overpowering the meal with a turmeric flavor. If you're making Indian food, though, be more generous. Vegan curries rock!

〜 **PURPLE CABBAGE**: Just submerge and boil a quarter head of chopped purple cabbage in a small pot. Once the water is deep purple, turn off the heat. (This usually takes about 10 minutes.) Remove ¼ cup of the purple water, and place it in a small dish. Add a scant ½ teaspoon of baking soda, and voila! Blue! All thanks to purple cabbage juice being a great pH indicator. If you add a base to it, like baking soda, it turns blue, but if you add an acid, such as lemon juice, it will turn pink. I love science!

Want more? For other cool combos that you can make at home, check out the entertaining little YouTube video "How to Make Natural Food Coloring—Concentrated Color Recipe."[4] It's cute! Or look for Color Garden pure natural food colors at the grocery store. They're 100 percent plant-based with no preservatives and GMO-free, too! They're not as bright as some artificial colors, but I'll take muted natural colors over the crazy chemical ones any day! Check out Colorgarden.net

2. *Now, it's time to start thinking about an entire weeks' worth of beautiful vegan meals.* See if you can avoid the last-minute frenzy of figuring out what you're going to eat when you're already ravenously hungry, and instead plan out a weeks' worth of food in advance. You won't always have the luxury of doing this, but if you can give a little forethought to your meals as often as possible, it should relieve a bit of "newbie vegan" stress.

On the next page is a sample of vegan meals for a week to help you on your way and, although this isn't a cookbook, I'm tossing in a few more recipes, too. Just remember, these are primarily for inspiration so you can see what a nice variety of food vegans eat. I'm hoping you'll try making one or two of them (especially the krautfleckerl!), but there's no need to make them all, and certainly not within a single week. That would be nutty! Try to keep things **as simple as possible** as you transition to becoming vegan. Even if you just figure out a way to make a yummy vegan smoothie you enjoy, and "veganize" a few of your favorite meals, that's a *huge* victory! You've got this, kind one.

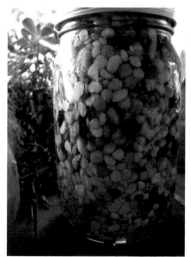

MONDAY

BREAKFAST: Bagel with avocado, tomato, onion

LUNCH: **Homemade Collard Rolls** (page 172)

DINNER: **Easy Tofu Veggie Stir-Fry** (see page 160) with brown rice and spinach salad

TUESDAY

BREAKFAST: Silk, Kite Hill, or Daiya vegan yogurt with fresh berries

LUNCH: Bean and Rice Burrito or Easy Black Bean Tacos (see **Tacos** page 173) with chips and guacamole.

DINNER: **Sweet Potato Split Pea Soup** (page 117) and salad

WEDNESDAY

BREAKFAST: Blueberry banana flaxseed smoothie (see **My Vegan Smoothie**, page 134)

LUNCH: **No Tuna–Salad Sandwich** (page 99) with celery and carrot sticks

DINNER: **Stovetop Ratatouille** (page 161) with salad and fresh bread

THURSDAY

BREAKFAST: **My Vegan Breakfast Scramble** (page 88) with hash browns, Sweet Earth Foods Benevolent Bacon, and a sliced orange

LUNCH: Avocado and Tofurky sandwich, whole grain chips, and an apple

DINNER: Grilled portobello mushroom burgers, or **Black Bean–Beet Burgers** (page 162) with corn on the cob and a salad

FRIDAY

BREAKFAST: **My Overnight Oats** (page 135) with fresh blueberries, maple syrup, and almond milk

LUNCH: Peanut Butter and Jelly sandwich with fresh fruit

DINNER: **Harvest Bowls** (see sidebar page 255) or **Farmers' Market Soup** (page 164)

SATURDAY

BREAKFAST: **Easy Peasy Pancakes** (page 158) with fresh fruit and Field Roast Grain Meat Breakfast Sausages

LUNCH: **Eggplant Hummus Veggie Burger Wrap** (page 168)

DINNER: **Seitan Veggie Kabobs** (page 160), spinach salad, and wild rice

SUNDAY

BREAKFAST: **Sweet Sunday French Crepes** (page 170)

LUNCH: **Eggplant Seitan Chili** (page 157) and fresh bread

DINNER: **Krautfleckerl** (page 159), roasted veggies, and a spinach salad

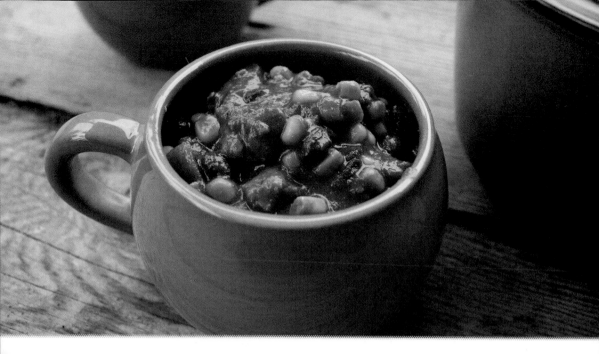

Eggplant Seitan Chili

SERVES 4 TO 6

Oil, for the pot (I like to use cold-pressed olive oil, but any will do)

½ onion, chopped

1½ teaspoons minced garlic

1 teaspoon salt

1 to 2 teaspoons chili powder

Freshly ground black pepper, to taste

1 cup grilled homemade or store-bought seitan pieces (about the size of nickles)

½ large unpeeled eggplant, chopped into small cubes (about 2 cups)

Two 15-ounce cans black beans, rinsed and drained

One 15-ounce can whole kernel corn, rinsed and drained

One 15-ounce can tomato sauce

1 cup water

1. Lightly film the bottom of a large pot with oil.

2. Add the chopped onions and garlic and sauté for 3 to 5 minutes on medium heat, stirring occasionally to prevent sticking, until the onions are translucent.

3. Add the pieces of seitan and sauté for a few minutes more until brown.

4. Add the eggplant, black beans, corn kernels, tomato sauce, and water and cook on medium heat for 15 minutes.

5. Reduce the heat to low and continue to cook for another 15 to 20, stirring occasionally. The longer you cook the chili, the softer and more flavorful the eggplant will become. This dish is especially good the next day, *if* you have leftovers.

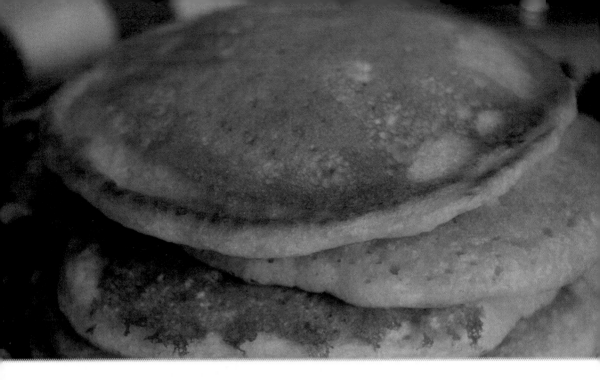

Easy Peasy Pancakes

SERVES 2

1 cup unbleached all-purpose flour

1 tablespoon brown sugar

1 tablespoon baking powder

⅛ teaspoon salt

1¼ cups almond milk (or any non-dairy milk of your choice)

1 teaspoon pure vanilla extract

1 tablespoon vegetable or coconut oil

1. In a bowl, mix together all the dry ingredients.

2. Add the liquid ingredients and mix the batter with a spoon until most of the large lumps are gone. You won't get all the lumps out, just try to at least smash the big ones with the back of the spoon.

3. Lightly coat a large pan or griddle with oil and set on medium heat. (Oil is not necessary if using a nonstick pan, but is suggested to help the edges of the pancake turn a nice golden brown.)

4. Using a ladle, scoop ¼ to ½ cup of the batter per pancake into the hot pan. When you see lots of bubbles forming on the top of the pancake, flip and cook on the opposite side.

5. Keep making pancakes until you've used up all the batter. Serve hot with jam and powdered sugar or vegan butter and maple syrup or even berries or chopped fresh fruit on top. Use your imagination, and enjoy!

Krautfleckerl

SERVES 2 TO 4

1 large head green cabbage

3 tablespoons vegetable or olive oil, or more as needed

One 16-ounce package vegan bow-tie pasta, or eggless ribbon pasta (see Note)

1 teaspoon freshly ground black pepper, plus more as needed

Bragg's Liquid Aminos, for serving

1. Cut the head of cabbage into quarters and remove the core. Cut the quarters into square pieces about the size of 50-cent pieces.

2. Warm the oil in a large pot on low heat.

3. Add the cabbage to the pot and season with the pepper.

4. Cook on low, stirring occasionally, until the cabbage cooks down, softens, and is browned. This should take approximately 1 hour.

5. Once the cabbage is cooked, turn off the heat, and set aside.

6. Bring a large pot of water to a boil, and add the pasta. Cook according to the package directions. Drain well, add to the pot with the cooked cabbage and mix to combine.

7. To serve, pass the pepper mill at the table, and encourage your guests to add Bragg's Liquid Aminos to taste; this is *essential* as the salty taste enhances the sweet taste in the cabbage.

NOTE: This dish may not sound fancy or flavorful, but everyone, and I mean *everyone*, I've ever made it for, has loved it! It's well worth the investment of time to cook down that cabbage. If you're worried it will taste like sauerkraut—it doesn't, the cabbage becomes sweet. I could eat Krautfleckerl every day! My mother used to make Krautfleckerl with homemade pasta. She would roll the dough out flat, and then cut it into square pieces, which is how it's traditionally done. I don't make noodles from scratch, so I've found that bow-tie pasta works best for me, but if you enjoy making your own pasta, this is a great dish to use it in. Just serve it up with a vibrant side salad, or anything else you enjoy, and BAM. Tummy satisfaction!

Seitan Veggie Kabobs

AS MANY SKEWERS AS YOU WANT

Grilled seitan pieces (see Simple Seitan recipe page 112)

Colorful veggies, cut into chunks (bell peppers, mushrooms, zucchini, and tomatoes, or whatever is in season)

Bamboo or metal skewers

1. If using skewers other than bamboo, soak in water first for 30 minutes so they are less likely to catch fire on the grill.

2. Carefully pierce the veggies onto the skewer, alternating the colors and placing a grilled seitan piece between every 3 to 4 veggies. Use softer veggies, as it's difficult (and can be dangerous) to pierce a hard piece of carrot, beet, parsnip, etc. There's plenty of softer veggies to make this dish super easy to make.

3. Place the skewers on the grill, turning them over every few minutes so they get nice grill lines, which should take 5 to 10 minutes. You'll know when they're done!

Easy Tofu Veggie Stir-Fry

SERVES 4

½ package of tofu chopped into cubes

3 to 4 cups chopped vegetables

2 teaspoons chopped garlic

1 teaspoon ginger (chopped fresh, or powder)

3 tablespoons tamari

2 teaspoons toasted sesame seed oil

2 teaspoons Sriracha

2 teaspoons sesame seeds (black or white)

1 tablespoon maple syrup, or sweetener of choice

Cracked pepper to taste

1. Coat large pan or wok lightly with oil and set to medium-high heat.

2. Add chopped tofu, garlic, and 2 tablespoons of tamari, and sauté for 5 minutes. Flip tofu pieces occasionally so they don't stick to the pan.

3. Add any firm veggies that you're using, i.e. carrots, celery, etc., Sriracha, sesame oil, ginger, and sesame oil. Sauté and flip pieces occasionally for 5 minutes.

4. Add any softer veggies, such as zucchini, bell peppers, etc. and the remaining 1 tablespoon tamari, sweetener, and cracked pepper. Sauté and flip pieces occasionally for 5 minutes.

5. Add any very soft, quick cooking veggies (mushrooms, spinach, etc.), and cook for one to two minutes.

6. Remove from heat, and serve on a bed of rice with condiments of choice. Yum!

Stovetop Ratatouille

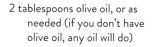

SERVES 4 TO 6

2 tablespoons olive oil, or as needed (if you don't have olive oil, any oil will do)

½ red or white onion, chopped

3 large garlic cloves, chopped (or 2 tablespoons garlic powder)

1 large unpeeled eggplant, cut into 1 to 1 ½ inch cubes

½ cup water

One 28-ounce can chopped tomatoes with juice

1 large bell pepper (any color), seeded and chopped

2 large zucchini or 3 small zucchini, sliced into ½-inch-thick pieces

1 cup chopped mushrooms

2 teaspoons sea salt (you can add less if your canned tomatoes are salted)

1 to 1½ teaspoons freshly ground black pepper

2 tablespoons Italian Seasoning (or a combo of dried basil, oregano, and thyme)

1. Lightly film the bottom of a large pot with oil and set on low heat.

2. Add the chopped onion and cook, stirring every minute or so, until slightly translucent and golden brown. This should take about 5 minutes and will bring out sweetness in the onion.

3. Add the water and tomatoes with their juice. Stir until incorporated.

4. Add the eggplant, garlic, bell peppers, zucchini, and mushrooms.

5. Season with the sea salt, black pepper, and Italian Seasoning. Mix gently to combine; the pot will be full.

6. Cook on low to medium heat for 45 minutes to 1 hour, stirring every 7 to 10 minutes. The mixture will slowly cook down and become stewlike.

7. Taste and adjust the seasonings, and add more water if needed. We're all different, you know!

8. Serve yourself a nice bowl of the ratatouille and relax with all the goodness of a colorful and tasty home-cooked meal. Just don't burn your tongue. After an hour on the stovetop, this rustic vegetable stew is *hot*!

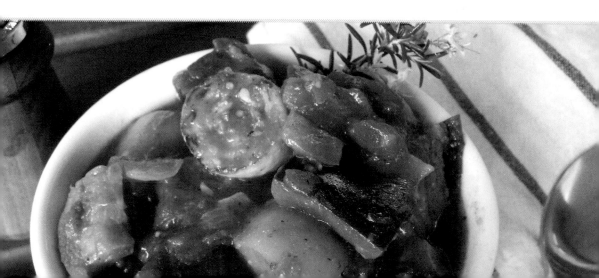

Black Bean–Beet Burgers

SERVES 2 TO 3

I encourage you to adapt this recipe to taste. Just start off with the black beans and go from there. Rice, mashed sweet potatoes, chopped nuts, quinoa, mushrooms, or spring onions are nice additions, too. Remember, a plant-based diet is one of abundance, so toss in all the flavors and textures you love! This is just *one* way to make a delicious bean burger.

½ cup boiled or baked beets (equal to about 1 small beet or half of a large beet)

One 15-ounce can black beans, rinsed and drained

⅓ cup bread crumbs (I use Trader Joe's Organic Bread Crumbs)

1 teaspoon sea salt

1 teaspoon crushed garlic (garlic powder works, too!)

½ teaspoon freshly ground black pepper

1 teaspoon favorite seasoning mix (I use Organic No Salt Seasoning, a mix of 21 organic spices, from Costco, but any will do)

Pinch of cayenne pepper (optional)

Oil, for the griddle or pan (olive or coconut oil works well)

1. Chop the beets into small pieces about the size of the black beans. Beets are softer once cooked. You can boil the beet pieces for 15 to 20 minutes, or bake a small beet in a toaster oven at 375°F for about 45 minutes; less if it's already chopped up. As the beet is cooking, you can move on to the next step.

2. Place the rinsed and drained black beans in a large bowl.

3. Add the bread crumbs, salt, garlic, black pepper, and seasoning mix of choice, and the cayenne if using.

4. Smash the mixture together with the back of your fork. You can use a potato masher if you prefer. It's OK if you still see a few whole beans; they don't all have to be completely smashed.

5. Add the chopped cooked beet pieces (without any liquid) to the bean mixture and continue smashing until it has a pasty texture with a reddish-pink color, and the beets are completely incorporated into the bean mixture. Again, small visible chunks are OK. (Reserve any vibrant beet juice to use later for soup stock or for color. It's too pretty and healthy to waste!)

6. Form the mixture into patties; you'll have enough to make 2 to 3 patties, or 8 to 12 small croquettes.

7. Lightly oil a stovetop grill or pan and place on medium heat. Add the patties to the pan and cook as you would

veggie burgers, but be gentle and patient when flipping them; bean burgers are softer and more fragile than most store-bought veggie burgers.

8. When browned and somewhat crispy, serve on a bun with your favorite condiments, or enjoy alone with yummy sides.

NOTE: Need ideas for vegan buns? Check out buns made by Bimbo (pronounced beembo) Bakeries USA and Nature's Own. The mono- and diglycerides in their products are derived from vegetable sources. (Hurray!) Just be sure to read the ingredients on the package, as some of their products aren't vegan. Pretzilla buns (soft pretzel buns) are vegan. They are a little bit pricey, but so good! There's Dave's Killer Bread Million Dollar Bun. And Trader Joe's sells Multigrain Slims—a round sandwich bread—that will do the trick. Or hey, just skip the bun and eat more homemade sides; they'll likely be healthier. That's what I usually do!

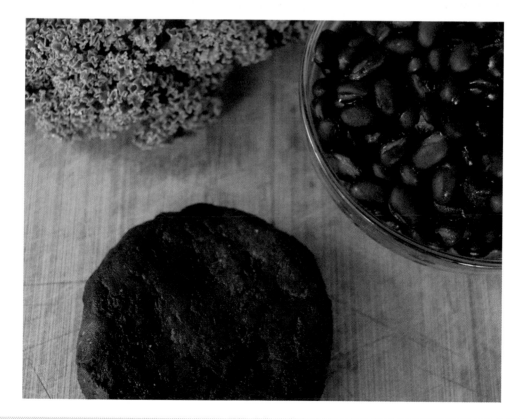

Farmers' Market Soup

SERVES 6

As I mentioned earlier, my local farmers' market is held on Saturday mornings, and I look forward to it all week. The only problem is that I often have veggies left over on Thursday or Friday that need to be eaten quickly to make room for all the fresh produce I will buy on the weekend. My solution? I make a big pot of soup! The recipe changes slightly each time depending on what I have in the fridge; variety is the spice of life, you know! So here's the template. All you have to do is adjust it to what you have handy, and you'll be good to go.

Oil, for the pot

1 chopped onion

2 teaspoons crushed or freshly chopped garlic

2 teaspoons spice mix (I use Kirkland's Organic No Salt Seasoning, a mix of 21 organic spices, from Costco, but Mrs. Dash and others work well, too)

Freshly ground black pepper

7 cups water

1 cup grain or legume of choice (rice, lentils, quinoa, etc.)

1 teaspoon sriracha sauce

1 chopped beet

4 to 5 cups chopped veggies of your choice (I always include a potato or sweet potato for texture)

⅛ cup tamari or Bragg's Liquid Aminos

1 teaspoon sea salt (optional)

1. Lightly film the bottom of a large soup pot with oil. Add chopped onion and cook on low heat until slightly translucent and the edges are lightly golden.

2. Add the garlic, spice mix, and black pepper to taste. Cook just until fragrant.

3. Add the water and bring to a boil. Add the grain or legumes of choice and reduce to a simmer.

4. Add the sriracha sauce, chopped beet, and other chopped veggies, making sure to leave *at least* 1 inch of space from top of pot so the soup has room to simmer without overflowing. Remember to add a chopped potato or sweet potato if you have one handy.

5. Season with the tamari or Bragg's Liquid Aminos; you may need more than ⅛ cup depending on your taste buds. If so, just don't add too much all at once as it will get too salty *fast*. Just add it little by little, sample it, and stop when it tastes good to you! Add sea salt to taste if you wish, but it probably won't be necessary. As your veggies cook, the soup will become more flavorful on its own.

6. Simmer the soup for 1 hour, stirring every 10 minutes or so. As the potato or sweet potato softens, gently smash the pieces against the side of the pot with a wooden spoon. This will give the soup a denser texture.

Depending on the type of veggies you used, your soup should be done in 60 to 90 minutes.

7. Enjoy your supercolorful and flavorful soup! And feel good knowing that you didn't let those nutritious veggies go to waste. And now there's room in your fridge for another fresh haul of produce from the farmers' market!

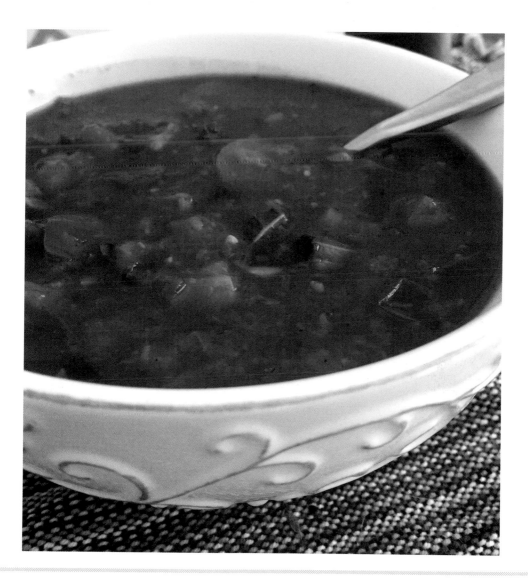

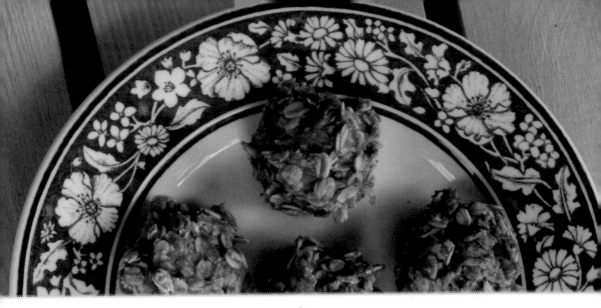

Healthy Snack-Attack Cookies

MAKES 8 TO 10 COOKIES

These are perfect when you just need a little something sweet to enjoy while you're watching a movie or working on the computer, or need a healthy snack to tide you over until dinner. You can pop them in a bag for an easy hiking snack, too. There's *no* added oil, and *no* added sugar, and you can make 'em in your toaster oven. Ready for some easy directions? OK!

1 large ripe banana

1 cup old-fashioned rolled oats

2 tablespoons nut butter (peanut butter or almond butter work great)

¼ teaspoon pure vanilla extract

¼ teaspoon ground cinnamon or pumpkin pie spice mix

Pinch of sea salt (optional)

1. Preheat a toaster oven to 350°F.

2. Break up the banana into pieces and place them in a bowl. Smash gently with a fork.

3. Toss in all of the remaining ingredients and mash with your fork until you have a sticky, well-blended mixture. (Feel free to add other items you enjoy, i.e., raisins, dried cranberries, chopped dates, chia seeds, chopped nuts, etc. The more, the merrier!)

4. Form the mixture into 8 to 10 balls, flatten slightly, and place on parchment paper–lined baking sheet.

5. Bake 15 to 20 minutes in your toaster oven. (A regular oven works fine, too!) They'll be fairly firm, and lightly browned when done. OK, that's it! It's SO easy to be vegan!

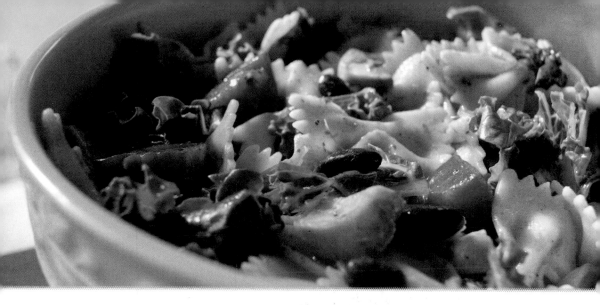

Kale, Avocado, and Bean Pasta Salad

MAKES 4 SIDE SALADS

This is a flavorful, inexpensive pasta salad that's perfect for summertime picnics!

One 16-ounce package vegan bow-tie pasta

½ bunch curly leaf kale, tough stems removed, leaves chopped into bite-size pieces

1 large tomato, chopped

1 avocado, pitted, peeled, and chopped

One 15-ounce can beans, rinsed and drained (I think kidney beans look pretty in this salad, but any type of beans will do)

1 recipe My Dressing (page 139)

1. In a large pot of boiling water, cook the pasta just until *al dente* (no one likes overcooked, mushy pasta salad). Turn off the heat, and just before you strain the pasta, toss the fresh kale into the pot and mix in. Once all of the kale pieces have been submerged, drain the pasta and kale. Don't let the kale sit in the pot more than a minute; you want it to stay vibrant. Rinse with cold water and drain again. Transfer to a large bowl.

2. Add the tomato, avocado, and beans to the pasta and kale and mix gently. Add the dressing to taste, and gently mix to coat.

3. Transfer the salad to the refrigerator and chill thoroughly.

4. Just before serving remix gently, serve, and chow down.

Eggplant Hummus Veggie Burger Wrap

SERVES 1

If you have a veggie burger you like, here's another way to enjoy it. The last time I made this wrap I used a Trader Joe's Masala Burger (it's packed with veggies and Indian spices) and it was perfect, but any vegan burger you enjoy will work. Use whatever suits your fancy!

1 large piece lavash (Middle Eastern flat bread)

1 scoop eggplant hummus (homemade or store-bought)

Oil, for the frying pan

1 vegan burger of choice

1 handful shredded veggies (you can grate your own, or use Trader Joe's shredded broccoli and carrot mix)

Sriracha sauce (optional)

1. Lay out a sheet of lavash on a board or clean work surface. (Trader Joe's has vegan lavash made with stone-ground whole wheat flour, but it's easy to find elsewhere, as well, especially at international grocery stores)

2. Spread the lavash with the eggplant hummus (or any hummus of choice)

3. Lightly oil a frying pan. Add the veggie burger and cook, breaking it into small pieces with the spatula, as it gets warm.

4. Stir in the grated veggies and cook, stirring occasionally, until warm. Once everything is warm (not hot) remove from heat and spread the mixture across the hummus-covered lavash bread. If there's any other spices or dressings you enjoy (like sriracha sauce!), now is the time to add those little yummies.

5. Roll up the lavash, slice the wrap in half, and enjoy!

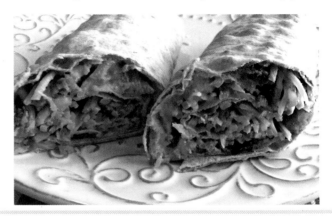

Three Sisters Chili

SERVES 4 TO 6

This recipe was inspired by the brilliant crop-growing strategy of Native Americans who planted beans, corn, and squash together because they were so beneficial to one another. The corn provides the structure for the beans to grow (no need for poles), the beans provide nitrogen for the soil, and the big squash leaves create shade, which helps prevent weeds from growing. Harmony and cooperation in the garden: I love it!

2 tablespoons oil

1 onion, chopped

1 teaspoon crushed or chopped fresh garlic

2 medium to large zucchinis, sliced and quartered (2 to 3 cups)

1 cup chopped mushrooms (5 or 6 mushrooms)

1 teaspoon sea salt

½ teaspoon freshly ground black pepper

1 teaspoon ground cumin

1 teaspoon cayenne pepper

One 15-ounce can kidney beans

One 15-ounce can black beans

One 15-ounce can corn kernels

One 15-ounce can tomato sauce

One 15-ounce can diced tomatoes

½ cup water

1. Lightly film the bottom of a large pot with oil. Add the onion and sauté on low to medium heat until the onion becomes slightly translucent and golden brown on the edges. Add the garlic and cook until fragrant.

2. Add the chopped zuchinni and mushrooms. Season with the salt, black pepper, cumin, and cayenne. (If you like your chili extra mild, start with a smaller amount of cayenne and work your way up. One teaspoon of cayenne will give this chili "medium" heat. At least to my taste buds!)

3. Add all of the canned ingredients. Stir in the water and simmer on low heat for 45 minutes to 1 hour, stirring every 10 minutes or as needed to make sure nothing sticks to the bottom of pot.

4. Taste to see if it's as spicy as you like your chili—if not, adjust as needed. Enjoy!

Sweet Sunday French Crepes

MAKES 4 TO 6 SMALL CREPES

Oooh, la laaah, these are so good! I created this recipe with the novice crepe maker in mind, so they're a tiny bit thicker, and slightly smaller than traditional French crepes, making them easier to flip. If making crepes is old hat for you, feel free to add a bit more nut milk to make them thinner. And don't fret if the first one doesn't turn out perfect. It's called the "chef eats first" rule: gobble it up, and move on to the second! Nom, nom, nom.

Be sure to read through the directions before beginning to make these, so you're not caught off guard by the "wait" time.

1 cup unbleached all-purpose flour

2 teaspoons sugar

1⅛ cups almond milk

¼ cup fresh orange juice

¼ teaspoon sea salt

1 tablespoon aquafaba

1 teaspoon pure vanilla extract

Oil or vegan butter, for the pan

Warm jam or fresh berries, for the filling

Melted vegan chocolate chips and powdered sugar, for topping (optional)

1. In a large nonreactive bowl, mix together the flour, sugar, milk, orange juice, salt, aquafaba, and vanilla. Try to get out as many lumps as possible. Now here's the hard part: let the batter sit for at least 15 minutes. The reason this is necessary is so that the liquid permeates into any remaining lumps of flour. No one wants lumpy crepes.

2. Once the batter has "rested" for 15 minutes, give it another mix, and heat up a little bit of oil or vegan butter in a 12-inch nonstick pan on medium heat.

3. Gently add about ⅓ to ½ cup of the batter to the center of pan, then lift, tilt, and rotate pan immediately to create a thin, even circle of batter. It's good to leave about an inch or so of space around the crepe so you'll be able to get a spatula underneath to flip it.

4. Once the crepe has a few bubbles, and is lightly golden on the edges, gently move around the crepe with the spatula. Once loose enough around the entire circle, gently flip it to the opposite side. The second side will likely only need about a minute or less to cook.

5. Gently lift the crepe out of the pan and place on a plate. (If your plates are cold, I recommend placing them in the oven on "warm" before you begin so your crepes stay

warm as you make more. Just make sure they're oven-safe plates and that the oven is at the lowest setting.)

6. Continue making crepes in the same manner until you use up the batter.

7. To serve, spread warm jam on the crepes, and then roll up. Or fill each crepe with fresh berries, and fold. Drizzle the crepes with melted vegan chocolate chips (Trader Joe's has vegan dark chocolate chips) and/or dust with powdered sugar if desired. Bon vegan appétit!

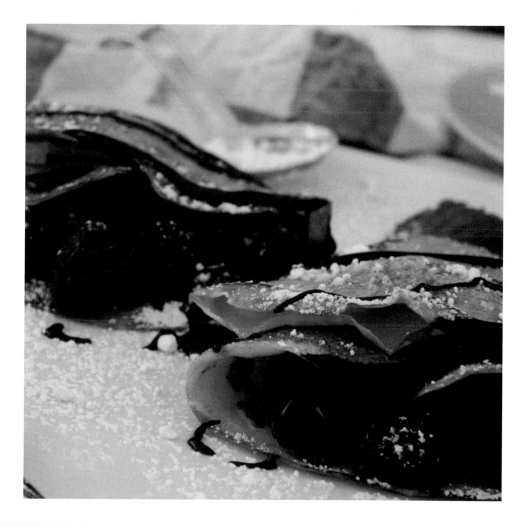

Homemade Collard Rolls

SERVES 1

These are super healthy, and fun to make when you find particularly large-leafed collard greens at the farmers' market!

1 to 2 collard leaves

1 scoop hummus of choice

A variety of colored vegetables, cut into long strips

Fresh herbs or sprouts

1. Cut the stem off of one very large collard leaf, or off of two smaller ones. You'll still notice that the white stalk goes into the leaf, so you'll either need to cut it out (without going too far into the leaf), or carefully shave it down with a small knife so that it's flat. If you don't, it will break when you roll it up later.

2. Blanch the leaf/leaves in a pan of hot water for 30 to 45 seconds. We're not really cooking them; we're just making them more pliable so they are easier to roll.

3. Lay the leaf flat on a work surface (or two leaves, slightly overlapping if they're small), and spread with the hummus.

4. Add the strips of vegetables, keeping in mind that when you cut the collard roll in half, you'll want it to show all the pretty colors, so think strategically as you're placing them.

5. Add any fresh herbs or sprouts you enjoy.

6. Carefully roll up collard leaf/leaves like you would a burrito, tucking in the ends on the sides, then slice the roll in half. If it is not holding together, insert a toothpick. Serve with your favorite dipping sauce, or hot sauce, and chow down!

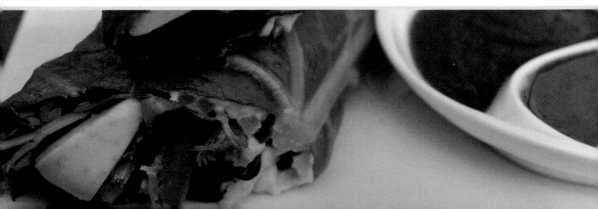

Need *more*? Here are a few more fast and easy meals you can whip up in a snap: Tacos, Pizza, and Zucchini Noodle Salad.

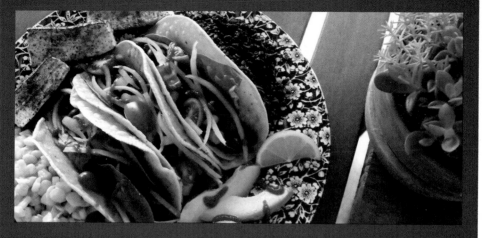

TACOS

Making vegan tacos couldn't be easier. In lieu of meat, just use beans, lentils, or vegan beefless crumbles from the store. Or you can even use jackfruit. (Did you know jackfruit is the largest tree-born fruit in the world? One fruit can weigh 100 lbs!)

I like using black beans as a taco filling, along with avocado, a squirt of sriracha, and all the traditional fixings. If you want to make them *extra* healthy, substitute a little shredded carrots for the vegan cheese.

PIZZA

Sure, you can make your own dough and sauce, which I do once in a blue moon, but did you know you can buy vegan pizza dough already made in the bag at Trader Joe's and Whole Foods Market? That's probably the easiest option for you as you're transitioning to becoming vegan. And you can snag vegan pizza sauce at mainstream supermarkets, too. Then all you have to do is just slather it with vegan cheese and all the grilled veggies you enjoy. Or you can do what I do: grill mushrooms, pineapples, and onions for the topping, skip the packaged cheese, and sprinkle homemade Parmesan cheese on top instead. The recipe on the next page is an easy-peasy vegan cheese recipe.

Vegan Parmesan Cheese

MAKES ABOUT 1 CUP

½ cup cashews

½ cup nutritional yeast

¼ teaspoon sea salt

1. Put the cashews, nutritional yeast, and sea salt in the bowl of a food processor and blend until it has the consistency of Parmesan cheese. The ratio of nuts to nutritional yeast is simply 1:1, so you can make more, or less, super easily!

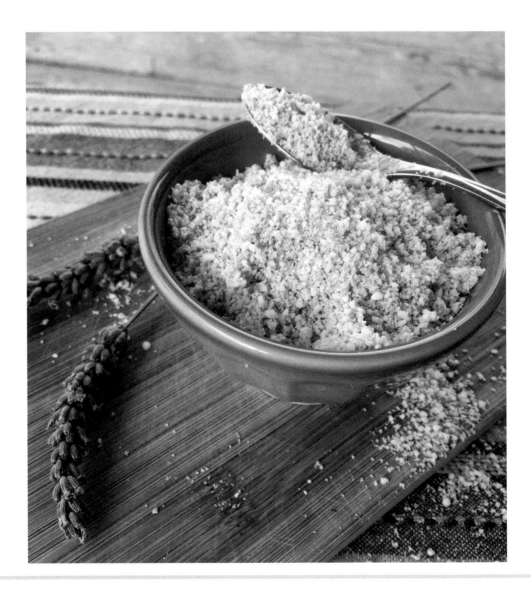

Zucchini Noodles with Citrus Peanut Sauce

SERVES 2

This quick-and-easy recipe calls for a spiralizer, which is a pretty nifty gadget for making salads. If you don't have one, you can easily use this sauce on rice noodles. The sauce might seem thick at first, but that's because zucchini noodles ooze lots of water, so not to worry—it becomes the right consistency once mixed.

1 large (or 2 medium) zucchini spiralized into noodles

1 handful chopped cherry tomatoes

SAUCE

¼ cup peanut butter

Juice of ½ lime

1 tablespoon tamari

2 tablespoons fresh orange juice

1 teaspoon fresh ginger, chopped

1 tablespoon maple syrup

¼ teaspoon crushed garlic (or garlic powder)

A few dashes black sesame seeds

1 teaspoon toasted sesame seed oil

Dash of red chili pepper or a squirt of sriracha sauce

1. In a small bowl, blend all the ingredients for the sauce with a spoon until creamy.

2. In a large bowl, gently mix the zucchini noodles and cherry tomatoes with the sauce. Serve.

NOTE: Short on time? Just pick up a bottle of Trader Joe's Asian Style Spicy Peanut Vinaigrette. It's super yum!

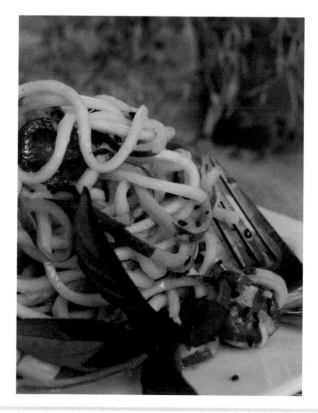

Checklist

- ☐ Did you create a beautiful meal that's colorful with a variety of shapes?

- ☐ Did you plan out what you're eating for the week ahead?

- ☐ Did you drink enough water today?

Thought FOR THE Day

"Every meal should be a small celebration."

—MARION CUNNINGHAM

DAY 11

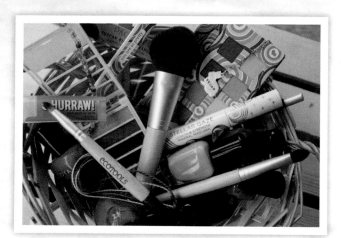

Because Bunnies DON'T HAVE Tear Ducts

GOAL FOR THE DAY: Go through your cosmetics and toiletries and separate what's vegan and what's not.

Bunnies don't have tear ducts. And researchers like the late United States FDA Toxicologist, Dr. Draize, think that's just fantastic. You see, if bunnies can't cry, you can restrain them in boxes, clamp their eyes wide open so they can't blink, and jam whatever the hell you want in there, and they can't do a damn thing about it. With no tears to cry out the chemicals, corrosive products will just sit there and burn—sometimes *for days*, without any pain relief—while folks in white coats take notes.[1] Can you imagine someone pouring shampoo into your eyes, and not being able to wash it out? There's also a skin version of the "Draize" test, too. Researchers shave the bunny's fur, rip off several layers of skin, and slather on whatever they want to test. Hair Removal Cream. Perfume. Nail Polish Remover. Soap. You name it. For over seventy years, researchers have been performing this gruesome experiment, documenting the ulcers and other injuries that develop, to allegedly ensure cosmetic items are "safe" for consumers to use. At the end of the Draize test, the animals are usually killed by asphyxiation, neck-breaking, or decapitation, without any pain relief, while others are subjected to more chemicals over and over again, until they meet the same sad fate.[2]

The crazy thing is, we already have over five thousand cosmetic ingredients that have been established as "safe" in the United States, and Europe has a list of over eleven thousand! We also have artificial human skin that's grown in labs, as well as test tube toxicology methods, that many believe give more accurate results when it comes to testing. Even the FDA, which *does NOT require animal testing on cosmetics*, states, "companies may rely on combinations of scientific literature, non-animal testing, raw material safety testing, or controlled human-use testing to substantiate their product safety."[3] The Draize test is so outdated and unnecessary that it's banned in all twenty-eight countries in the European Union, as well as India, Israel, New Zealand, and Norway, too. South Korea has a five-year plan to end cosmetic testing, with other countries poised to follow. And yet despite 73 percent of Americans supporting a ban on cosmetic testing, along with more than half stating that they think the *most important* packaging claims on cosmetics are: "no animal products" and "not tested on animals," the horrifically cruel and antiquated experiments continue on.[4]

An act to end cosmetic testing in the United States was introduced in Congress, but just as with the right to know what's in natural flavors, the law never came to be.[5] Another sound policy tossed in the trash, despite resounding public support. Your brain should be swirling with the questions, "Why?" While you're pondering, I'll go ahead and cue the O'Jay's "For the Love of Money."[6]

Whenever something involving the government doesn't make any sense, I just follow the money trail. Animals can't vote and they don't have any money to support campaigns. But those who line their coffers with profits from lab equipment sales and breeding animals sure can, and do. Experimenting on animals is a multibillion-dollar industry, with hundreds of thousands killed each year testing cosmetics alone. And if you're wondering how many rats and mice are killed, you'll just have to keep guessing. Just as birds are excluded from the Animal Welfare Act, the sweet little mice and rats are, too, which means no one has to keep a tab on how many are killed, or in which manner they do the grisly deed.[7]

So, if the government doesn't mandate testing cosmetics on animals, and companies still keep doing it despite the public's outrage, let's just stop buying their products, and switch over to cruelty-free cosmetics. Ready to use the power of our pocketbook and change the world? Let's do it!

1. *Open those cosmetic cases and bathroom cupboards and let's see what we can do to help the animals.* I told you I'd never skirt the truth, and I'd always let you know the facts, but most important, I'd never leave you hopeless. Here's what you need to do. On large sheets of paper, create a label for each of the following categories:

   A. Use Up and/or Give Away

   B. Not Tested on Animals

   C. Not Tested on Animals AND No Animal Ingredients (This is what we're aiming for, folks!)

Now place your labels on the floor. You're going to use them to organize the products you have. Just follow these steps:

STEP #1: See if the product is labeled VEGAN. If it is, you hit the jackpot! Ding, ding, ding!!! Straight to pile C it goes! If not, move to the next step.

STEP #2: Does it have a cruelty-free label on it? Look for a Leaping Bunny (blue and black), the PETA Bunny (pink and black), the words "cruelty-free," or the words "not tested on animals." If your cosmetics are from Australia, you also might see a black "Choose Cruelty-Free" logo. If you see any of those on your label, no animals were harmed in the making of the product as far as testing goes, so toss it in pile B. Keep in mind, though, it doesn't ensure that there are no animal ingredients in it. We'll get to that conundrum in just a second! No cruelty-free label? Move to the next step.

STEP #3: Is the company that manufacturers it on a well-respected, cruelty-free list?

Sometimes you can't tell if a product has been tested on animals just by looking at the label, since there's a chance it's not marked even if it is cruelty-free. If you didn't see the language or logo, look the company up on the following lists to see if they're cruelty-free: leapingbunny.org/guide/brands, and features.peta.org/cruelty-free-company-search, or http://www.choosecrueltyfree.org.au/cruelty-free-list-by-category if you buy products from Australia. All three have pocket-sized lists, too, that you can download. PETA has a pocket-sized one they will send you for free if you want to keep one in your wallet, and there's even an app for your phone as well. If it's on the list, great! Put it in pile B with the others. If you discover it's tested on animals, put it in pile A.

STEP #4: There's always a chance that it's not tested on animals despite being unmarked, *and* not being on any list. If you still can't determine if it's been tested on animals or not, call the manufacturer to find out. You can usually find their contact information on the product or on their website. If you send them an e-mail, it may take them a few days for them to get back to you. If you still need to do more investigative work, set the product aside by your computer or phone.

STEP #5: Now you need to figure out which products in pile B are actually vegan. Just because they don't test a cosmetic on animals doesn't mean it's not packed with animal by-products. Nail polish and eye shadows often contain fish scales, lipstick can contain crushed bugs, and lotion often contains grease from the wool of sheep. Of course, they don't actually list the names like that, or you'd never buy the stuff—sneaky little devils. Well, we're on to them! Evaluate your cosmetics and toiletries ingredients by perusing this list: peta.org/living/beauty/animal-ingredients-list, and then place in the appropriate pile. This is also an opportune time for me to remind you of something I've been telling you from the onset, and I bet you can guess what that is. You can never, ever, be a perfect vegan my warmhearted friends, so just do the best that you can!

2. *Learn how to replace your non-vegan products.* Hopefully a few of your favorites managed to make their way to victory pile C. But if you're finding you're now a little short on the goods, just know it's not difficult to find vegan cosmetics. So many companies are not only going vegan, they're darn proud of it. Look!

Wet *n* Wild	"We're proud to say we have never and will never test on animals. We also make it a point to work with cruelty-free, third-party vendors. Wet *n* Wild loves our furry, scaly, and feathery friends! While not all our products are 100% vegan, we are striving towards making them all vegan friendly."[8] You can find a complete list of their current vegan cosmetics under the FAQ section of their website: wetnwildbeauty.com
e.l.f. Cosmetics	"All ingredients used in e.l.f. cosmetics are vegan friendly, safe, and meet F.D.A. requirements. Ingredients are listed on our website as well as on the packaging of our products. We are proud to say that we do not test on animals or endorse such practices."[9]
Obsessive Compulsive Cosmetics	"In a time when many cosmetic companies make the claim that their products are "Cruelty-Free" simply because Animal Testing has become unfashionable and less cost-effective, OCC felt it was necessary to raise the bar on this issue. We pledge never to use animal-derived ingredients (including Lanolin, Beeswax, Carmine, and more) in our products and accessories. Beyond any personal convictions, we simply believe that it's unnecessary, especially when there are alternatives that are just as readily available, and equally effective in the formulation of our products."[10]

Isn't that awesome?

Once again, I'm trying to keep your budget in mind when it comes to suggestions as well as make things as easy to access as possible. It doesn't do much good if there's a nifty vegan mascara that's fifty bucks and only available in Malibu, right? So I've compiled a partial list of cosmetics that don't have any animal ingredients in them, and were not tested on animals. You should be able to find them at familiar places, like Target, Walmart, Ulta, Sephora, and Urban Outfitters. Buying vegan cosmetics has never been easier, my friends!

COSMETICS THAT ARE BOTH CRUELTY-FREE AND CONTAIN NO ANIMAL INGREDIENTS

FOUNDATION, CONCEALERS, AND TINTED MOISTURIZERS

bareMinerals Original Foundation Broad Spectrum SPF 15

e.l.f. Essentials Tone Correcting Concealer

Juice Beauty Correcting Concealer

Kat Von D Beauty Lock-It Foundation

NYX Concealer Wand

Pacifica Dreamy Cover Bare-Faced Serum Foundation SPF 20

Too Faced Absolutely Flawless Concealer

Too Faced Tinted Beauty Balm

Too Faced Born This Way Foundation

Urban Decay Naked Skin Weightless Ultra Definition Liquid Makeup

POWDERS

Juice Beauty PHYTO-PIGMENTS Flawless Pressed Powder

Physicians Formula Super BB All-in-1 Beautify Balm Powder

Too Faced Amazing Face SPF 15 Powder Foundation

Too Faced Primed & Poreless Powder

Pacifica Perfect Lotus Powder

Pacifica Golden Lotus Highlighting Powder

PRIMERS

Jordana Eye Primer

Juice Beauty PHYTO-PIGMENTS Illuminating Primer

SheaMoisture Cosmetics Primer

Too Faced Lip Insurance Lip Primer

Too Faced Primed & Poreless Primer

EYELINERS AND EYEBROW PENCILS

Anastasia Beverly Hills Brow Wiz

e.l.f. Eyeliners

Jordana Fabuliner Bold Felt-Tip Liquid Eyeliner

Juice Beauty Defining Eyeliner

Too Faced Cosmetics Metal Eyed Eyeliners (Blackout, Hand Cuffs, Twilight, Get Lucky, Plum Crazy, Brown Sugar, Dirt Bag, Shotgun)

NYX Auto Eyebrow Pencils

NYX Push-Up Bra for Your Eyebrow
NYX Super Fat Eye Marker
Physicians Formula Shimmer Strips Custom Eye Enhancing Eyeliner Trio
Too Faced Liquid Lava Eyeliner (vegan color: Lava Matte)
Too Faced Perfect Eyes Eyeliner
Urban Decay 24/7 Velvet Glide-On Eye Pencil

MASCARA

e.l.f. Studio Eye Enhancing Mascara
Ecco Bella Flowercolor Natural Mascara
Jordan Best Length Extreme Lengthening Mascara
Juice Beauty Lash Defining Mascara
LUSH Eyes Right Mascara
Milani Total Lash Cover Mascara
Pacifica Stellar Gaze Length & Strength Mineral Mascara
Pacifica Dream Big Lash Extending 7 in 1 Mascara
Tarte lights, camera, Lashes Double-Ended Lash Fibers & 4-in-1 Mascara
Two Faced Better Than Sex Mascara
Urban Decay Mascara Resurrection
Wet *n* Wild Mega Length Mascara
Wet *n* Wild MegaPlump Mascara
Wet *n* Wild MegaVolume Mascara

EYE SHADOW

Pacifica Shadow Palettes (all colors are vegan)
Runway Eyes Palette, by Milani (vegan colors: Designer Browns, Couture in
    Purples, and Backstage Basics are vegan)
e.l.f. Eye Shadow Palettes (all colors are vegan)
Too Faced Duo Eye Shadows (vegan colors: Ooh & Aah, Fantasy Island, Skinny
    Dip, Lucky Charms, Shamrock Chic, Rich Bitch)

BLUSH AND BRONZERS

100% Pure Fruit Pigmented Lip & Cheek Tint
e.l.f. Blushes and Bronzers (all are vegan)
Juice Beauty Glowing Cheek Color
Milani Bronzer
NYX Powder Blush (all 27 shades!)

Too Faced Full Bloom Powder (vegan colors: Sweet Pink, Coca Rose)

Two Faced Chocolate Soleil Matte Bronzer

Wet *n* Wild Mega Glo Illuminating Powder (all are vegan except for #345 and #347)

LIPSTICK, LIPGLOSS, AND LIP BALM

ButterLONDON LIPPY Liquid Lipstick

e.l.f. Lipsticks

Circa Color Absolute Velvet Luxe Lipstick

Gabriel Cosmetics ZuZu Luxe Lipstick

Juice Beauty Lip Colors

Kat Von D Beauty Studded Kiss Lipstick

Lime Crime Lipsticks and Glosses

LUSH Liquid Lipsticks

LUSH None of your Beeswax

NYX Cosmetics Xtreme Lip Cream and Butter Lipstick

Obsessive Compulsive Cosmetics Lip Tar

Pacifica Enlightened Gloss

Urban Decay Sheer Revolution Lipstick

FIGHT CLUB SOAP

Blah! Who want's *that*? Sadly, most soap contains animal fat disguised as the word "tallow" mixed with a bunch of other letters or words, i.e. "sodium tallowate." It's leftover fat from the slaughterhouse because, you know, nothing says "squeaky clean" like rubbing the fat of a dead animal all over you. Go figure. Vegan options include Kiss My Face and Dr. Bronner's, or if you prefer fancier suds, check out Trader Joe's Bisous de Provence Lavender Triple Milled Soap. Vegan shampoo and conditioner? No problem. Check out Trader Joe's Nourish Spa line, Whole Foods 365 Everyday Value line, Desert Essence, Pureology, Nature's Gate, and Avalon Organics—just to name a few. Or, if money is no object, LUSH sells a few indulgent vegan hair care products and soap with ingredients like cinnamon, cocoa, and nutmeg—they smell good enough to eat!

Valana Minerals Sparkie Lips Color Sticks

Wet *n* Wild Mega Slicks Lip Gloss (Colors 560A-578 are vegan, with the exception of 564A) and Wet n Wild Silk Finish Lipsticks

COSMETIC BRUSHES

100% Pure (all brushes are vegan)

e.l.f. (all brushes are vegan)

Eco-Tools Brushes (all brushes are vegan)

Juice Beauty (all brushes are vegan)

Too Faced Kabuki Brush

Too Faced Powder Pouf Brush

Too Faced Shadow Brushes

Wet *n* Wild (all brushes are vegan)

NAIL POLISH

100% Pure Nail Polish

Beauty Without Cruelty (BWC)

ButterLONDON

e.l.f.

TO WEAR OR GO BARE

You're beautiful without makeup. You're perfect when you wake up! And no, I'm not pulling an Amy Schumer boy band trick on you here (although admittedly, that song is now stuck in my head![11]) Going bare is a great option, especially when you want to let your skin breathe and create some Vitamin D (stay tuned for vegan sunscreens around the bend). You might also want to lighten up knowing that everything you put on your skin goes directly into your bloodstream; it's like eating through your pores. Just because it's vegan doesn't mean it's healthy. If you want more information, check out the Environmental Working Group's "Skin Deep" search engine (www.ewg.org/skindeep) where you can look up thousands of cosmetic products to see what toxins or carcinogens might be in that pretty lipstick of yours that you just swallowed while sipping your latte.

LVX

    Tish & Snooky's Manic Panic

    No Miss

    Pacifica

    Obsessive Compulsive Cosmetics

    Priti NYC

    SpaRitual Nail Lacquer Collection

    Wet *n* Wild MegaLast Nail Color (colors 201B-218 are vegan)

    Zoya

Need *more*? Mosey on over to LogicalHarmony.net and VeganBeautyReview.com. Both have long lists of vegan cosmetics that are updated as new products become available.

And a few ideas for the Dapper Man . . .

CRUELTY-FREE, VEGAN SHAVING SUPPLIES

The Body Shop Men's Synthetic Shaving Brush

Every Man Jack Premium Shave Brush

Jack Black Pure Performance Shave Brush

Aubrey Organics Aftershave

Kiss My Face Moisture Shave

Herban Cowboy Natural Grooming Shave Cream for Men

Herban Cowboy Natural Grooming After Shave Balm for Men

Crabtree & Evelyn Shave Cream

Bold For Men Dry Shave Gel

Bulldog Original Shave Gel

3. *Learn to avoid the slick tricks.* Watch out for companies that claim they don't test on animals but actually do pay for mandatory testing on their products that are sold in China. China doesn't require that "ordinary" cosmetics *made in their country* be tested on animals; that's why e.l.f. and Wet *n* Wild cosmetics are cruelty-free, despite being made in China. However, if an outside company wants to sell their cosmetics over there, they have to first test them on animals. Sounds crazy, I know. Some U.S. manufacturers, such as Paul Mitchell, have passed on the lucrative opportunity, assuring consumers they have no interest in selling in China. (Thank you, Paul Mitchell!) Whereas, Avon, Estee Lauder, MAC, Victoria's Secret, Stila

Cosmetics, Boscia, Benefit Cosmetics, Organix, and Revlon have all jumped off the beautiful cruelty-free ship, and have set sail to cash in with Chinese consumers— yet *another* reason why we need to join so many other countries in their decision to outlaw the testing of cosmetics on animals. Oh, how I long for the day someone reads this paragraph and says, "Wow, this book must be really old!"

ARE YOUR COSMETICS OLD?

If you bought a cosmetic a really long time ago, or it smells a little odd, you might want to toss it. Just like food, cosmetics expire, and no matter how much you treasure that last bit of color or scent, it's probably not wise to use it if it's past its prime. Look for an expiration date or a Period After Opening (PAO) date to help guide you.

CRUELTY-FREE HAIR

Looking for a cruelty-free hair salon? Check out the Paul Mitchell store locator search engine: PaulMitchell.com. Not only will it find the nearest Paul Mitchell Salon near you, it will also find other hair salons that carry Paul Mitchell products, too! Almost all of Paul Mitchell's products are vegan and none have been tested on animals. Another option is Aveda, a company that proudly proclaims they're "Changing the world, one snip at a time!" A few of their products contain beeswax and/or honey, but the vast majority are vegan, and they are not tested on animals: visit Aveda.com. Just want to goof around with color at home? LUSH Henna, Herbatint, Good Dye Young, and Tish & Snooky's Manic Panic have some vegan, cruelty-free hair colors to play with. Have fun!

Checklist

☐ Did you sort through your cosmetics and toiletries?

☐ Did you find vegan cosmetics to replace those that are tested on animals, or contain animal ingredients?

☐ Did you find any vegan soap, shampoos, or conditioners you'd like to try?

Thought FOR THE Day

"Dear intelligent people of the world, don't get shampoo in your eyes.

It really stings.

There. Done.

Now fucking stop torturing animals."

—Tweet by **RICKY GERVAIS**, actor and comedian

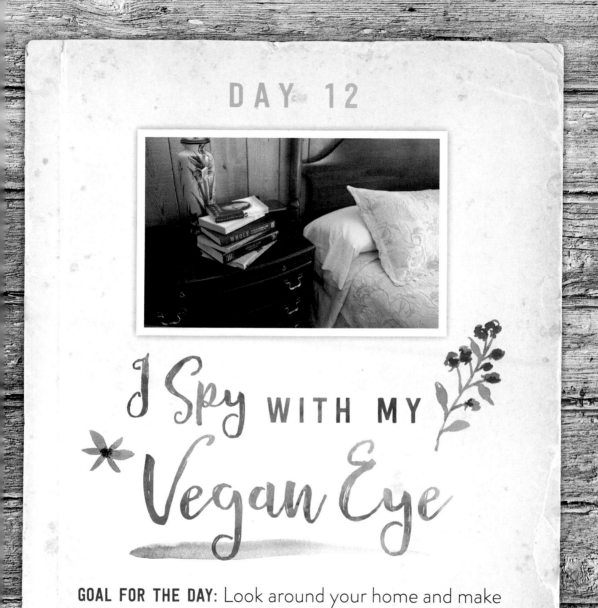

I Spy WITH MY Vegan Eye

GOAL FOR THE DAY: Look around your home and make note of any non-vegan products.

Today is super easy! You can even stay in your PJs and slipper socks, since you'll just be bopping around the house. We're going to look at two main categories: household items, and household cleaners. By the end of the day, you'll know which are vegan (hurray!), and which have been created with the undue suffering of others (boo!). Again, it's really up to you as to how quickly you discard, donate, or regift non-vegan items in your home. You can even choose to use them until they're used up or wear out, the goal being simply not to buy them again, creating a home that's filled with everything you need to live comfortably and compassionately.

OK, are we ready to stroll around the house? Grab your vegan cocoa, and let's go!

1. *Create a compassionate living space.*

PILLOWS, COMFORTERS, AND DUVETS: Check your bedding for feathers. When it's time to replace any pillows, duvets, or comforters, look for synthetic alternatives, which will likely have the added bonus of being hypoallergenic as well. I prefer those lined in organic cotton so they're cooler against the skin.

MATTRESS: When it's time to buy a new mattress, look on the tag or ask the salesperson if the mattress contains wool or "other fibers," which might be wool. Non-wool mattresses are easy to find. We bought a non-wool mattress at IKEA for a great price, and when we upgrade, we'll likely look into a nontoxic, eco-friendly one. As Walter Bader, author of *Sleep Safe in a Toxic World: Your Guide to Identifying and Removing Hidden Toxins from Your Bedroom*, says, "Mattresses are like cigarettes were in the 1930s, completely unregulated, and everyone thinks they're safe."[1]

BLANKETS: Check for wool fibers. No need to toss Aunt Marge's hand-knit woolen blankie, but a box full of cruelty-free yarn might be a good idea for next year's holiday gift.

LAMPSHADES: Look for silk or skin lampshades, and just switch them out for synthetic or plant fibers such as cotton the next time.

FURNITURE: Leather, silk, wool, and other animal fibers abound on couches, chairs and footstools. Just switch them out for cruelty-free options when you're ready to let go of them. They're easy to find. They'll likely be cheaper and easier to keep clean, too. Bonus points? Skip buying furniture made from tropical rainforest trees, such as teak or mahogany. Rainforestrelief.org has a nice list of which woods are best to avoid, as well as great suggestions if you'd like to buy wood from sustainable sources.

CARPETS AND THROW RUGS: Check for wool and other animal fibers. "Oriental" carpets are notorious for having wool in them, but I've seen beautiful ones without. IKEA, Amazon, and Overstock.com have them; they're usually made from an olefin/polypropylene blend. Or better yet, go the natural route and seek out hemp, sisal, or organic cotton rugs. Stone, bamboo, and hardwood flooring are nice wall-to-wall options, too. Whatever suits your little vegan tootsies!

DECORATIONS: Vegans avoid ornamentation that is made of feathers, bones, abalone and other doodads made from animal bits and pieces. When you're out and about shopping, just try to think about whether or not an animal was used to make whatever you're buying. And if you see something with a coating that's particularly shiny as though someone painted it with a frosted nail polish—heads up—it might be fish scales.

CURTAINS AND DECORATIVE PILLOWS: Just be on the lookout for silk, wool, and other non-vegan fibers. When it's time to replace, consider making them yourself, and go explore a fabric store. You'll find that there are all sorts of beautiful cruelty-free fabrics. You can turn pretty sheets into curtains and pillows with very little effort, too. Channel that Martha Stewart in you, and have some fun!

2. *Learn how to clean without cruelty.*

Sadly, just as with cosmetics, many household cleaning products are tested on animals before being sold. I don't need to make rabbits drink bleach to know I'm not supposed to, or put oven cleaner in their eyes to know that's a bad idea. Every time I'm at the store and see a "toxic" label on a cleaner, I always think about the animals who were forced to swallow the poison before it made its way to the store shelf. Thankfully, we don't need to wait for laws to change in order to do the right thing. Ready to clean with compassion? Here's how to do it!

Let's take a peek . . .

UNDER THE KITCHEN SINK: Windex, Easy-Off, Joy, Ivory, Cascade, Mr. Clean, Swiffer, Pine-Sol, Orange GLO, Oxiclean, Pledge, Resolve, Renuzit, and Comet are just a few of the household cleaning items that are made by companies that test on animals. Boo! If they're under your sink, use them up or give them away, and replace them with cruelty-free versions. OK? OK!

UNDER THE BATHROOM SINK: Lysol, Comet, Soft Scrub, Tilex, Kaboom, Scrub Free, and Scrubbing Bubbles are all made by companies who jam their products into the stomachs, eyes, and/or skin of animals. Let's push these products aside, too. Good-bye, and good riddance!

LAUNDRY ROOM: Tide, Cheer, Febreze, Oomph, Downy, Oust, Woolite, Gain, Bounce, Clorox, and Shout are all made by companies that test products on animals. Too bad the animals can't shout, "Let me out!" Until they leave the animals alone, these cleaning supplies are off our shopping list. There's no need to make someone bleed just to get our laundry clean.

EVERYWHERE ELSE: Here's a handy database where you can see a list of products that are tested on animals, and those that are not: http://features.peta.org/cruelty-free-company-search/index.aspx. If you have other cleaning products in your home that I didn't list above, just plug the name of them into the search engine to find out if they're cruelty-free. Easy peasy!

And now for the fun part! Replacing household cleaners with cruelty-free products has never been easier. On the next page is a list of companies to consider as you make your "clean break" from products stained with antiquated animal

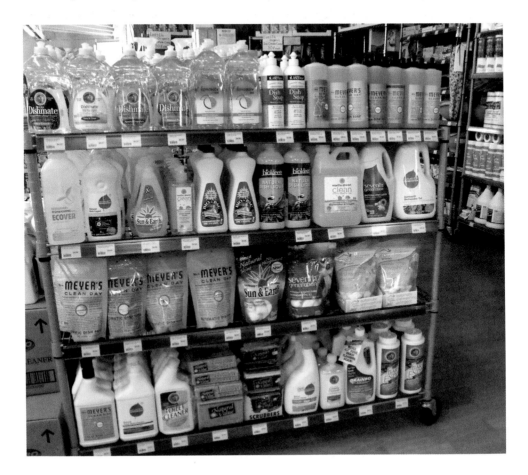

experiments, to compassionate cleaning. Just a heads up, though, sometimes a "parent" company may still test products on animals, while one of the smaller companies it owns does not. For example, Mrs. Meyer's Clean Day is owned by S. C. Johnson & Son, a company that not only tests on animals, but also boldly defends doing so. However, Mrs. Meyer's not only *does not test* its products on animals, it does not use any animal ingredients either (nice!). It also does not use any chlorine bleach, ammonia, petroleum distillates, parabens, phosphates, or phthalates. I'll leave it up to you to decide what you're comfortable with. It's a fine line with vegans. Some feel that if you boycott *all* of the products of smaller cruelty-free companies with parent companies that test, then you're sending the wrong message by not encouraging the big guys to follow suit. If cruelty-free products don't sell well, what's the parent company's incentive to stop testing? Others feel as though the money all goes into the same big pot, so they steer clear of any cruelty-free companies that are owned by a parent company that tests. It's a bit like the conundrum we talked about regarding miniscule ingredients back when we were sorting through our pantry. When it comes to purchasing cosmetics, toiletries, and household cleaners, just follow your heart, and do what you think is best.

CRUELTY-FREE, VEGAN CLEANING, DISHWASHING, AND LAUNDRY PRODUCTS

Dr. Bronner's Pure-Castile Liquid Soaps

Seventh Generation

Method Products (branded as Method)

Earth Friendly Products

Ecover

ECOS

Whole Foods Market 365 house brand

Bar Keepers Friend (soft cleanser and powder)

Mrs. Meyer's Clean Day

The Good Home Co. Glass and Surface Cleaner

Trader Joe's

Citra Solv Natural Cleaner and Degreaser

Biokleen

Or . . . make your own!

If you want cruelty-free cleaners that are inexpensive and easy to make, you can find an array of simple household cleaner recipes online. It's amazing what a little vinegar and water can clean, or the scrubbing power of lemon juice with baking soda or salt. Just search "eco-friendly homemade cleaners" and you'll find all sorts of nifty, natural cleaning tricks!

I know cleaning isn't as much fun as baking cupcakes, but chin up, buttercup! We're over halfway there. Congratulations! Now sit back, relax, and we'll muddle through the closet tomorrow!

Checklist

- ☐ Did you walk around the house and figure out which decorative items, bedding, and furniture aren't vegan? And give a little thought on how to replace them with cruelty-free alternatives when the time comes?

- ☐ Did you separate your vegan cleaning items from the non-vegan items under your sinks?

- ☐ Did you find new vegan cleaning items to replace the non-vegan items as you use them up or set them aside?

- ☐ Did you consider making a homemade cleaner?

Thought FOR THE Day

No one should have to bleed to get our laundry clean.

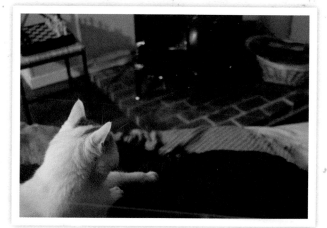

The Skeletons
IN YOUR *Closet*

GOAL FOR THE DAY: Organize your closet and separate your vegan clothes from those made with animal products so you can gradually phase out wearing non-vegan items.

Well, I have some fantastic news for you, chickadees. Most vegans get a lot of the familiar queries like "But don't you miss eating bacon?" and "How do you live without cheese?" from those who haven't quite made the connection yet, but we seldom, if *ever*, get asked if we miss wearing wool, leather, silk, angora, down, reptile skins, or a host of other body parts of animals. And do you know *why* no one asks? Because everyone knows there's so many darn tootin' cool and functional alternatives these days; we're not missing a thing! And that's great for you, *and* the animals! Tossing those skins, furs, feathers, hair, and cocoons out of your closet, and slowly replacing them with comfortable, feel-good fabrics is going to be a breeze.

But first, let's turn on the closet light (click!) and take a look at what some of our clothes, shoes, and accessories are made of, so we can see exactly what we've been schlepping around town, and why we're leaving the animal bits and pieces all behind.

WOOL

Most folks seem to think sheering sheep is a calm and necessary process, akin to men shaving beards when they've grown too thick. Or simply a kind gesture from ranchers who are just doing sheep a big favor; after all, no one likes to be too hot in the summertime, right? I used to picture the wool-gathering process as an old man sitting on a bench in a big field shaving a cuddly sheep for an hour or so. Once finished with the shave, I imagined the sheep springing lightly into the air and going about his way to frolic with his friends in the field. Bounce, bounce, bounce. But I was wrong.

Similar to the storybook picture of happy dairy cows grazing in green pastures, our blissful image of gentle sheep gladly giving up their wool for us to wear is a fairy tale, too.

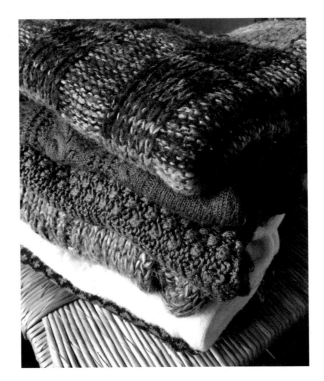

There's nothing relaxing or generous about a stranger punching a hole in your ear for a tag at a few weeks old. There's nothing nice about having your tail chopped off with a hot blade, or being castrated without anesthesia. Even Patagonia, a clothing store well-known for its financial contributions to make the world a better place, was shocked to learn that their wool supplier abused animals. Undercover film footage revealed lambs being stabbed in the neck, and at least one being skinned alive.[1] It's rare that the process is filmed, so who knows how often the abuse occurs.

In Australia, the largest producer of wool in the world, ranchers breed merino sheep in such a way that they'll have extremely wrinkled skin; after all, it's all about the money, and the more skin they have, the more wool ranchers can get. Sadly, this overabundance of skin also creates folds, which attracts flies, particularly around their bottoms, pro-ducing maggots that eat them alive. To curtail the infestation, ranchers perform what's called "mulesing." It's a crude process of cutting large areas of skin and flesh from around the animals' anus, and for the girl sheep, their vulvas, too, all of which happens without any law requiring anesthesia, nor even a veterinarian. In response to the public outcry, Australia's wool industry agreed to ban the practice in 2010, but they changed their mind, and it continues today.[2]

Making matters worse, most shearers aren't paid by the hour, but rather by how many sheep they shave. This can be up to 200 sheep per day, giving them a measly two to three minutes to remove the hair from each animal.[3] As you can imagine, the fast pace doesn't bode well for the sheep. This is how people treat animals, far away, where we can't see them. We see the price tag on the sweater, and the sale sign on the scarves, but what we *don't* see is the price the *animal* had to pay to have those clothes wrapped beneath the Christmas tree. How much did it really cost to get those woolen clothes to hangers in our closet? It's far too high a price for me. Thankfully, it doesn't have to be this way. We don't need wool to make us stylish or warm, and today, you're putting wool aside. And when you count those sheep as you fall asleep, you can rest assured they're grateful.

SILK

Have you ever watched a caterpillar slowly cross a leaf, or had the good fortune of one gently crawl across your hand? They're so cute. The word *caterpillar* can be traced back to the 1500s where it likely arose as a combination of the Old French words for "cat" and "hairy."[4] The incredible transformation of these tiny "hairy cats" has provided fodder for poets, storytellers, and artists since first sight. Knowing that one of these little guys can build a cocoon and transform his soft and pudgy little body into a glorious butterfly, and then flutter away to the sky, makes the mind swirl with wonder. And mine certainly has, ever since I was a kid.

As I mentioned earlier, I grew up in Pacific Grove (PG), California, a coastal community that's aptly know as "Butterfly Town, USA." Beautiful monarch butterflies make a stop here each autumn as part of their three-thousand-mile journey from Canada to Mexico. It's true; a delicate little butterfly can fly three thousand miles, and up to twenty-five miles per hour in speed. My mind drifts off to daydream just thinking about the grandeur of it all. The residents of Pacific Grove have welcomed the arrival of the bright orange and black butterflies with a big a parade since 1939. Butterfly signs, paintings, and photos adorn the city and there's even an annual "Butterfly Ball." PG sure loves Monarch butterflies, and they honor their visit in the most spectacular way.

Sadly, there's no pomp and circumstance for caterpillars used for silk, who are killed before they even get a chance to spread their wings. Silk caterpillars are kept in large rooms where they're fed mulberry leaves, increasing their weight by ten thousand times within just one month. Once they have enough energy, they spend three to four days spinning a cocoon with thread that can be over half a mile long.[5] To ensure the lengthy thread isn't damaged, most moths used for silk aren't allowed to emerge on their own: they're steamed or boiled alive while they're still in their cocoon. The beautiful transformation they work so hard for is halted by death because someone, somewhere, wants a silk tie. Someone wants a silk dress. And another wants a silk scarf. All of which are woven with strings of sadness, from a life cut short out of tradition, rather than necessity. There are no parades for a silk moth.

LEATHER

For those of you who haven't seen *The Texas Chainsaw Massacre*, it's based upon the real life story of a Wisconsin man named Ed Gein. Ed was a tanner by profession, amongst other things, who spent a great deal of time exhuming bodies in the late '40s and early '50s. He made belts from female nipples. He used skin to craft leggings, upholstery, masks, and a wastebasket, too. He even made a lampshade using the skin from someone's face. When I first read the long list of horrors, I had to take a moment just to sit and breathe. It's jarring, to say the least.

It comes as no surprise that Ed Gein was diagnosed with schizophrenia: a severe mental illness in which someone cannot think or behave "normally."[6] After all, who would use someone's skin as a garment, or for decorating their home, unless they had

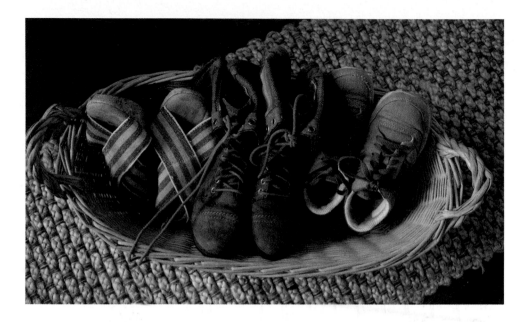

the severest of mental aberrations? I think you know where I'm going with this. That leather coat. That leather belt. Those leather shoes. All made with skin peeled from bodies, and yet in our twisted world, they're described as "fine fashion," while human skin-wearing Ed is described as a freak, and is sentenced to a mental institution for life. While I know most leather-wearing folks aren't as crazy as Ed Gein, the irony of it all is certainly worth thinking about.

Most leather comes from third world countries where there are usually no laws to protect animals used for clothing. They are dehorned, castrated, and have their tails cut, all without any anesthesia. Once the animals can no longer give milk, or no longer have the strength to pull heavy carts, they are thrown onto truck beds with their legs bound, and smuggled thousands of miles into Bangladesh. Upon arrival at the slaughterhouses, their throats are slit while conscious, and they're skinned—many while still alive.[7] Two million animals meet this same, sad fate each and every year. Let's face it: we may know where our shoes, jacket, wallet, or handbag was assembled, but when is the last time we were able to figure out *where*, or *how*, the animal was killed? Today, we're separating skin from our clothes and accessories, for the animals, and for our own mental well-being.

ANGORA

About 90 percent of all angora comes from farms in China, and even if your clothing says "Made in USA" or elsewhere, there's still no guarantee they didn't get the bunny fur from China, and simply assemble the garment somewhere else. It would be nice if all sweaters, scarves, hats, and accessories that are made with angora came from hair that's naturally shed when someone gently pets a bunny. But, sadly, nothing could be further from the truth. Chinese ranchers have been filmed ripping the fur off of their live bodies, because this method produces longer hairs, and in China there are no laws to stop them.[8] Bunnies are often left naked and bloody until they do it again in a few months' time. The practice is so horrific, that upon learning the truth about how bunnies are treated, Robert Redford removed all items made from angora from his clothing company's website, joining over one hundred other companies who have done the same.[9]

As with the fate of so many other animals who are used and abused, it comes as no surprise that there's no happy retirement home for bunnies who have outstayed their visit on the angora farm. As they age, the quantity of fur they produce diminishes, and they're simply not worth their keep to those who profit from their fur. Their throats are slit, the ranchers move on to younger bunnies, and the cycle of abuse marches on. It's a mad, mad world.

DOWN

The majority of down comes from China (again), where it's legal to pluck the feathers off of live ducks and geese. Workers have been filmed flipping frightened birds on their back and locking them between their knees as they pluck their feathers out.[10] It's possible that the filling for your down coat, comforter, sleeping bag, or pillow came from a bird that was killed prior to plucking, but as you can imagine, it's difficult to prove. Even if you could, the down would still likely be the by-product of equally abusive circumstances, such as the production of foie gras pâté, or duck meat. Birds need their down feathers for insulation; we don't. There are far better options. Today, we're leaving the feathers on the birds where they belong.

FUR

I think most of us are already familiar with the sadness that looms on a fur farm. With little legal protection, it's pretty much an "anything goes" industry. Animals are often anally electrocuted, which basically means they're killed from the inside out; after all, who wants to chance damaging the "goods" with blood. Other animals are caught via leghold traps; the few "lucky" ones chew off their own paws to escape.

What you may not know, however, is that "faux" fur is sometimes mislabeled, so as you're out and about on your next shopping spree, you might want to not only avoid fur, but *skip the fake fur, too*. And if you already have a few faux fur items, check them out closely. There are many mislabeled fake fur items floating around. A Marc Jacobs coat was recently advertised as having "faux fur" trim, but it was actually made from "raccoon dog" fur.[11] These beautiful animals, who are in the same family as the domestic dog, live in horrible conditions and have been filmed being skinned alive, among other atrocities, and investigators have documented the use of fur from domestic dogs and cats, too.[12] If you have time—and plenty of tissues—you can check out the full report on the Care for the Wild website: www.CareForTheWild.com. Another Marc Jacobs coat had a tag that described the item as "faux fur," but after taking it to the lab, investigators determined it was really rabbit fur. If you think it's just labels that say "Made in China" that are false, you'd be wrong. Another jacket had a "Made in Italy" tag and once again, the real rabbit fur was mislabeled "faux fur."[13] In a separate investigation, clothing samples sent to a lab revealed Neiman Marcus boots that were labeled "faux fur, 55% polyester, 45% acrylic" turned out to be rabbit fur, and so was a "faux fur trimmed sweater" from Nordstrom Rack.[14] I could go on and on, but I think you get the point. There's a lot of false advertising out there, and I think most folks, vegan or not, would be pretty outraged to know they're slipping into someone else's skin every time they put on what they thought was a compassionate "faux fur" coat.

Ready to make *compassion* your fashion? OK, *mon petit chéri* , let's do it!

1. *Create a cruelty-free closet.*

   Here's a list of words that describe vegan materials. This should help guide you as you peruse your closet and drawers. You'll find them listed on the tags of clothes, just inside the neck or the inside seam. If you're looking at shoes, the tag should be on the inside of the tongue, or inside the back of the shoe on the heel.

VEGAN

Faux Leather	Fleece	Rayon
Microfiber	Acrylic	Modal
Cork	Denim	Nylon
Cotton	Twill	Denim
Linen	Microfiber	All Synthetic Materials
Hemp	Viscose	All Man-made
Polyester	Tencel	Materials

And here are the items to avoid. Good riddance!

ANIMAL PRODUCTS

Wool	Suede	Shearling
Down	Angora	Kangaroo Skin
Silk	Mohair	Alligator, or any other
Fur	Pashmina	reptile skin
Leather	Alpaca	Cashmere

2. *Make your jewelry box cruelty-free.*

   PEARLS: We all know how bothersome it is to have a tiny grain of sand in our eye. Imagine having that sand bothering you for an entire year. That's how pearls are formed. Pearl cultivators open up a mollusk's shell and stick an irritant inside, to which the mollusk responds by coating it over and over until it becomes a pearl. Considering most mollusks have a heart that beats, eyes that see, as well as a central nervous system, vegans skip wearing real pearls. We let the scientists bicker over whether or not they feel pain, while we err on the side of caution. If you still want to wear pearl jewelry, you can easily find beautiful fake pearl accessories for a fraction of the price, and use all that money saved to buy a month's worth of vegan cupcakes. Sounds like a good trade to me!

SHELLS: Massive shell gathering throughout the world has taken a great toll on the environment.[15] We also don't know if anyone was killed in the process of gathering them. Considering some shells, like the Hawaiian "Sunrise Shell," can fetch thousands of dollars *per shell*, it's safe to assume that some folks might not care too much about whether or not someone still considers a shell their home if selling shells is how they make their money.[16] When it comes to jewelry, let's leave the sea shells by the seashore.

BONE: Sure, some jewelry made from bones might actually be from roadkill, or maybe an animal who died of natural causes, but how can we really be sure, and who wants to wear someone's bones, anyhow? That's just creepy. Let's put those kneecap necklaces and pinky toe earrings aside, shall we? Blah.

Now that you've sorted through your wardrobe and accessories, I'm going to take a wild guess that you've discovered that you actually still have *plenty* to wear that isn't a product of animal suffering. There might be an old pair of comfy leather shoes you might miss for a bit, or a warm woolen coat that might be hard to part with, but chances are, there's already a heck of a lot in your closet, dresser, and jewelry box that you can still wear, and feel good about.

3. OK! It's time to decide what to do with your non-vegan items, and maybe score a few new ones. Just as with the refrigerator, freezer, and pantry food, it's probably best to not be wasteful. You can either wear the items until they wear out, or donate them to friends, family members, or your local charity, church, or shelter. You could even hold a garage sale to earn a little extra money (I'm thinking cash for cupcakes again). Whatever you decide to do, I'm sure someone can make good use of them, and donating clothes and accessories makes *you* feel good, too. For now, just set them aside and think about the next steps; there's no rush. We're taking things nice and easy here.

And now for the fun part: picking out vegan clothes! Even if you don't need to shop today, just go online and check out all of the cool clothes that are out there that are completely cruelty-free.

> If you're interested in learning about regulations involving wildlife that's used for jewelry, such as coral, sea turtles, and ivory, visit "Wildlife in the Jewelry Trade" on the U.S. Fish and Wildlife Services website: https://www.fws.gov/le/pdf/Wildlife-in-the-Jewelry-Trade.pdf

From dress shoes that look like the finest of Italian leather, to fashionable peacoats for an autumn pub-crawl, vegan fashion has never been easier. I've compiled a long list in the resource section with all sorts of websites that have vegan garments, but even local stores have tons of cool vegan things to wear. H&M, Forever 21, and Target are just a few that have loads of inexpensive vegan accessories, shoes, and clothes. You can check out your local thrift shops, too. I've found lots of supercute vegan sweaters at Goodwill in great shape, some of which were brand new, with the original price tag on them. For higher-end attire, check out Brave GentleMan (bravegentleman.com) where they use vegan "future wool," "future leather," and "future suede" to make the most impressive fine menswear. Seriously, the quality of the clothes and shoes will knock your socks off. For higher-end women's attire, check out the coat selection at Vaute Couture (vautecouture.com), and the shoes and boots at Mooshoes (mooshoes.com). If you think vegans just shop at those pleather-filled punk rock shops in the malls, you're in for a big surprise. Vegan clothing has come a long way, baby!

Need more? Check out the resources section at the end of this book. You'll find everything you need, from vegan bowling shoes and ballet slippers to wallets and baseball gloves. Vegan everything for everyone!

Checklist

☐ Did you separate your vegan clothes from your non-vegan clothing?

☐ Did you separate your vegan jewelry from your non-vegan jewelry?

☐ Are you still enjoying a nice variety of fresh produce every day?

☐ Have you spent a little "mindful" time with an animal recently?

Thought FOR THE Day

"Teaching a child not to step on a caterpillar is as valuable to the child as it is to the caterpillar."

–BRADLEY MILLER

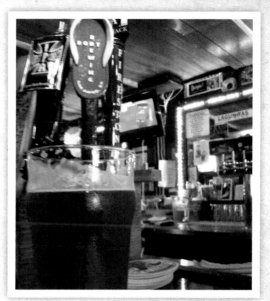

Excuse me, Waiter,

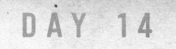

THERE'S A FISH IN MY BEER!

GOAL FOR THE DAY: Find a vegan beer, wine, champagne, or favorite type of liquor for you, or a loved one, to enjoy!

What animal parts could possibly be in beer, wine, and champagne? Fish bladders, eggs, gelatin, and even blood have all been used to help clarify booze during the "fining" process. Most folks don't want to see particles floating in their mug of beer or flute of champagne, so they toss in weird animal parts that will bind with them, making the particles larger and allowing them to precipitate out.

Thankfully, some wineries use minerals, such as bentonite clay, to clarify wine and beer, or they simply let the particulates float to the bottom and bottle their wine without fining at all. When I used to enjoy a glass of port, I'd buy it unfined because honestly, I don't mind if a few grape skins settle to the bottom of the bottle. (Yes, I'm in one of those phases, you know, where you drink too much one night, and swear you'll never drink again.) The problem is, wine and beer manufacturers don't have to disclose their fining agents on the bottle, nor even list if it was fined at all. Who knows what's in that wine or beer? Usually, the only way for consumers to find out is to ask. A few producers are starting to take the lead on their own, though, disclosing all the ingredients on their labels, including what the fining agents are: "[W]hatever has been added in production or to the finished wine, even in the minutest fraction, will appear on our labels," says Bonnie Doon Winery owner Randall Grahm.[1] Here's what's on Bonny Doon's 2007 Muscat label: "In the winemaking process the following were utilized: indigenous yeast, organic yeast hulls, bentonite, cream of tartar," which means, this particular wine is vegan, as are all of their current red wines. I sure wish every winemaker and beer master was that transparent about production.

But don't you worry. Most vegans know the perfect place to go to find out the scoop when it comes to vegan spirits (don't be scared; they're friendly!): Visit Barnivore at www.barnivore.com. They've meticulously researched over twenty-six thousand different wines, beers, and liquors throughout the world to find out which ones are produced *with* animal products, and which ones *aren't*. It's such a helpful website. I can't count how many times I've pulled it up on my cell phone while meandering down the aisles at BevMo! or the grocery store. You can either search by category, or if you already have a wine or beer you enjoy, you can just search it by name and it will pull up vegan options (green squares), and non-vegan options (red squares), made by that company. There are plenty of vegan beers, wines, and liquors to choose from, so head on over to Barnivore and see what's on tap!

BEERFESTS AND OKTOBERFESTS GO VEGAN!

If wine isn't your thing, and you're in the mood to party, consider heading out to a Vegan Beerfest! They're getting more popular every year. I've watched the one in L.A. grow from festivities that fit in a little area the size of a small patio, to taking over the Rose Bowl stadium. How awesome is that? If you'd like to get a flavor for one, check out the video: veganbeerfest.com. Vegan beer is here!

You can also find plenty of vegan beer at Vegan Oktoberfests around the world. Here's the scoop for the one that's held annually in Los Angeles: veganoktoberfest.com.

Even the granddaddy of them all, Oktoberfest in Munich, Germany, has introduced vegan food and beer! Yes, amidst all of those split roasts and pork sausages, a new world of vegan booze and food awaits you. German festival goers have found *Herzkasperl*, made with soy "pork" medallions and sautéed chanterelle mushrooms, and the traditional cheesy egg noodle bake known as *Käsespätzle* prepared without the egg or dairy cheese.[2] And as for vegan German beer, the Reinheitsgebot of 1516 has your back. Thanks to this old purity law, which is still on the books, German beer can only be made with water, barley, and hops.[3] I'm sure the eight hundred thousand vegans living in Germany are happy about that![4]

And here are a few vegan tips to wet your whistle:

ᕦ Guinness beer is set to become 100 percent vegan by the end of 2016, so keep your ears peeled for the big announcement. After 256 years of making beer using isinglass, Guinness decided to ditch using fish bladders and instead use a vegan "state-of-the-art filtration system." What's extra cool is that this change isn't due to finding a cheaper ingredient, nor a desire to improve the taste; it's all thanks to so many Guinness fans simply asking for a vegan option. So, don't be shy; if you want something that makes the world a better place, speak up! That's how change occurs. In the meantime, you can still celebrate Saint Patty's Day with a fine glass of Irish brew right now. These beers will bring a bit of the ole' Irish luck to you, and the animals, too!

George Killian's Irish Red
Samuel Smith's Imperial Stout
Magners Irish Pear Cider
Harvest Moon Paddy's Irish Stout
Samuel Adams Irish Red

ᕦ Other beers that are vegan: Heineken, Amstel, Corona, Pacifico. Pass the chips and guac!

ᕦ Eager to enjoy a good glass of cruelty-free wine without breaking the bank? Check out Trader Joe's Charles Shaw Red Wines. All of TJ's red wines under the Charles Shaw label are vegan. The reason you'll find that more red wines than white wines are vegan is because you can't see as much of the particulates in dark wine, so winemakers aren't as worried about leaving them there. So cheers to Charles Shaw's red, but leave their non-vegan white wines on the shelf.

✤ Need a little champagne to ring in the New Year? You can fill your flutes with these vegan bubblies: Domaine Ste. Michelle, Moët Champagne, and Domaine Carneros Sparkling Wines (which is even labeled vegan!). Or if you'd like to enjoy what every newly elected president sips, grab a bottle of Korbel Natural sparkling wine. It's been the champagne of choice at the past eight presidential inaugurations, and it's vegan. Just don't call it Champagne, like I did, unless you put the word "California" in front of it. Champagne can only be labeled as such if it's made in the Champagne region of France, and this one's from California. And this is why there are Wine Lawyers.

✤ Red Truck Wine, White Truck Wine, and Pink Truck Wine are all vegan. Vroom vroom!

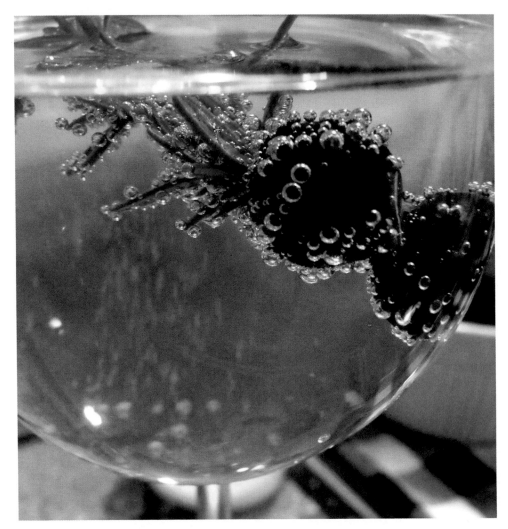

- The Vegan Vine wine is, you guessed it: Vegan. They list all of their ingredients, too. It's made by Clos LaChance Winery and owned in part by NBA champion, John Salley, who not only drinks vegan wine, but also only eats vegan food. I'll cheers to that!
- Martinis anyone? Ketel One, Grey Goose, and Hangar One vodkas are all vegan.
- Need some gin for that tonic? Tanqueray and Gordon's Gin are vegan.
- A little rum for that fruity beach drink? Just party hearty with some Bacardi.
- Considering a trip to Napa Valley? Here are a few Napa wineries that *only* sell vegan wine, just to get you started: O'Brien Estate: www.obrienestate.com; Thumbprint Cellars: www.thumprintcellars.com; Mason Cellars: www.masoncellars.com

. . . AND THEN THERE'S THE PARTY POOPERS

Sometimes someone can seem so wonderful until you really get to know them, and the manufacturers of booze are no exception. I'll leave it up to you as to whether or not you want to support the following companies. Their products may be vegan, but their values sure make their drinks stink.

Absolut, Stolichnaya, Dow's Vintage Port, Cockburn's Vintage Port, Beefeater, Malibu rum, and Perrier-Jouët Champagne are all vegan, but their owners are major funders of bullfighting. They get their kicks watching animals get stabbed.

Yellow Tail red wine is vegan, but the Casella family, who owns the winery, is the largest corporate sponsor of the Sporting Shooters Association of Australia, which organized the national park hunting trials in Australia. They shoot a lot of animals, just for the hell of it.[5]

Budweiser and MillerCoors beer are vegan, but they support rodeos. They love watching folks drag frightened animals around by their necks with tight ropes. MillerCoors loves hunting, too. They even donated fifty thousand dollars to Whitetails Unlimited, an organization that "celebrate[s] North America's premier big-game animal, the whitetailed deer" and is "dedicated to conservation, education, and the preservation of the hunting tradition."[6] Why, people, *why?*

I'm telling you, ditching animal products in alcohol is a breeze, as long as you give it some thought and choose wisely. And don't forget: drink, drive, and karaoke responsibly. Designate a non-drinking driver before you head out, and let the merriment begin!

Checklist

☐ Did you explore www. barnivore.com?

☐ If you drink alcohol, did you find a vegan beer, wine, or spirit you enjoy?

Thought FOR THE Day

"Unless someone like you cares a whole awful lot, nothing is going to get better. It's not."

—DR. SEUSS, *The Lorax.*

Keeping THE Happy IN THE Holidays

GOAL FOR THE DAY: Look ahead to the next holiday and make a plan so that your holiday is vegan and enjoyable for everyone around your table.

The holidays can be stressful enough without throwing a new way of living into the mix, especially when you're surrounded by friends and family who may be south of enthusiastic about your newfound love and empathy for all beings. But that's OK, bring on the nog and mistletoe! We're ready to celebrate!

The two "biggies" when it comes to holidays and being a newbie vegan are Thanksgiving and the December mix of festivities: Christmas, Chanukah, Kwanzaa, and the rest. No surprise there, right? First you need to figure out if you'd like to host a holiday feast at your own home, or accept an invitation to someone else's dinner table. If you're staying in, there are all sorts of creative ways to celebrate the season with a host of vegan fare.

Ready for a festive season that's filled with compassion and joy for *all*? Then bring on the good tidings and cheer; let's go!

1. *Figure out a plan for celebrating the holiday at home.* What can be festive and vegan for the holidays? First, take a look online and you'll discover loads of free recipes there. Just search what you normally love to eat around the holidays, along with the word *vegan* and be prepared to have your holiday socks knocked off. There are so many to choose from. One good place to start is on PETA's Vegan Holiday page: www.peta.org/living/food/celebrate-vegan-holiday. There are beautiful cooking videos and loads of vegan entree recipes—everything from Almost "Beef" Wellington with Madeira Sauce to Wheatmeat Roulade with Chestnut "Sausage" Stuffing. The major magazines and newspapers often list special vegan recipes throughout the holiday season, too. You can get creative with the Simple Seitan recipe on page 112, if you're in the mood. Make a roast with it! And if you enjoy traditional British holiday fare, The Vegan Society has a long list of vegan recipes from Haggis to Yorkshire Pudding (popovers).[1] Pinterest is loaded with vegan holiday recipes, too. Vegan Sticky Toffee Pudding, anyone? There's a recipe for that, too! Just hop online and watch the holiday cooking video by North Londoner Ava Szajna-Hopgood.[2] She's adorable!

HOLIDAY COOKING TIP

As you make a few switch-a-roos in recipes, just know that if you're making something savory, like mashed potatoes or gravy, don't use a sweetened vanilla nut milk. Use plain and unsweetened! I can't tell you how many times vegans, myself included, have grabbed that vanilla almond milk, just because it was handy dandy, and ruined a perfectly fine dish. Once you pour it in, there's no getting that sweet vanilla flavor out. Consider yourself warned.

After you've gone through the online options, peruse vegan holiday cookbooks, like Lindsay Nixon's *Happy Herbivore Holidays and Gatherings*, or *The Superfun Times Vegan Holiday Cookbook: Entertaining for Absolutely Every Occasion* by Isa Chandra Moskowitz. Go to the bookstore or your local library and see what's on the shelf. Even if you just flip through a few, you'll get some new ideas.

Looking for a way to avoid spending all day in the kitchen? Check out the premade options at a grocery store! These are best if you want something fast and easy for the main dish, allowing you more time to focus on the delicious sides. Just pop them in the oven and you're done! Here's a quick snapshot of main dish options to give you a taste:

- Trader Joe's Turkey-less Stuffed Roast
- Gardein's Savory Stuffed Turk'y
- Gardein's Holiday Roast
- Vegetarian Plus Vegan Whole Turkey
- Field Roast Grain Meat Hazelnut Cranberry Roast en Croute
- Field Roast Grain Meat Celebration Roast
- Field Roast Grain Meat Smokey Forager's Roast with Pineapple Mustard Glaze
- Tofurky Holiday Vegetarian Roast and Gravy

And don't forget the stuffing! You can easily grab a bag of it at the store. You can make it from scratch, of course, but if this is your first vegan holiday season, and you're looking for something easy, just pick up a bag of any of these. (Some store-bought stuffing mixes are far healthier than others, so read the ingredients carefully and try to make the best choice possible.)

- Pepperidge Farm Herbed Seasoned Stuffing
- Mrs. Cubbison's Focaccia Bread Stuffing
- Whole Foods Everyday 365 Organic Vegan Stuffing

As you get closer to the holidays, you'll notice that the selection of festive foods for your vegan holiday will increase. The more the merrier!

You can also explore local vegan restaurants and grocery stores to see if they're creating any special meals for the holidays. Whole Foods Market creates a vegan holiday plate each year that you can order in advance. Ditto Native Foods. They usually have Native Wellingtons, vegan pumpkin pies, and pumpkin cheesecakes to go, too. Vegans are happily, and *heartily*, celebrating the holidays across the world. See what's cookin' in your neighborhood.

Tofurky makes a yummy Savory Gravy that's easy to find around the holidays, but if you have a little bit of time, consider making your own. It's easy!

Easy Vegan Gravy

Here's how I make basic gravy. Feel free to adjust it to taste. You can easily use vegetable stock in lieu of the Bragg's Liquid Aminos and water. And you can add sautéed mushrooms, thyme, or whatever else your holiday heart desires!

¼ cup nutritional yeast

¼ cup unbleached all-purpose flour

2 cups water

⅛ cup Bragg's Liquid Aminos

2 teaspoons garlic powder

1 teaspoon onion powder

½ teaspoon sage

¼ teaspoon freshly ground black pepper

2 teaspoons cornstarch

1. In a small pot, combine the nutritional yeast and flour. Add the water, Bragg's Liquid Aminos, garlic and onion powders, sage, and pepper and mix together over low heat.

2. In a separate small bowl, combine the cornstarch with just enough water to dissolve it (1 to 2 tablespoons). When completely dissolved, pour it into a pot while whisking slowly. The goal is to avoid any clumps, but if your cornstarch dissolved completely in the water, this shouldn't be a problem.

3. Bring the mixture to a boil, reduce heat to medium, and cook, whisking occasionally, for 5 minutes. Pour the gravy into a pretty gravy boat, and drench those mashed potatoes and stuffing. Enjoy!

2. *Figure out what to do if you choose to spend the holiday at someone else's home.* Unless someone has invited you over for the holidays with the understanding that you're doing all the cooking (how nice of you!), you'll likely have a lot less control over what's on the table. But here's the beauty of it all: going to someone else's home gives you the opportunity to bring over a vegan dish or two for all to enjoy. This kind gesture will not only provide you with the certainty that you'll have something good to eat, it will also:

- Give you the chance to show everyone that you really do eat delicious food. (Deflecting those "poor you" looks!)
- Demonstrate that you're not expecting anyone to go out of their way for you. (You're still polite and sweet as pumpkin pie!)
- Provide an easy platform to talk about your decision to go vegan with the rest of the family. (Because it will come up, even if you don't say a peep, so it might as well happen while everyone's enjoying your vegan candied yams!)

I like bringing homemade cranberry sauce and gravy since most folks can enjoy those no matter what else is on their plate, and if you're having any plain homemade sides at someone's house, they'll provide you with something flavorful to slather them with. I bring lots of other yummy stuff, like vegan stuffing, and a main dish, too. I'm not a fan of laborious meal-making throughout the year, as you've probably gathered by now, but when it comes to the holidays, I get the cooking bug like no other!

The recipe that follows is a little treat I like to make that's impressive around the holidays, or any time of the year, and it makes a great gift for your hosts, your friends—well, anybody—including yourself!

Easy Cashew Date Balls

MAKES 18 TO 20 PIECES

1 cup pitted dates

1 cup raw cashews

¼ teaspoon sea salt

Sesame seeds, powdered sugar, and cocoa powder for decoration (optional)

Just toss the pitted dates, cashews and salt into a food processor and blend until they have a sticky consistency. Roll the mixture into balls the size of giant marbles and place on a plate. They taste great just like this, but I go one more step and roll a few in white sesame seeds (my favorite combo!), and a few in powdered sugar and cocoa powder, too.

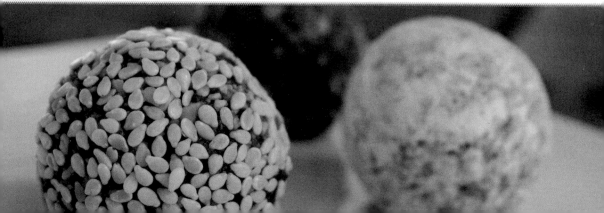

3. *Keep in mind that although your first holiday as a vegan might not be easy, keeping things in perspective will really help* . . . and with this thought, I'm interrupting our celebration for a tiny reality check so we're not completely blinded by the lights and glitter. Holidays are difficult for most newbie vegans, no doubt about it. You're likely going to miss a few traditional meals you've come to love over the years until you make a few adjustments, and you'll probably upset a few friends or family members, too, who just won't understand. Folks are already a little stressed and cranky around the holidays, so you'll be an easy target. But take a beat to think about what the holidays are *really* all about. We all know they're to inspire peace and joy to the world, but go beyond the words, and reflect. Take these thoughts in and let them nestle in your heart for a moment.

- Someone is missing their parent, sibling, spouse, or child, who for the first time isn't sitting at the table.
- Someone is falsely imprisoned this holiday season, without any freedom in sight.
- Someone is living under a freeway ramp, not realizing it's a holiday at all.

When you take a step back and look at the big picture, it's really not the food that makes us happy. It's our loved ones and companionship, or simply being at peace with ourselves. No matter what happens during your first holiday as a vegan, just remember to be grateful for what you have, enjoy the company of those you love, and realize that going vegan hasn't made you give up anything that truly matters. Your heart is filled with compassion and your actions are making the world a better place for all. And that, my friends, will carry you through the season, no matter how many times Uncle Ned asks, "Want some turkey?" or Aunt Marge says, "You're going to die without your protein!" Just love them as you always have, and enjoy your holiday meal. 'Tis the season, my sugarplums! You're going to be A-OK.

JACKIE'S HOLIDAY TIPS

Although this isn't a cookbook, I'm going to share a few tasty tidbits to help keep your holidays merry and bright.

Do you want to make vegan gravy or desserts and need cruelty-free thickeners? Holiday food is often thickened with things vegans don't eat, but fear not. Here's a list of common thickeners that you can use for sauces and desserts in lieu of eggs and cream:

- Flour
- Arrowroot
- Cornstarch
- Agar-agar

Do you need a quick festive holiday meal? "Veganize" a shepherd's pie, one of my favorite meals as a kid; it's perfect comfort food for the holiday season. To "veganize" your traditional recipe, just use a vegan butter in place of dairy butter for the mashed potato topping, and for the underlying filling, use chopped mushrooms, or vegan beef crumbles, in lieu of the ground meat and you'll be good to go!

Are you looking for some colorful and healthy vegan "Sides?" Here are a few suggestions:

HOLIDAY BEETS

Did you know you can bake a beet just like you bake a potato? Just wash and trim a large beet, without removing the skin, and wrap it in aluminum foil. Be sure you wrap it well so that the beet juice doesn't leak everywhere. If you prefer to avoid cooking with aluminum, you can bake it in an oven-safe dish, too. Just pop in your oven, or toaster oven, and bake at 375°F for 1 hour. After you let it cool for a bit, you can easily remove the skin, but I prefer to gobble it up as is. Slice, or serve whole, and season to taste with a dash of sea salt and freshly ground black pepper, and, if you're like me, a splash of balsamic vinegar. If you're serving beets at the holidays, toss a little green herb on top, like fresh dill, for an extra-festive look. Simple, tasty, and healthy, too!

OKINAWAN SWEET POTATO

These are vibrant purple inside, packed with antioxidants, high in fiber, and super delicious! Keep your eyes open for them around the holidays. Some folks just prepare them as they would regular potatoes, but others enjoy taking advantage of their slightly sweet taste by baking and then mashing them with coconut milk and a dash cinnamon or curry powder. The Okinawan sweet potato isn't even related to potatoes; it's part of the morning glory family. But who cares? They're beautiful and tasty!

POMEGRANATE SEEDS AND GREENS

I love that pomegranates are in season during the holidays because, as I mentioned in Day 10, Culinary Arts, I love to sprinkle them on sides that are green! Consider tossing them on everything from spinach salads to roasted Brussels sprouts. They're so festive, and healthy, too!

Need a topping for that holiday dessert?

If you're in the mood for a dollop of whipped cream for that hot cocoa or pumpkin pie, So Delicious makes a yummy CocoWhip! from coconut milk, or you can just make your own!

Vegan Coconut Whipped Cream

ENOUGH FOR 1 TO 2 PIES

One 15-ounce can unsweetened regular coconut milk (not the "low fat" or "light" type)

1 teaspoon pure vanilla extract

2 teaspoons organic sugar

1. Place the can of coconut milk upside down in the fridge overnight.

2. The next day get your pie out and ready to top. Or you can be extra healthy and prepare a bowl of fresh fruit!

3. Open the can and scoop out the thick part, leaving the really liquidy part behind. You'll notice a really nice hard clump on the top of the can, and a decent amount on the bottom, too!

4. Place the liquid in a bowl and add vanilla and sugar to taste. We're all different, so add what you think you'll like!

5. Blend! After about 1½ minutes or so, you will see a nice consistency.

6. Top your cake, pie, fresh fruit, hot cocoa, vegan ice cream, or whatever else suits your fancy with your vegan whipped cream, and enjoy!

VEGAN SWEETS FOR THE HOLIDAYS

If you're looking for candy for Easter or Halloween that's a bit "healthier" than what I posted on the *I Can't Believe It's Vegan* list, check out Surf Sweets Candy (vegan gummies!), Tree Hugger Bubble Gum (gumballs!), JJ Sweet's Cocomels (caramels!), and Torie and Howard's Chewie Fruities (similar to Starbursts!). These treats have no high fructose corn syrup, no artificial colors, and no artificial flavors. And two vegan thumbs up for Amy's "Sunny" Candy Bar (made with coconut and toasted almonds), and their "Dreamy" Candy Bar (made with a creamy nougat). They're organic, and *crazy* good!

Need marshmallows without gelatin for your hot cocoa or gingerbread house? Check out Sweet & Sara, Dandies, and Trader Joe's Marshmallows. Just keep them away from me, *please*. I have no self-control when it comes to vegan marshmallows—they are *so* good. Looking for the sweetness of condensed dairy milk for sweet holiday treats? Nature's Charm and Let's Do Organic have you covered. You can heat their condensed coconut milk up to make a smooth caramel sauce, or keep going and make homemade caramels!

VALENTINE'S DAY

There's no shortage when it comes to vegan chocolate on Valentine's Day! xoxo

- Green & Black's Organic Dark Chocolate
- Whole Foods Organic Dark Chocolate with Almonds
- Chocolove Almonds & Sea Salt in Dark Chocolate (check out their other vegan flavors, too!)
- Newman's Own Organic Super Dark Chocolate Bar
- Endangered Species Natural Dark Chocolate Squares

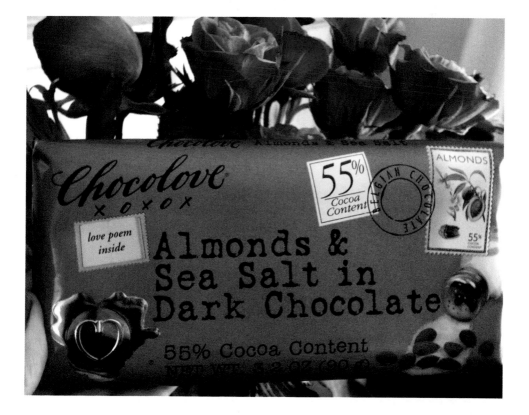

Valentine's Day Chocolate-Dipped Strawberries

SERVES 2

½ cup Trader Joe's chocolate chips (any plain vegan chocolate will do!)

1 tablespoon coconut oil

1 pint basket strawberries (chilled)

Parchment paper

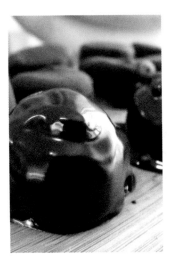

1. Place the chocolate chips in a microwave-safe bowl and add the coconut oil on top. Microwave for 30 seconds. Carefully remove the bowl, stir, return to the microwave, and continue to melt for another 10 to 15 seconds. Remove from the microwave, stir, making sure the mixture is completely melted, and set aside.

2. Place the parchment paper on a plate or a tray; just make sure the plate or tray is a size that can fit in your refrigerator. Carefully dip each strawberry into the bowl of melted chocolate, covering about two-thirds of each strawberry, and carefully transfer to the parchment paper–lined plate.

3. Once you've dipped all of the strawberries, place them in the fridge so the shell can set, and feed them to your lucky valentine.

NOTE: This chocolate shell coating also works well for dipping frozen banana slices. I like to put a dollop of peanut butter on top of each slice, then dip, then freeze. Voilà—frozen peanut butter–banana bites! Deeeelicious!

AND HERE'S MORE SWEETS, MY SWEET!

A can of garbanzo beans walks into a bar . . . There's no punch line here folks, but what I'm about to tell you is so amazing that when people first heard it, many thought it was a joke! Aquafaba has taken the world by storm, and it's just aqua = water, and faba = beans. As I mentioned on Day 5, it's simply the brine from a can of beans; the liquid you usually strain out! But you can easily make marshmallow fluff, meringue cookies and pies, chocolate mousse, buttercream frosting, nougat, and all sorts of yummy things with it that were a wee bit difficult to do before this crazy discovery! It's the perfect substitute for egg whites, so get that mind of yours thinking about what you want to create with it. You can visit aquafaba.com and the aquafaba "hits and misses" Facebook page for a few ideas!

Easy Meringue Bites

MAKES 70 TO 80 SMALL BITES

There are so many variations. By all means, don't stop here; just use this recipe as a base. Get creative, and make something spectacular! I'm just learning how to work with aquafaba myself. It's a whole new world!

Brine from one 15-ounce can garbanzo beans (Great Northern bean or cannellini bean brine works well, too)

½ cup sugar

1 teaspoon pure vanilla extract

1. Preheat the oven to 250°F

2. Pour the brine into your mixer bowl and blend on high for 10 to 15 minutes. (You might need to give your mixer a minute to rest now and then as you're doing this so it doesn't overheat.) You'll know when it's done because you'll see the brine form nice peaks. Theoretically, you should be able to turn the mixer bowl upside down and it won't fall out.

3. Once you see peaks, slowly add the sugar and vanilla and blend until well mixed. Again, you should still see peaks.

4. Place very small dollops of the whipped aquafaba onto a rimmed baking sheet lined with parchment paper.

5. Bake in the preheated oven for approximately 90 minutes. Let cool completely while in oven. When the meringues are cooled, they will be hard to the touch. Store in an airtight container.

NOTE: Want to make buttercream frosting? Just blend in some vegan butter and sugar once the peaks have formed, and frost away. Need a little marshmallow fluff to go with vegan s'mores or on ice cream? Just use powdered sugar instead of granulated and pile it on. Craving some vegan chocolate mousse? After the peaks have formed, just add a little melted chocolate, whip, refrigerate, and serve. The possibilities are truly endless. Go explore some recipes online and have some fun! Just remember: Sweet treats are OK now and then, but don't overdo the sugar, sugah! You are plenty sweet enough. As they say, with every bite of food we're either fighting disease, or feeding it, and I'm pretty sure we all know which role processed sugar plays. Phooey!

And now back to that can of beans that walked into the bar. You're not going to just let him get away, are you? Get back here, you can of beans! Let's make hummus!

Sun-dried Tomato–Kalamata Hummus

MAKES ABOUT 1 CUP

Always a great dip for a party, this hummus makes good of those leftover beans when you've been making something with aquafaba.

One 15-ounce can garbanzo beans (chickpeas), drained

Juice of ½ lemon (you can add a little water, or more lemon juice, if you want your hummus to be thinner)

1 to 2 tablespoons olive oil

1 heaping tablespoon sun-dried tomatoes

1 teaspoon garlic powder (or chopped fresh garlic)

1 teaspoon onion powder (or chopped fresh onion)

½ teaspoon sea salt (skip the salt if your beans have salt added already)

6 pitted Kalamata olives

Freshly ground black pepper

OK, here's how simple this recipe is: Put everything into a food processor, and blend until smooth! Just use your own judgment for the proper amount of olive oil. And you can use water in lieu of oil, if you prefer. The main ingredient is simply garbanzo beans (chickpeas); the rest is up to you! Experiment with the foods you love, or those you have handy. Other fun additions to consider: tahini, capers, cooked eggplant, avocado, or artichoke hearts. Dips are so easy and fun!

Checklist

☐ Did you figure out where you're spending the next big holiday?

☐ Did you make a game plan for what food you'll be enjoying?

☐ Did you find a store that will have the items you need for your holiday meal?

☐ Did you experiment with aquafaba?

Thought FOR THE Day

Life goes by fast. Walk, run, swim, and skip while you can.

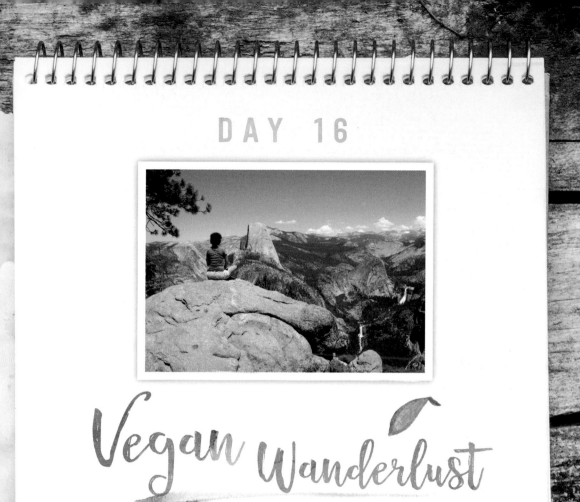

Vegan Wanderlust

GOAL FOR THE DAY: Grab a map and pick a place you'd like to go. Then, plan out the meals for your next travel adventure so you can see just how easy it is to be vegan when you're away from home.

Road trip time! Aaaah, today is a fun day. So many places to go and things to do. Traveling vegan style has never been easier. If you've got the travel bug, but you're worried you'll fall off the vegan wagon because you'll have nothing but desert cactus pears to eat, have no fear. With a little knowledge and a pinch of planning, it will be smooth sailing.

Ready? Then, let's go!

1. *Consider your vegan fast-food options.* Imagine traveling across the country on Route 66, and your buddy Jim suggests pulling over for some KFC Chicken Pot Pie. He likes the five-dollar "fill up" deal that includes a medium coke and a chocolate chip cookie, too. And Jim's not alone. The "fill up" deals are what's being hailed as the reason for KFC's boost in business this year.[1] They've even created the "family fill-up" for twenty dollars, so mom, pop, and the kids can all fill up together, and sales are strong. How much do you get for your money? Let's take a look at the ingredient list for a KFC Chicken Pot Pie:

KFC'S CHICKEN POT PIE *Chicken Stock, Potatoes (with Sodium Acid Pyrophosphate to Protect Color), Carrots, Peas, Heavy Cream, Food Starch Modified, Contains 2% or Less of Wheat Flour, Salt, Chicken Fat, Dried Dairy Blend (Whey, Calcium Caseinate), Butter (Cream, Salt), Natural Flavor (Salt, Natural Flavoring, Maltodextrin, Whey Powder, Nonfat Dry Milk, Chicken Fat, Ascorbic Acid [to Help Protect Flavor], Sesame Oil, Chicken Broth Powder), Monosodium Glutamate, Liquid Margarine (Vegetable Oil Blend [Liquid Soybean, Hydrogenated Soybean], Water, Salt, Vegetable Mono and Diglycerides, Beta Carotene [Color]), Roasted Garlic Juice Flavor (Garlic Juice, Salt, Natural Flavors), Roasted Onion Juice Flavor (Onion Juice, Salt, Natural Flavors), Gelatin, Chicken Pot Pie Flavor (Hydrolyzed Corn, Soy and Wheat Gluten Protein, Salt, Vegetable Stock [Carrot, Onion, Celery], Maltodextrin, Flavors, Dextrose, Chicken Broth), Sugar, Mono and Diglycerides, Spice, Seasoning (Soybean Oil, Oleoresin Turmeric, Spice Extractives), Parsley, Citric Acid, Caramel Color, Yellow 5. Enriched Flour Bleached (Wheat Flour, Niacin, Ferrous Sulfate, Thiamin Mononitrate, Riboflavin, Folic Acid), Hydrogenated Palm Kernel Oil, Water, Nonfat Milk, Maltodextrin, Salt, Dextrose, Sugar, Whey, Natural Flavor, Soy Lecithin, Citric Acid, Dough Conditioner (L-Cysteine Hydrochloride), Potassium Sorbate and Sodium Benzoate (Preservatives), Colored with Yellow 5 & Red 40. Fresh Chicken Marinated with: Salt, Sodium Phosphate and Monosodium Glutamate. Breaded with: Wheat Flour, Salt, Spices, Monosodium Glutamate, Corn Starch, Leavening (Sodium Bicarbonate), Garlic Powder, Modified Corn Starch, Spice Extractives, Citric Acid and 2% Calcium Silicate added as an Anticaking Agent. Or Fresh Chicken Marinated with: Salt, Sodium Phosphate and Monosodium Glutamate. Breaded with: Wheat Flour, Salt, Spices, Monosodium Glutamate, Corn Starch, Leavening (Sodium Bicarbonate), Garlic Powder, Natural Flavorings, Citric Acid, Maltodextrin, Sugar, Corn Syrup Solids, with not more than 2% Calcium Silicate added as Anticaking Agent. Or Fresh Chicken Marinated with Water, Seasoning (Salt, Modified Corn Starch, Sodium Phosphates, Monosodium Glutamate, Potassium Phosphate, and Carrageenan.) Seasoned with: Maltodextrin, Salt, Bleached Wheat Flour, Partially Hydrogenated Soybean and Cottonseed Oil, Monosodium Glutamate, Spice, Palm Oil, Natural Flavor, Garlic Powder, Soy Sauce (Soybean, Wheat, Salt), Chicken Fat, Chicken Broth, Autolyzed Yeast Extract, Extractives of Turmeric, Dehydrated Carrot, Onion Powder, and not more than 2% each of Calcium Silicate and Silicon Dioxide added as Anticaking Agents. Or Fresh Chicken Marinated with: Salt, Sodium Phosphate and Monosodium Glutamate. Breaded* with: Wheat Flour, Sodium Chloride and Anticaking agent (Tricalcium Phosphate), Whey, Nonfat Milk, Egg Whites, Corn Starch, Potato Starch, Maltodextrin, Triglycerides, Natural Flavoring (Milk), Gelatin (from Chicken), Colonel's Secret Original Recipe Seasoning. Or Chicken Tenderloins or Chicken Breast Strips, Seasoning (Modified Potato Starch, Salt, Onion Powder, Natural Chicken Flavor [with Maltodextrin, Autolyzed Yeast Extract, Chicken Fat, Dehydrated Cooked Chicken], Spice Extractive), with not more than 2% Silicon Dioxide added as an Anticaking Agent, Potassium and Sodium Phosphates. Breaded with: Wheat Flour, Salt, Spices, Monosodium Glutamate, Corn Starch, Leavening (Sodium Bicarbonate), Garlic Powder, Modified Corn Starch, Spice Extractives, Citric Acid and 2% Calcium Silicate added as an Anticaking Agent. Or Chicken Tenderloins or Chicken Breast Strips, Seasoning (Modified Potato Starch, Salt, Onion Powder, Natural Chicken Flavor [with Maltodextrin, Autolyzed Yeast Extract, Chicken Fat, Dehydrated Cooked Chicken], Spice Extractive), with not more than 2% Silicon Dioxide added as an Anticaking Agent, Potassium and Sodium Phosphates. Breaded with: Wheat Flour, Salt, Spices, Monosodium Glutamate, Corn Starch, Leavening (Sodium Bicarbonate), Garlic Powder, Natural Flavorings, Citric Acid, Maltodextrin, Sugar, Corn Syrup Solids, with not more than 2% Calcium Silicate added as an Anticaking Agent. Or Fresh Chicken Marinated with: Salt, Sodium Phosphate, Monosodium Glutamate, Salt, Spices, Mono and Diglycerides, Spice Extractives, Garlic Powder and Calcium Silicate. Breaded with: Wheat Flour, Salt, Spices, Monosodium Glutamate, Corn Starch, Leavening (Sodium Bicarbonate), Garlic Powder, Modified Corn Starch, Spice Extractives, Citric Acid and 2% Calcium Silicate added as an Anticaking Agent. Or Fresh Chicken Marinated with: Salt, Sodium Phosphate, Monosodium Glutamate, Salt, Spice, Mono and Diglycerides, Spice Extractives, Garlic Powder and Calcium Silicate. Breaded with: Wheat Flour, Salt, Spices, Monosodium Glutamate, Corn Starch, Leavening (Sodium Bicarbonate), Garlic Powder, Natural Flavorings, Citric Acid, Maltodextrin, Sugar, Corn Syrup Solids, with not more than 2% Calcium Silicate added as Anticaking Agent. Fresh Chicken Marinated with: Salt, Sodium Phosphate and Monosodium Glutamate. Breaded with: Wheat Flour, Salt, Tricalcium Phosphate, Whey, Nonfat Milk, Egg Whites, Corn Starch, Potato Starch, Maltodextrin, Triglycerides, Natural Flavoring (Milk), Gelatin (from Chicken), Colonel's Secret Original Recipe Seasoning. Or Fresh Chicken Marinated with: Salt, Sodium Phosphate and Monosodium Glutamate. Breaded with: Wheat Flour, Salt, Spices, Monosodium Glutamate, Corn Starch, Leavening (Sodium Bicarbonate), Garlic Powder, Modified Corn Starch, Spice Extractives, Citric Acid and 2% Calcium Silicate added as an Anticaking Agent. Or Fresh Chicken Marinated with: Salt, Sodium Phosphate and Monosodium Glutamate. Breaded with: Wheat Flour, Salt, Spices, Monosodium Glutamate, Corn Starch, Leavening (Sodium Bicarbonate), Garlic Powder, Natural Flavorings, Citric Acid, Maltodextrin, Sugar, Corn Syrup Solids, with not more than 2% Calcium Silicate added as Anticaking Agent. Or fresh Chicken Marinated with: Salt, Sodium Phosphate and Monosodium Glutamate. Seasoned with: Maltodextrin, Salt, Bleached Wheat Flour, Partially Hydrogenated Soybean and Cottonseed Oil, Monosodium Glutamate, Spice, Palm Oil, Natural Flavor, Garlic Powder, Soy Sauce (Soybean, Wheat, Salt), Chicken Fat, Chicken Broth, Autolyzed Yeast Extract, Extractives of Turmeric, Dehydrated Carrot, Onion Powder, and not more than 2% each of Calcium Silicate and Silicon Dioxide added as

Anticaking Agents. Or Fresh Chicken Marinated with: Salt, Sodium Phosphate, Monosodium Glutamate, Spice, Mono and Diglycerides, Spice Extractives, Garlic Powder and Calcium Silicate. Breaded with: Wheat Flour, Salt, Spices, Monosodium Glutamate, Leavening (Sodium Bicarbonate), Garlic Powder, Natural Flavorings, Citric Acid, Maltodextrin, Sugar, Corn Syrup Solids, with not more than 2% Calcium Silicate added as an Anticaking Agent. Or Fresh Chicken Marinated with: Salt, Sodium Phosphate, Monosodium Glutamate, Spice, Mono and Diglycerides, Spice Extractives, Garlic Powder and Calcium Silicate. Breaded with: Wheat Flour, Salt, Spices, Monosodium Glutamate, Corn Starch, Leavening (Sodium Bicarbonate), Garlic Powder, Modified Corn Starch, Spice Extractives, Citric Acid, and 2% Calcium Silicate added as Anticaking Agent. Or Chicken Breast Tenderloins or Chicken Breast Strips with Rib Meat Marinated with: Seasoning (Modified Potato Starch, Salt, Onion Powder, Natural Chicken Flavor [with Maltodextrin, Autolyzed Yeast Extract, Chicken Fat, Dehydrated Cooked Chicken], Spice Extractive), Potassium and Sodium Phosphates. Breaded with: Wheat Flour, Salt, Spices, Monosodium Glutamate, Corn Starch, Leavening (Sodium Bicarbonate), Garlic Powder, Modified Corn Starch, Spice Extractives, Citric Acid and 2% Calcium Silicate added as an Antcaking Agent. Or Chicken Breast Tenderloins or Chicken Breast Strips with Rib Meat Marinated with: Seasoning (Modified Potato Starch, Salt, Onion Powder, Natural Chicken Flavor [with Maltodextrin, Autolyzed Yeast Extract, Chicken Fat, Dehydrated Cooked Chicken], Spice Extractive), Potassium and Sodium Phosphates. Breaded with: Wheat Flour, Salt, Spices, Monosodium Glutamate, Corn Starch, Leavening (Sodium Bicarbonate), Garlic Powder, Natural Flavorings, Citric Acid, Maltodextrin, Sugar, Corn Syrup Solids, with not more than 2% Calcium Silicate added as Anticaking Agent.)[2]

I know. I couldn't believe it, either.

I think you get the point: Food that's easy to grab while you're on the road can be pretty darn disgusting. The good news is, when you're *vegan*, you tend to make better choices just by default, even at fast-food joints. So if you're in a pinch, vegan fast-food will do. And no matter how "bad" it is, your choice will certainly be healthier than Jim's Chicken Pot Pie and a host of other Standard American Diet (SAD) menu items. So let's make a run for the border and see what's out there! First stop? Taco Bell!

I don't eat at Taco Bell anymore, but if you get what I call "shaky hungry" while you're on the road, and you're nowhere near healthier fare, Taco Bell can save the famished newbie vegan. Check out the "What's Vegan at Taco Bell" list and get creative. Even their guacamole is vegan. Score! And don't feel like you're being unusually difficult by customizing your order; over 60 percent of Taco Bell customers already do![3]

WHAT'S VEGAN AT TACO BELL (Certified by the American Vegetarian Association)

Black Beans

Border Sauce (Fire, Hot, Mild, Verde)

Cantina Salsa

Cilantro

Flatbread

Green Chili Sauce

Green Tomatillo Sauce

Guacamole

Jalapeños

Lettuce

Mexican Pizza Sauce

Onions

Pico de Gallo

Premium Latin Rice

Rainforest Coffee

Red Sauce

Refried Beans

Romaine Lettuce

Salsa del Sol

Taco Shells

Tomatoes

Tortilla

Tostada Shell

And here's a quick snapshot of a few other vegan fast-food ideas for when you're getting your kicks on Route 66, or any other highway across the country.

- **DEL TACO:** You can "veganize" the Jacked Up Value Bean and Cheese Burrito with red or green sauce, the 8-Layer Veggie Burrito, or the ½ lb. Bean & Cheese Burrito. Just ask for no cheese, no rice, and no sour cream.

- **EL POLLO LOCO:** To "veganize" the BRC Burrito, just ask for no cheese. The pinto beans and corn on the cob are vegan, too.

- **JACK IN THE BOX:** The black beans, potato wedges, seasoned curly fries, and their breakfast blueberry muffin oatmeal are all vegan.

- **WHITE CASTLE:** Check out the veggie sliders. Even the buns are vegan!

- **DUNKIN' DONUTS:** In a breakfast mood? Grab a bagel or some hash browns.

- **IN N OUT:** It's the one thing I'll still eat at a fast-food restaurant if I'm "shaky hungry" and feel like I'm going to pass out: In N Out french fries! They only have three ingredients: potatoes, oil, and salt. And you can even ask them to leave off the salt if you want. This little snack has saved me more than once on late-night road trips, when I'm driving alone and don't want to get out of the car.

And a sample of what you can order at mainstream restaurants while you're on the road, too!

- ❧ **CHEESECAKE FACTORY**: Vegan cobb salad

- ❧ **OLIVE GARDEN**: Tri-colored vegetable penne with kids' tomato sauce, steamed broccoli, and breadsticks

- ❧ **JOHNNY ROCKETS**: Streamliner burger with American fries

- ❧ **SUBWAY**: Veggie sub on Italian or sourdough bread with spicy mustard dressing and avocado, with Minestrone soup

- ❧ **CHIPOTLE**: Sofritas bowl, taco, and burrito

- ❧ **P.F. CHANG'S**: Orange-peel tofu and Chang's vegetarian lettuce wraps

- ❧ **ZPIZZA**: Berkeley vegan pizza

- ❧ **DENNY'S**: Veggie burger and fries, with a side salad

- ❧ **OUTBACK STEAKHOUSE**: Plain baked sweet potato, steamed fresh seasonal mixed vegetables (hold the seasoned butter), and house bread.

- ❧ **CHILI'S**: Fresh guacamole with flour tortillas and a side of black beans and citrus-chili rice

VEGAN FAST-FOOD HEAVEN!

Organic burgers, shakes, fries, mac 'n' cheese, pizza, burritos, chili—Amy's Drive Thru has vegan versions of it all. See www.amysdrivethru.com. This solar powered fast-food restaurant is a great stop if you're ever road trippin' it near Petaluma, California. My favorite roadside snack-a-roos? The vegan vanilla shake, "The Amy" burger ("veganized"), and the fresh lemonade! All organic! Business is booming, so fingers-crossed Amy's Drive Thru's spread across the nation. Times they are a changin'!

- **LITTLE CAESAR'S PIZZA**: Veggie pizza with no cheese

- **PIZZA HUT**: Thin and crispy pizza with marinara sauce (no cheese) and veggies

- **MELLOW MUSHROOM PIZZA BAKERS**: They have an entire vegan menu, with three types of vegan hoagies, too!

- **PIZZAREV**: Original crust pizza with daiya cheese and veggies

- **PIZZA NOVA**: Veggie pizza with daiya cheese

- **PANERA**: Low-fat vegetarian black bean soup or soba noodle bowl with edamame

- **UNCLE MADDIO'S**: Build your own pizza with 3 vegan crusts, 6 vegan sauces, vegan cheese, and 22 vegetable toppings!

This is by no means all-inclusive. There's a whole lot more that you can enjoy so don't worry, you'll be in great shape! (Well, I can't guarantee you'll be in great "shape" if you eat junk food, but you know what I mean. Wink.)

OK, now let's see what happens if we plan ahead. After all, when we don't, we're more likely to make eating choices by impulse rather than intention, and that can lead to very unhealthy habits. If you want to go vegan and *stay* vegan, a little bit of forethought goes a long way!

2. *Learn to plan ahead.* There's probably no better piece of advice I can give you about planning your trip in advance than these three words: **Use Happy Cow!** Need I say more? HappyCow.net is amazing and an essential tool for the happy vegan traveler. It's a fantastic first step. Just plug in the name of the city you're traveling to or through, and it will pull up an array of vegan options available. Check out the newly launched website vegantravel.com, too. It's very cool!

READ REVIEWS: Explore the comments on TripAdvisor.com and Yelp.com. If you go to their websites, you can search any location and enter the keyword *vegan* and not only find vegan options, but also all of the comments left by folks who mention the word *vegan*. This will help you see if guests had a good or bad experience with a particular vegan meal or stay. You'll also find good experiences at non-vegan establishments as well, which I think is very helpful. Just keep in mind that people with bad experiences tend to post more often than those with good ones. When people have a positive experience, they tell eight people on average, but when it's a bad experience, they blast it out to about sixty-four.[4] Misery loves company.

CALL IN ADVANCE: Whether it's the airline, hotel, restaurant, cruise, or *any* aspect of your vegan adventure, make sure you call in advance to see if they have the food and amenities you want, and if they don't, you'll know to make arrangements of your own. If you're calling a restaurant or a conference venue, you might want to politely ask to speak with the chef or someone who's in the kitchen, as whoever answers the phone might not know how the food is actually prepared. If you're calling a hotel, instead of speaking with the front desk, you might want to politely ask for the hotel manager, guest services, or the concierge, as they're used to accommodating our crazy, *ahem*, I mean *special*, requests. It's pretty common these days for hotels to provide a mini refrigerator or microwave, too, if you request one in advance. If hotel or restaurant menus seem lacking when it comes to vegan food, you can usually just combine vegan sides to make your own meal, just ask them to leave off the butter or any other animal products they might add. Don't forget to call your airline, too, as most offer vegan meals to those who request them. Just be sure to give them at least 72 hours' notice.

SPEAK UP: Ask and you shall receive. I recently went to a restaurant at DisneyWorld that didn't look like it would have much to offer in terms of vegan fare, but I was pooped and hungry, so I took a chance and asked the hostess if they had any vegan food. And you know what? She reached into the podium, and pulled out an entire vegan menu! Appetizers, entrées, desserts, the works! I couldn't believe it. And I'm not alone; this has been happening to a lot of people, at a lot of unexpected places. A friend of mine recently had the same experience at an ice cream shop; she was presented with a full *vegan* ice cream menu! But if you don't ask, you'll likely never know.

Hotels and restaurants often have nut milks on hand, too, even if it's not on the menu, or missing from the complementary breakfast bar or buffet, so be sure to ask. Once I called a hotel in advance and expressed my concern about having access to enough vegan food during my three-day stay, and when I arrived I was given two keys: one to my room, and one highly unexpected key to the special "club" room, where the more affluent guests get freebies all day long. I had access to as much fresh fruit, French bread, hummus, crudités, nuts, and beverages as I wanted, all for free, and all just because I asked politely. Vegans still get the super-confused *"huh?"* reaction now and then, but hey, it's thanks to everyone asking politely that things are getting easier. So don't assume something's not available. Ask. You might be pleasantly surprised!

MAKE A QUICK STOP INTO A GROCERY STORE: Every grocery store has *something* you can eat while you're traveling. When my husband and I got hungry on the road recently, we ran into Trader Joe's, bought two bags of butterleaf lettuce and a bottle of their Goddess Dressing and took it back to the hotel. We poured the dressing straight into the bags, which served as our bowls, and gobbled the good stuff up. So easy! Cheap and delicious, too. Get creative. You've got this!

BRING YOUR OWN FOOD: Bringing your own food not only gives you peace of mind, it's usually a lot cheaper and healthier, too. A variety of nuts, sandwiches, Clif Bars, Larabars, dried fruit, fresh fruit and veggies make great traveling food. And if you have access to hot water (which is as simple as asking nicely at a Starbucks), you can even enjoy a cup of instant soup or a ramen bowl. Heck, you can even just pack up a few cans of baked beans, or any other canned goods you like, as long as you bring a can opener; just pick one up at the Dollar Tree for a buck, and you're good to go. Or even easier, grab canned beans or veggies that have pull tops. Some folks even carry around a portable plastic cutting board that rolls up, along with a small knife so they can chop fresh produce or tofu. A spoonful of peanut butter with Trader Joe's chocolate chips on top makes for a nice road trip snack. So good! And you might want to toss a plastic jar of spices in your purse, too, just in case you need to give a little zip to any bland steamed veggies. You know, that unfortunate work conference "veggie platter" of overcooked carrots, string beans, and cauliflower, that despite being different shapes and colors, all taste exactly the same? Yep, we've all been there at least once. 21 Seasoning Salute to the rescue!

You've been bringing your own food places since you smashed that brown lunch bag into your elementary school backpack. I think you know what to do here, kids. You'll be just fine!

3. *Consider using the most vegan-friendly airports whenever possible.* If you're traveling by plane, you might want to fly in or out of one of these airports, if you can. According to the Physicians Committee for Responsible Medicine's annual Airport Food Review, the following airports have the most healthful plant-based

food in the United States, offering all sorts of vegan goodies, from black bean burgers and tempeh sandwiches, to Pad Thai and vegan sushi.[5] LAX even has a 100 percent vegan restaurant, Real Food Daily. Yes, at the airport. And it's good!

- ⚜ Los Angeles International Airport
- ⚜ Newark Liberty International Airport
- ⚜ San Francisco International Airport
- ⚜ Philadelphia International Airport
- ⚜ Denver International Airport
- ⚜ Ronald Reagan Washington National Airport
- ⚜ Salt Lake City International Airport
- ⚜ Washington Dulles International Airport
- ⚜ Baltimore/Washington International Airport
- ⚜ John F. Kennedy International Airport

Even if you can't fly in or out of one of these, you should still be OK, as 71 percent of airport restaurants nationwide offer *at least* one fiber-packed, cholesterol-free, plant-based entrée.[6] You won't be stuck with a bag of pretzels, my friend. It's a great time to be vegan!

And there's vegan-friendly cruises, too. All aboard!

- ⚜ Vegan River Cruise: VeganRiverCruises.com
- ⚜ Vegan Cruise Planners: VeganCruisePlanners.com
- ⚜ Holistic Holiday at Sea: atasteofhealth.org/vegan-cruise.htm

And when the tired traveler needs to rest, here are a few vegan-lodging options if you're lucky enough to be near one:

STANFORD INN BY THE SEA, MENDOCINO, CALIFORNIA: The Stanford Inn is the only vegan eco resort in the country and it really sets the bar for those to follow. It's decked out with a serene pool, hot tub, sauna, great views, luscious gardens, fine vegan dining, and a few resident animals to play with, too. And if you're in the mood for a bike ride or canoe adventure along Mendocino's Big River, rentals are just a hop, skip, and a jump away. We went for an easy bike ride along the salt water (it travels over eight miles up from the ocean before reaching fresh water!) on a beautiful path lined with trees, wild sweet peas, and spectacular views of the river. The Stanford Inn has cooking, tai chi, and yoga classes, too. The resort is truly life-changing, and the staff couldn't be more helpful and friendly. Be sure to swing by and say hello to Sid Garza-Hillman, the resident nutritionist, and author of *Approaching the Natural: A Health Manifesto*. He'll wow you with all sorts of helpful tidbits for newbie vegans. You'll have a blast!

ADDITIONAL VEGAN ACCOMMODATIONS:

- Vero Bed and Breakfast, Eugene, Oregon
- Someday Farm Vegan Bed and Breakfast, Whidbey Island, Washington
- The Guesthouse at Woodstock Sanctuary, Woodstock, New York
- The Ginger Cat Bed & Breakfast, Rock Stream, New York
- Whisper's Ranch Bed & Breakfast, Elgin, Arizona
- Deer Run Bed & Breakfast, Big Pine Key, Florida Keys

If you're off to explore other countries and are wondering how you'll order vegan food in other languages, just search "Plant Foods Only, Please" at TranslateGoogle.com and it will translate the phrase for you. And if you'd like some nifty translation cards, in over ninety languages, here's a website where you can download and print them for free: www.maxlearning.net/HEALth/V-Cards. The Toronto Vegetarian Society has some handy translation cards, too: http://veg.ca/2013/01/17/vegetarian-travel-translation-cards. Or, you can buy a "Vegan Passport" from The Vegan Society. It's a multilingual vegan phrasebook that's small enough to fit in your pocket, that not only provides translations in eighty-five different languages, but has pictures to help folks understand, too.[7] *Fantastique!*

TRANSLATION OF "PLANT FOODS ONLY, PLEASE"[8]

- Croatian: *Biljne namirnice samo molim*
- French: *Les aliments végétaux seulement, s'il vous plaît*
- Spanish: *Los alimentos vegetales por favor solamente*
- Chinese (simplified): 只有植物性食物, 请 *Zhǐwù xìng shíwù zh⬚ néng q⬚ng*
- Japanese: 植物性食品のみお願い*Shokubutsu-sei shokuhin nomi onegai*
- German: *Nur pflanzliche Nahrungsmittel bitte*
- Russian:только растительные продукты, пожалуйста (*Tol'ko rastitel'nyye produkty, pozhaluysta*)
- Italy: *Solo cibi vegetali per favore*
- Korean: 식물성 식품 만 하시기 바랍니다 (*Sigmulseong sigpum man hasigi balabnida*)
- Norwegian: *Matplanter bare kan*

VEGAN SUNSCREENS FOR FUN IN THE SUN

- Kiss My Face Natural Mineral Sunscreen SPF 40
- Ocean Potion Protect & Nourish SPF 50
- Nature's Gate Aqua Vegan Sunscreen SPF 50
- Alba Botanica Very Emollient Sunscreen Pure Lavender SPF 45

Checklist

☐ Did you check out Happy Cow, Vegan Travel, and Trip Advisor to explore vegan-friendly restaurants and accommodations for your next adventure?

☐ Did you think about what you'd pack to eat for your next road trip?

☐ Did you figure out where you'd stop for a quick bite should you forget to pack your own food?

Thought FOR THE Day

Every bite you take, and every thing you buy, casts a vote for the kind of world you wish to live in.

DAY 17

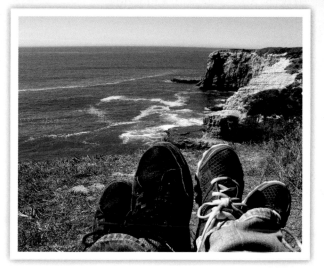

Now, THAT'S *Entertainment!*

GOAL FOR THE DAY: Plan out an adventure that doesn't involve the abuse of animals.

Watching an orca do tricks while living his entire life in an area that to him is the size of a bathtub isn't entertainment; it's sadistic. Watching lions jump through rings of fire, or lonely elephants do stunts thanks to the prod of sharp bull hooks isn't fun, it's depressing. Thanks to the efforts of advocates, and films like *The Cove* and *Blackfish*, the dark side of animals in entertainment is slowly losing its veil. People may have felt duped by slick marketing campaigns showing smiling dolphins who seemingly want to swim with you. Some may have been temporarily swayed by the industries' insistence that the "educational" nature of zoos and animal parks outweigh any tragedies that occur. But the days of blissful naivete have passed now. The word is out, and we all know cruelty *isn't entertaining*. So skip the zoos, the animal circuses, the aquariums, the rodeos, the fishing contests, and the hunting trips. And let's pass on gawking at those lonely animals at roadside attractions, too. Check out all of these great ideas instead. Remember, good entertainment is "all for fun, and fun for *all*," and when you're vegan, that means everyone.

All right, let's have some fun!

1. *Instead of going to the zoo, pony rides, or a roadside animal attraction, consider an animal sanctuary.* If you've never been to an animal sanctuary, you're in for a real treat, especially if you go on Thanksgiving. I went one year and instead of eating a turkey, I found myself kissing one. Smooch! They're as cute as cute can be. And so soft, too! The three animal sanctuaries that I've been lucky enough to visit are: Animal Place, Farm Sanctuary, and 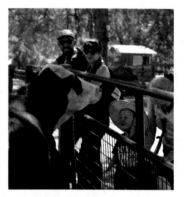 the Gentle Barn. All are unique, highly educational, and full of inspiration. And they're run by the sweetest volunteers ever! Most have picnic areas, where you can enjoy your vegan lunch from home, and bask in the sunshine knowing that everyone around you is eating vegan food, too. And the *best* part? You get to cuddle with the animals! Check out the list of animal sanctuaries in the Resource section (page 284) and see if there's one near you. Some even have special events, such as the Celebration of the Turkeys at Farm Sanctuary, where you get open-barn time to meet the Farm Sanctuary animal residents and experience their famous turkey-feeding ceremony where you help them treat the beloved turkeys to a feast of squash, cranberries, and pumpkin pie! They even have bed and breakfast cabins if you want to make a vacation out of it. These events generally sell out well before the date, so plan ahead. Whenever I visit a sanctuary, I never want to leave. No offense, Mickey, but to vegans like me, an animal sanctuary is the happiest place on earth.

2. *Instead of going to a circus that has animals, consider one without.* Thank goodness countries across the world are banning the use of animals in circuses.[1] It's about

time! Just waiting until the good ole' U.S. of A does, too, but until then, cities across the country are taking action independently and putting their foot down. San Francisco not only bans all exotic animals from performing in the city, but from motion pictures, too.[2] And it makes sense. If you were a wild animal, where would you rather

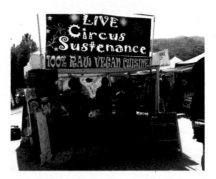

be? On a scorching hot film set where the director just can't get the shot right, so you have to perform a trick for the umpteenth try, just so a movie producer can make the big bucks? And then back to your cage? Or would you rather be out in the wild, free to roam on the land where you were born, enjoying life with your friends and family? When you push profits aside, the choice is clear.

Once folks know the truth about how animals are stolen from their families, and then poked, prodded, and shocked into doing tricks just for kicks, most don't want any part of it. I once helped PETA organize a peaceful protest when Ringling Brothers came to town in San Diego, and when I explained to the circus goers who were proceeding to the door how the animals were treated, an entire family of ten gave me their tickets, walked back to the parking lot, and drove away. People really do want to do the right thing. It's just a matter of getting the truth out there and letting them know there are other, far better ways to enjoy the day. Lucky for us, there are still lots of animal-free circuses that are full of excitement! Cirque du Soleil, anyone? Check out the list of Animal-Free Circuses on page 285 in the Resources section, and pick out one that sounds like fun to you!

3. *Instead of a horse-drawn carriage ride, consider a bike ride.* Nine hours a day, seven days a week, in boiling hot weather or the freezing cold, horses schlep carriages full of people around the city because folks think it's romantic. Yep. Nothing says "I love you" like a horse with four tootsies on frost or boiling-hot cement, lungs full of car

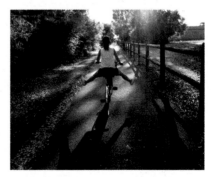

exhaust, and a back burdened by heavy weight as they drag lovebirds around town to the sound of honking horns and screeching cars. When the exhausted horse is done hauling the duo and their box of See's chocolate about Manhattan, the horse goes back to her tiny city stall, never setting foot on grass or enjoying the world as most other horses do.[3] And as you've probably guessed by now, there's no idyllic retirement home for a horse once the man holding the control reins is done with her. I'm pretty sure you've noticed a pattern by now, and know exactly what happens next.

May I interest you in a bike ride, milady or fine gent? When's the last time you rode a bike just for fun? I started riding mine again a few years ago and it's a blast! There's an abundance of countryside paths, and routes along the ocean, too. Our most recent bike ride was along Big River in Mendocino, California, which I raved about in "Vegan Wanderlust." Amazing! And you don't need a fancy bike, either. I have a hand-me-down beach cruiser, which works just fine for easy trails, and if you don't have a bike, you can easily find one at a garage sale, or you can rent one. You can also rent tandem bikes for you and your sweetheart, or a surrey for the whole family. My bike has an awesome little bell (Ring! Ring!) to let passersby know how happy I am, and it also has a big basket, which makes it easy to bring along a yummy vegan picnic and blanket, too. So drop that stale box of See's, let the horses be, and hop on your wheels and have some heart-healthy fun! It's a beautiful world; go out and enjoy it!

4. *Instead of a marine park or aquarium, consider an aquatic ecotour, sea life sanctuary visit, or snorkeling.* My best advice for kicking the perverse obsession with watching captive ocean animals in small tanks is to watch *Blackfish*, which streams on Netflix. And if you're up to a double feature, you can follow it up with *The Cove* on Netflix, too. Every 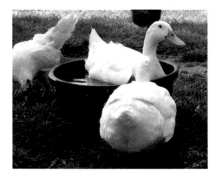 time I learn more about how sea life is treated and confined for entertainment purposes, I get teary eyed and sick to my stomach. I couldn't make it through either film, and if you can't, either, I completely understand. But if you're not aware of what happens to these animals, you should at least give it a shot. Watching the footage will inspire you to create change, and that's always a good thing.

Let's think of the beautiful ocean for a moment. I know you can't see the vastness of it all very well from land, but imagine huge mountains, only turned upside down and filled with salt water and beautiful aquatic life all swirling about in the mysterious depth of the sea. At 35,837 feet, the Pacific Ocean is *far* deeper than the highest mountain is tall, by a long shot. Just try to get your mind around that for a moment. Now envision the animals being captured and dropped into the tiny tanks at the aquariums and pools. No one I know of is willing to be sacrificed and held captive in the name of research before they're dead. Any volunteers? No one wants to live in an area that to them is the size of a tub, performing tricks for their entire lives, either. While it's believed there are thousands of orcas and dolphins still in captivity, cities and entire countries are starting to ban the practice, with India's ban going as far as referring to dolphins as "non-human persons."[4] There's hope my friends, truly there is. As my father's good friend and chess partner Jimmy used to say whenever anyone was down, "This, too, shall pass." And it will.

In the meantime, there's still lots of fun to be had! How's about snorkeling? Or a day out on a kayak? There are often guided tours so you'll know where to look for the animals. Or perhaps consider visiting a sanctuary. One that I really enjoy, and have been to often, is Piedras Blancas, just above San Simeon in California. You can watch hundreds of elephant seals being absolutely adorable, lounging around as they rest on the sand twice each year, after swimming thousands of miles. Can you imagine sticking one in a tank? And then paying to watch them float in it? Boggles the mind.

In the 1800s elephant seals were thought to be extinct, so it's a real treat to be able to watch so many of them enjoying the freedom and protection they deserve. And unlike pricey SeaWorld and aquariums, watching the elephant seals is free. Just bundle up, grab your camera, and be prepared to be wowed. If it's too far away from you, the Friends of the Elephant Seal website has a "Seal Cam" you can watch: www.elephantseal.org. I'm also posting a link to "SENSE-able" whale watches in the Resource section, which lists responsible whale watching tours, if that floats your boat. Bon voyage!

5. *Instead of going to a rodeo, go watch humans duke it out.* Although I'm not a fan of people getting their kicks watching other people hurt each other, at least the participants at a mixed martial arts (MMA) match have a choice to refrain from the abuse. Bulls at rodeos aren't afforded the same luxury. Amongst the horrors is the practice of making the animals seem more aggressive by using a "hotshot,"

an electric prod used on the animal while captive in the chute.[5] Bulls also have to endure a "bucking strap" that's placed tightly around their abdomen, along with metal spurs, causing so much pain that they buck, just as intended.[6] After all, no one paying good money to go to the rodeo wants to see a calm and happy animal.

Calf roping is self-explanatory. Why someone would want to pay to watch a guy whip a rope around a baby cow's neck and slam her to the ground is beyond me. That's not talent, that's misplaced anger. Seek help, Mr. Rodeo Man, *stat*. Unless there's a state or local law, the treatment while transporting the animals isn't much better. They can truck them around for twenty-four hours without a morsel of food or a drop of water, because yet again, the calves are exempt from the Federal Animal Welfare Act.

6. *Still looking for more fun? Head out to a Veggie Festival!*

CALIFORNIA

WorldFest Los Angeles
Animal Place's Music in the Meadows benefit
Farm Sanctuary Hoe Down!
Eat Drink Vegan (formerly Los Angeles Vegan Beer & Food Festival)
Oakland Veg Week
SacTown VegFest
San Diego Veg Festival
San Francisco's World Veg Festival
SoCal VegFest
Sonoma County VegFest

DISTRICT OF COLUMBIA

DC VegFest

FLORIDA

North Florida VegFest
Central Florida Veg Fest
Northeast Florida Veg Fest
Tampa Bay Veg Fest

GEORGIA

Atlanta Veg Fest

ILLINOIS

Veggie Fest Chicago

Chicago VeganMania

Chicago Veggie Pride Parade

LOUISIANA

New Orleans Vegan Food Festival

MAINE

Maine Animal Coalition's Vegetarian Food Festival

MARYLAND

Baltimore VegFest

MASSACHUSETTS

Boston Vegetarian Food Festival

New England (formerly Worcester) VegFest

MICHIGAN

Michigan's VegFest

Grand Rapids VegFest

MINNESOTA

Twin Cities Veg Fest

NEW MEXICO

Red and Green VegFest Albuquerque

NEW YORK

Farm Sanctuary Celebration for the Turkeys

Farm Sanctuary Hoe Down!

NYC Vegetarian Food Festival

Veggie Pride Parade NYC

WNY VegFest

Woodstock Fruit Festival

NORTH CAROLINA

Asheville VeganFest

Charlotte VegFest

Triangle VegFest

OHIO

Cleveland VegFest

OREGON

Eat Drink Vegan

Portland VegFest

PENNSYLVANIA

Bethlehem VegFest

Philly VegFest

Vegetarian Summerfest

TEXAS

VegFest Houston

Texas VegFest

Texas Veggie Fair

HealthFest

VIRGINIA

Hampton Roads VegFest

WASHINGTON

Seattle VegFest

Spokane VegFest

WISCONSIN

Mad City Vegan Fest

INTERNATIONAL
AUSTRALIA

Cruelty Free Festival

World Vegan Day

BELGIUM

Ieper Hardcore Fest

CANADA

VegFest Guelph (Ontario)

Halifax VegFest (Nova Scotia)

VegFest Hamilton (Ontario)

VegFest London (Ontario)

Montreal Vegan Festival

Niagara VegFest

VegFest Vancouver

Victoria, Vegan Fest (Victoria BC)

Toronto Vegetarian Food Festival

ENGLAND

West Midlands Vegan Festival (veganmidlands.org.uk/festival/home.html)

Cheltenham Vegan Festival (cheltveganfair.moonfruit.com)

Kent Vegan Festival (www.facebook.com/KentVeganFestival)

Lancaster Vegan Fayre

Newcastle Vegan Festival (veganfestival.co.uk)

Northern Vegan Festival (northernveganfestival.com)

VegFest London (london.vegfest.co.uk)

HONG KONG

Hong Kong Veg Fest

ISRAEL

Vegan Fest

SCOTLAND

VegFest Scotland

Checklist

☐ Did you select a way to enjoy animals and the outdoors without harming anyone?

☐ Are you still enjoying a nut or seed milk in lieu of dairy milk?

☐ Are you trying to increase the amount of fresh produce in your meals?

Thought FOR THE Day

"Of all the creatures ever made, Man is the most detestable. He is the only creature that inflicts pain for sport, knowing it to be pain."

—MARK TWAIN

DAY 18

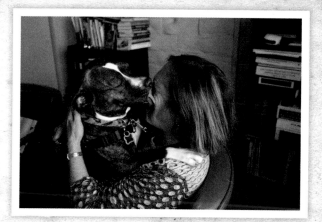

Adopt, DON'T Shop

GOAL FOR THE DAY: To understand why and how to help solve our feline and canine overpopulation problem, and put a few emergency numbers on the fridge.

The United States Humane Society estimates that roughly 2.7 million healthy, adoptable cats and dogs, *about one every 11 seconds*, are killed in U.S. shelters each year. This is one reason why vegans don't buy animals at "pet" stores, and instead rescue homeless animals that are either abandoned on the streets, or available for adoption at local shelters and rescue organizations. By the time you finish reading this paragraph, another healthy dog or cat will have been put to sleep. And just like that, they're gone.

What most folks don't seem to realize is that when you let one dog or cat run around without being "fixed" it doesn't trigger just one new batch of puppies or kittens, but potentially hundreds or thousands of them, as each newborn grows up and goes on to reproduce puppies or kittens of their own. The figures are shocking. According to the University of California Davis, School of Veterinary Medicine, in seven years, just one unspayed female and one unneutered male cat—along with their offspring, and all who follow—can produce up to 781,250 kittens.[1] Considering that there aren't enough good homes for all of them, when you spay or neuter a dog or cat, you're potentially saving thousands of lives just by that one small act. If your dog or cat goes outside, spaying or neutering also helps keep them close to home, as when mating season rolls around, they'll be less likely to wander and get into fights or hit by cars.

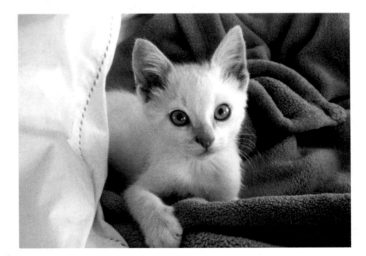

1. *Spay and neuter your companion animals.*

Some people don't think they can afford spaying or neutering animals, so they put it off until it's too late, and then before you know it kittens or puppies are on the way. But guess what? It is affordable, and in many cases even *free*. Check out the map at aspca.org/pet-care/spayneuter and enter your location to find an affordable spay and neuter clinic, or call your local SPCA or humane society. If your income is very low, ask if they can provide you with a free voucher. They also generally have cruelty-free traps that you can borrow to capture any feral kitties in your neighborhood who need to be spayed or neutered. We have skunks where we live, so when I caught our feral kitty Alfalfa, using a trap wasn't an option; I'm pretty sure Mr. Skunkie would have been upset with the contraption, and would have let me know just how much. Instead, I spent six long months coaxing Alfalfa into the house, and then shut the door. It wasn't easy, but now he's neutered, and with being FIV positive (aka kitty HIV), it's nice to know he's safe and sound, and not outside infecting any other kitties with the virus. He's also protected from coyotes. Peace of mind rocks.

2. *When you see or suspect animal abuse, report it.*

While in law school, I had the pleasure of meeting Nicole Pallotta, the student programs coordinator at the Animal Legal Defense Fund, and Teagan, the beautiful German Shepherd she adopted. Teagan was a victim of severe abuse and neglect before being rescued by Rocky Ridge Refuge in Arkansas, and as Nicole explains, it may be too late to get justice for Teagan, but her story will hopefully inspire others to be alert for animals who need our help, and to take action.

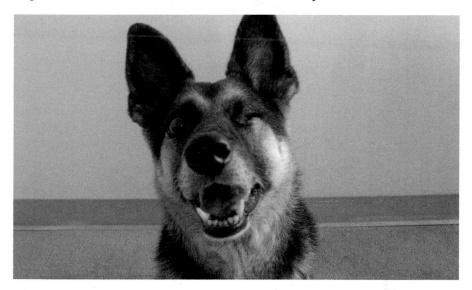

"Teagan was shot at close range and left for dead in central Mississippi. The bullet destroyed her left eye along with several teeth. Her front leg was trapped in her collar, creating a gash that cut deeper into her flesh with every painful step. Her back legs were crooked and deformed from being in a cage that was too small for her. She was starving and upon rescue weighed only fifteen pounds. Teagan is now a healthy thirty-eight pounds, but she will always be a tiny Shepherd, her growth likely stunted by early malnutrition and neglect. It's a wonder Teagan survived, and if a kind stranger had not discovered her, she would have died unknown and alone. Teagan's abuser was never found and the crimes against her were never reported. Despite the cruelty she suffered, Teagan has an amazing spirit and is gentle, sweet, and trusting. In the 7 months she has been with me, I have watched her truly blossom. Although it's too late to get justice for Teagan—she is one of the lucky ones, she was saved—I hope that Teagan's story can raise awareness and somehow create a ripple of positive change for animals everywhere, all of whom deserve to live a life free of cruelty and neglect."[2]

If you see an animal in immediate danger, always call 911.

Here are some other helpful references:
- United States Humane Society Dog Fighting and Cockfighting Hotline: 1-877-TIP-HSUS
- Washington D.C. Humane Society Animal Cruelty Hotline: 202-723-5730
- Humane Society of the United States Puppy Mill Hotline: 1-877-645-5847
- National Database for Lost and Found Animals: www.lostfoundpets.us
- PETA's Animal Abuse Hotline: 757-622-7382

You can also report abuse that you see by completing this form online: peta.org/about-peta/contact-peta/report-cruelty

And remember, if someone is abusing their companion animals, there's a good chance they're abusing people, too. Serial killer Jeffrey Dahmer used to decorate his front lawn with impaled cat and dog heads on sticks before moving on to eating people. Folks who like to hurt others don't always draw a line between species. In Wisconsin, a study revealed that 68 percent of battered women reported that abusive partners "had also been violent towards pets or livestock,"[3] too, mostly done in their presence to intimidate and control them. And women who seek safety at shelters are almost 11 times more likely to report that their partner has hurt or killed their animals than women who have not experienced domestic abuse.[4] So keep your eyes and ears open for the animals, *and* people, and if you suspect abuse, get help fast.

- National Domestic Violence Hotline: 800-799-SAFE TDD: 800-787-3224
- National Child Abuse Hotline: 800-4-A-CHILD
- National Center on Elder Abuse (Eldercare Locator): 800-677-1116

3. *Adopting an animal has mutual benefits, too.*

By adopting an animal, not only will your furry friend provide unconditional love, they often provide an incentive to get healthy, too. If you adopt a dog, you'll have inspiration to go on more walks, companionship to keep you company, and if you're alone, an extra reason to take good care of yourself; after all, there's someone who's depending on you to take care of *them*. You'll always have someone to snuggle with at night, and someone who will be waiting anxiously for breakfast. Animals are the best!

If you adopt a dog in need from a shelter or rescue organization you'll also feel good knowing you didn't fall prey to the allure of an animal produced at a puppy mill. Female dogs are kept in cages, often cramped and dirty, where they're bred over and over again to create seemingly "perfect" puppies. When the mother dogs are past their prime, they're discarded, dumped, or auctioned off. Most puppies at "pet" stores are the product of puppy mills, and are known for having multiple physical and emotional problems, including genetic defects.

If you'd like a furry addition, consider adopting a dog like Lucy. While Animal Legal Defense Fund's Vaughn Maurice was with the Red Cross on assignment in Korea, his wife was a volunteer at a vet clinic, which would take in homeless animals on the side. One of the rescued dogs had a litter of puppies, one of which was Lucy, and they adopted her. Vaughn explains, "That was fourteen years ago. She is vegan and eats *V-Dog* dog food. Lucy has traveled to thirty-four states and has visited more dog parks than she can count." Vaughn proudly notes Lucy can bark in fluent Korean, too! Woof Woof!

HOT CARS KILL

On a 78-degree day, the temperature inside a parked car can reach between 100 and 120 degrees in just minutes—even with the windows cracked.[6] On a 90-degree day, the interior temperature can reach as high as 160 degrees in less than 10 minutes. So if it's hot, leave your pup safely at home. If you see a dog in a car on a hot day, jot down the car's make, model, and license-plate number, then quickly ask the managers of any nearby stores to make an announcement to find the car's owner. If you can't find the owner, call the police or local animal control *immediately*. And don't forget: once the cold weather hits, be sure to keep your furry friends warm, too.

Checklist

- ☐ Did you put a few important phone numbers on your fridge and in your wallet?
- ☐ Did you drink enough water today?
- ☐ Did you eat an abundance of fresh fruits and vegetables?
- ☐ Did you wiggle your booty around for a little exercise?

Thought FOR THE Day

"People who say, 'Money can't buy happiness' have never paid an adoption fee."

—UNKNOWN

DAY 19

VEGAN 911!

Tips and Tricks to Stay on the
Vegan Wagon

GOAL FOR THE DAY: Fix any bumps on the road to "Veganville." If you're sailing smoothly, feel free to cruise on by, and just swing on back here should you need any help later on.

~~~~~~~~~~

OK, listen up, y'all!

There's only one big goal today: *to deal with the most common problems that knock people off the vegan wagon.* Don't worry; everything will be fine. Let's just debrief and see what went wrong so we can get you back on track. I need a little rest anyhow. After all, I'm the one pulling the wagon, not the horses; they're off in a field where they should be, eating fresh grass in the sunshine. OK—sit down, get cozy, and let's chat.

THOSE CRAZY COMPLICATED RECIPES

Did you veer off Easy Street and buy a fancy schmancy cookbook? Or find a post on Pinterest that inspired you to set off on your own to make a vegan Baked Alaska? I just read a recipe that called for fifteen ingredients to make a simple bowl of hummus. And get this: one of them was pumpkin-flavored vodka! Like we all have that handy, right? I also just went to the library and checked out a book written by an ultra-endurance athlete, which might be one of the most beautiful vegan cookbooks I've ever seen. I'll likely break down and buy it to ogle. But if I was just starting off on my vegan journey and someone handed me that book and said, "Here's some recipes to help you go vegan," I'd fall right over from fright! It's packed with unfamiliar, pricey, and hard-to-find ingredients. Delicious for sure, but my, oh my!

If you feel like you fell off the wagon because going vegan *just feels too complicated*, take a beat to reflect, and get back to the basics. A lot of the food you already ate and enjoyed was actually vegan. Spaghetti with marinara sauce, bean and rice burritos with guacamole and salsa, oatmeal with a little brown sugar, big salads, black bean soup, veggie stir-fries, fruit bowls, peanut butter and jelly sandwiches . . . I could go on and on. Just think back to the vegan food you *already* loved before you were trying to become vegan, and enjoy those foods for a little while. Instead of adding unfamiliar ingredients right off the bat, gradually enhance your meals with them as you feel more comfortable. Get back to your comfort zone, and keep things simple and familiar.

THOSE PESKY OUTSIDE FORCES

They can be brutal, I know. If you find that you're having trouble breaking a pattern while you're out and about, try mixing things up a bit. If you can't fight picking up that cheese pizza because you pass by the pizza parlor each day, just as I did walking back from CAL, take a different route home—out of sight, out of mind. If you find you can't resist the deep-fried mozzarella sticks at the bar where you and your friends meet each weekend, suggest trying out a new hot spot. Maybe a pub that has those thick "chips" with salt and vinegar? Or garlic fries! Now we're talkin'! If you regularly meet folks at a less-than-vegan-friendly coffee shop and can't resist those dairy cream–filled pastries, see if there's a different cafe where you can chitchat. None of this has to be permanent. Sometimes we just need a brief interlude from patterns that we follow, day in and day out, that make it really difficult for us to readjust any aspect of our lives. Familiar places often make us react out of impulse rather than acting with intentional thought. It's just something you've always done there, so you just keep doing it, without even thinking. Not to mention, it's *in your face*. Take a look to see if any patterns are causing havoc, and see if you can make a small change. Heck, if I never got nudged to try out a new pub, I would have never met my husband. Who, by the way, wasn't even at the pub, but that's a whole other story. Spice things up a bit. Go out there and do something new!

THE FOOD TASTES GROSS

Does vegan food taste less spectacular than what you were hoping for? Well, let me tell you a little story about our good friend water. Water is so important to our health. Our bodies are made up from about 60 percent of it; even our bones are 31 percent water. We need it to flush out toxins and regulate our body temperature, among other things, and without it, we go downhill fast! But for whatever reason, for almost my entire life, I just didn't like drinking it. I'd go weeks without a glass of water, no joke! Then one day I tried what I call "spa water," simply because it was the water they had at a spa, and I was intrigued. I tried it, and I loved it! And it was just water with sliced cucumbers floating in it! I still loathe plain water, but now I drink water that's infused with citrus or cucumbers every day. I usually just squeeze half a lemon into a glass, or make warm lemon water. I love it so much! Just this tiny adjustment has made a world of difference for me, and my health.

Try to look back and see if there's anything little that could make a difference in your transition to going vegan, and I mean really little, just like my spa water. Did you try one brand of almond milk, and now assume you don't like *any* nut milks? If so, try another! Maybe all you need is a good seasoning to toss on food, such as a spice blend like Costco's Organic No Salt Seasoning, Bragg's Liquid Aminos, or the lovely Mrs. Dash's salt-free seasoning mix. Or kick things up a notch with a splash of sriracha! Even vegans don't like bland food. Or perhaps just increase the creaminess of sauces by creating cashew, coconut, or cauliflower creams; wonderful variations abound! Maybe you didn't like something that was raw that you might enjoy cooked, or vice versa. One bad experience with tofu has ruined a lifetime of yummy vegan food for many. Did it taste disgusting to you? If so, maybe you need to give it another shot, when it's made with more flavor. Perhaps venture out to a good Asian restaurant so an experienced chef can prepare it for you, and see if you like it there. The wrong sweetener can be a doozie, too. Stevia ruins everything for me, but maple syrup? Now that's divine! As they say, sometimes the *little* things really are the big things, so go over what's gone wrong, and see if there's a small fix that will work for you. If so, make that minor repair and get back on the train!

TOO MUCH, TOO FAST

Did you try to flip that SAD diet into a healthy vegan one too quickly for your brain and belly to adjust? If you find yourself snatching a handful of your friend's Flamin' Hot Cheetos when they get up to grab a beer, or sneaking a spoonful of your lover's hot fudge sundae when they're focused on the game, maybe you need to have your *own* vegan junk food on hand for a snack-attack emergency? As we've learned, almost to the point of ad nauseum, a plant-based, whole foods diet is *best*, but sometimes folks need to take itsy-bitsy steps to get there. If you crave a little vegan junk food, have at it. Just try to balance it out with something healthy. If you want those vegan Joe Joe's, try to eat an apple or banana first. If you want those Spicy Sweet Chili Doritos, make yourself gobble up a raw carrot or celery stick prior. It's just like the old days when you had to clean up your room before you could go out and play. You know the drill. A little bit of temporary junk food might just do the trick to get you back on track to a lifetime of healthy eating, so give it a go!

YOU HAD NO CHOICE

Did you get "shaky hungry" when you were out and about? Or wind up eating dairy cheese at a business meeting because there was no other choice? It happens. But here's the trick: It's all about planning ahead. Have you ever seen a mom with a two-year-old pack up for a week of vacation? She has one suitcase for herself, and about a dozen contraptions and necessities for her toddler. The mama has to have the car seat, the stroller, the diapers, the cream, the snacks, the wipes . . . and don't forget the toys! It goes on and on. Just think of yourself as a baby vegan (aww, you're so cute!), and make sure to pack up all the little things you might need each day; I assure you, it will be a lot less cumbersome than what's on a new mother's list. Always have a Clif Bar or other snack bar in your purse or briefcase. Or even a bag of mixed nuts. Always call ahead to make sure where you're going has food for you to eat, too. And if you don't think they will, just take something with you, or fill up on something yummy before you go. I usually keep a bag of pretzels in the car. Remember, there's no shortage of vegan food, just plenty of the whoops-I-forgot. Plan ahead, and get back on track!

IT'S JUST TOO EXPENSIVE

Is vegan food draining your cruelty-free pocketbook? There's a quick fix for that, my friend, and we talked about it in Day 9: Fast, Cheap, and Easy. *Stop buying pricey processed foods.* They're so darn tasty, dang it, but they get even the best of us when it comes to keeping a tight budget. That means no more prepackaged veggie burgers, no more vegan cheese, no more veggie dogs, no more vegan cookies. Just buy whole foods (fresh or frozen): beans, rice, potatoes, carrots, lettuce, lentils, greens, oats, apples, etc., and try to cook at home whenever possible. You can find a lot of these foods at the Dollar Tree, too. You can gradually add back a few of the vegan goodies you enjoy, once the bucks roll in. I assure you if you stick to simple foods, and just buy a few spices and seasonings to jazz them up, you'll not only save tons of money, but you'll likely be eating healthier, too.

The money drain could also just be a result of poor fiscal management. Our couches are hand-me-downs and our curtains are made from sheets. I can't remember the last time I had a manicure, and after twenty-eight years of being vegan, I still don't own a Vitamix. But I don't think twice about spending a thousand dollars on my kitty's teeth to keep her happy, and our kitchen is always stocked with good food, no matter what the cost. It's all about priorities. Our furry kids and our wellness are at the top of my list. What's at the top of yours? Take a look at where your money goes, and see if you can make a few adjustments here and there. Maybe lower the ranks of entertainment, mall shopping, and pampering, and bring up the scrumptious vegan food a notch. Remember: Health is wealth!

HARVEST BOWLS

Some folks call them "Buddha Bowls" or "Rainbowls," but I call them Harvest Bowls because I envision them as a medley of simple but hearty seasonal food. Regardless of the name, they're quick to make, delicious to eat, and are packed with vitamins, minerals, antioxidants, and fiber! Depending on your preference, you can make one raw, roasted, steamed, or a combo of all three. Just think of the wide variety of colorful and fresh, whole foods, as we discussed in chapter 13, and create a deep, wide bowl full of your favorites, side by side, and top it with your favorite sauce and seasonings. One example would be to fill up a large soup or pasta bowl with chopped purple cabbage, tomatoes, baked sweet potatoes, steamed kale, brown rice, avocado, and black beans, drizzle with balsamic vinegar, add a sprinkle of nutritional yeast, sea salt, freshly ground black pepper, sesame seeds, and a small handful of chopped spring onions. Or maybe you'd prefer a sweet mix of tahini with maple syrup and lemon juice? Or perhaps toss on a few pumpkin seeds! Or you could top it with a simple cashew cream sauce: Just soak ½ cup of cashews for a few hours, rinse and drain, then blend with ¼ to ½ cup water or nut milk. Depending on your mood, you can then add sweet or savory additions to make your cashew cream just the way you like it. Enjoy!

IT'S JUST TOO DIFFICULT

I hear ya! A lot of things in life are. What's great is when something good becomes second nature to us. When that happens, we don't even have to think about it; it's just normal, and we can't imagine it being any other way. For most seasoned vegans, being vegan is exactly that: *natural*. And when something is natural, it's not difficult at all. It's as though a light switch flipped "on" in our head, and there's no turning back, and we couldn't be happier. We saw, we learned, we know. And barring a brain injury, what we know is here to stay. If you can shift *your* mind-set, I assure you, it will make going vegan a heck of a lot easier.

Imagine a plate of grilled newborn baby fingers, with a spicy BBQ newborn baby dipping sauce. Disgusting, I know, and it goes without saying, but you're *not* eating them. And neither am I. But what if there are no other options on the menu that you like? *Nope, not eating them.* But what if everything else is too expensive? *Nope, not touching that plate of newborn baby fingers. Get it away!* But what if you're really hungry, and there isn't any other food for one hundred miles. *No, still not eating them.* But what if someone told you that the baby was really happy, and could crawl around wherever she wanted before they cut off her fingers? *Disgusting. Still not eating them!* But what if the cook just uses bits and pieces of the baby, and the baby doesn't die? *Not eating them.* What if the cook was really resourceful and assured you they're using all of the other baby parts, so nothing is going to waste? *Gross! Not eating them.* What if every recipe in your cookbooks calls for newborn baby fingers, and you don't know how to cook without a recipe? *Who cares! Still not eating them.* What if you don't have time to go find something else to eat? *No! Still not eating them.* But what if you really loved the taste because you had unknowingly been eating them for years, and thought they were delicious? *I don't care how good they taste! Not eating them.* What if Aunt Marge has been making them at

KICK UP THE FLAVOR!

If you want to spice up your meal in a quick and easy way, consider adding a dollop of an über flavorful condiment to your plate! Salsa, chutney, sauerkraut, pickled ginger, and kimchi (made without fish stock) really pack a punch when it comes to taste. My mouth is watering just thinking about 'em!

the holidays for your entire life, and you'll hurt her feelings if you suddenly stop eating them? *Well, too bad for wacky Aunt Marge. I am NOT eating grilled newborn baby fingers!*

I think you get the point. When we think of cute newborn baby fingers, followed by the thought of eating them with BBQ sauce, these words and thoughts come to mind: disgusting, depressing, cruel, vile, sad, horrific, insane, etc. In fact you're probably thinking, "*What in the hell did I just read in the above paragraph? That was gross!*" All you read was exactly how most vegans feel when they think about eating animal products. Unless they have a crazy self-destructive lapse, like I did momentarily when I ate those Reese's Peanut Butter Cups fifteen plus years ago, most vegans don't eat animals or their by-products, because just like the newborn baby fingers, it's just something we would never do, and we don't even have to give it any thought. We don't want to eat something that's a product of cruelty, pain, or suffering, and with so many other delicious and healthy options, why would we? If you're really struggling and none of the tips above seem to help, I highly suggest watching one, or more, of the following films if you haven't already done so, because for most seasoned vegans—who have gone vegan and *stayed* vegan—visuals are what flipped the switch, sealed the deal, and made things *easy:*

- *Cowspiracy* (streaming on Netflix)
- *Speciesism* (streaming on Amazon and Vimeo)
- *Earthlings* (you can watch this one right now for free on YouTube)

And I'd top one of those off with the short video *The Best Speech You Will Ever Hear* by Gary Yourofsky, or Phillip Wollen's powerful ten-minute speech at the "Animals Should Be Left Off the Menu" debate. So articulate and inspiring! Both are available on YouTube. Not in the mood for a movie? Read *Eating Animals* by Jonathan Safran Foer.

It's highly praised for helping lots of folks make the switch. There aren't any graphic photos, but pages 117 through 121 will leave quite an impression, I assure you. Check it out.

IT'S YOUR MIND-SET

Once you change your mind-set, you'll realize it was never the recipes, the fancy kitchen gadgets, the money, or the time that you needed in order to go vegan. With a flip of a switch the light comes on, and you see the world in a whole new way, and you recognize your proper place in it. You walk away from the greed and sadness, and start marching toward justice, health, and compassion for all. Instead of causing problems, you strive to become part of the solution. You shed the guilt and start basking in the beauty and wonder of the world. You know that you're not perfect, and that you'll never be, but you do your best to be kind, each and every day. And this brings you joy. Now dust off those knees, take my little hand, and hop back on.

Checklist

- ☐ Did you pinpoint what your stumbling block is?
- ☐ Did you make a minor adjustment or two and get back on track?
- ☐ Did you envision how you would create your own Harvest Bowl?

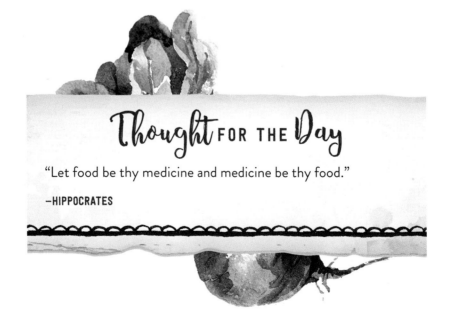

Thought FOR THE Day

"Let food be thy medicine and medicine be thy food."

—HIPPOCRATES

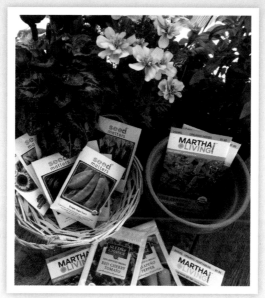

Planting SEEDS OF Compassion

GOAL FOR THE DAY: Help kindness grow throughout your community and beyond.

1. *Consider being an armchair activist.*

There are so many easy ways to make a huge difference in the world in the comfort of your own home, even if you have very little time to spare. It might sound lazy, but it's not; you can be very efficient and effective without even setting foot out the door! Here are a few ideas for inspiration:

- Start a vegan-themed blog. If you're lucky you can find a domain for ninety-nine cents, grab a Wordpress template for free, and start writing the same day!

- Start a vegan-themed Facebook page, Pinterest page, Instagram or Twitter account and start spreading the word.

- E-mail cosmetic companies and household product manufacturers and politely ask them to stop testing on animals. Thank-you notes to those who don't test are nice as well, as they encourage them to stay the course.

- E-mail restaurants and politely ask them to offer more vegan options.

- E-mail coffee shops and politely ask them to offer nut milks and vegan snacks.

- E-mail your school library or public library and ask them to carry more vegan books (like this one!).

- If you see a TV show that appears to involve or promote abuse toward animals or people, or is destructive toward the environment, send the producer an e-mail to voice your concern. (Consider notifying an animal rights organization, too.)

- Write a letter to the editor regarding any current vegan issues in the news, e.g., if there's an article about a drought, write a letter expressing that folks could save a lot of water by going vegan, far more than taking shorter showers or watering their lawns less.

- Write or call your elected officials and urge them to vote for pro-vegan legislation, and against any bills that harm human health, the environment, or animals. You can call, e-mail, or even reach out through social media. According to a recent poll, it takes less than thirty posts in response to a lawmaker's Facebook or Twitter post to cause a congressional office to take notice of the public feedback.[1] To find out who your elected officials are, go to the League of Women Voters: lwv.org and select the "contact elected officials" tab. Just enter your zip code, and you'll see them all: local, state, and national. Not sure what bills are up for vote? Check out the list at the Humane Society Legislative Fund: hslf.org. Just select the "View Current Bills" tab and you'll see a nice list. You can also check the "Action Alerts" page on the Animal Legal Defense Fund's website: aldf.org. They also have a selection of current petitions that you can sign, too.

- Read books and watch movies that add to your knowledge of vegan issues. Peruse the resource section at the end of this book for some great ideas.

- Make positive, informative comments on social media. You can easily request to see more vegan meal ideas on the major food pages (Food Network, etc.) or go to the social media pages for magazines and ask that they feature more vegan recipes and cruelty-free fashion. You can go to your favorite grocery store's social media pages and ask that they carry more vegan food and cruelty-free products, too.

൭ Ask your school, your child's school, or your local hospital to offer more vegan options. If they're hesitant, ask if they'd be interested in at least trying out the Humane Society of the United States' Meatless Monday program.[2] It's a great start!

൭ Post an inspirational quote in your e-mail signature that encourages folks to go vegan, or provide a link to a video or website that's inspirational.

These involve getting out of your chair, but still, very little effort is needed and you can still make a world of difference.

൭ Wear your heart on your sleeve, as they say, and toss on a T-shirt that encourages folks to go vegan. One of my favorites is my "Kale Yeah, I'm Vegan" shirt. Or you can pin a little button on your shirt, purse, or backpack. These are a great way to strike up a conversation while standing in line at the grocery store, or awaiting that morning cup of Joe at the coffee shop!

൭ Put a bumper sticker or two on your car. They even have magnetic ones if you're worried about sticker residue. I can't tell you how many times I've seen passengers in cars behind me take photos of my bumper stickers, or how many times passersby in parking lots and gas stations have struck up a conversation with me thanks to them. A few of my favorite stickers are: "Violence Begins with Your Fork," "Peace Begins in the Kitchen: Go Vegan" and "Love Animals, Eat Plants."

൭ Leave pamphlets and Vegan Starter Kits[3] in doctors' office waiting rooms, libraries, hair salons, and anywhere else folks casually sit down with time to spare (unless prohibited, of course). You can also post flyers on many community bulletin boards, too.

2. *Choose your words carefully and use the power of language to create a more compassionate world.*

Words are powerful, no doubt about it. They can make us feel loved or loathed in a heartbeat. Words can also manipulate good folks into doing some pretty crappy things. Throughout history people have strategically used language to foster the oppression of others, enabling factions of society to feel as though certain populations are less worthy of being treated fairly. Native Americans were referred to as "dogs" and "snakes," Chinese immigrants were called "rats," African Americans brought over as slaves were called "gorillas" and "baboons," and Jews were labeled as "vermin" and "insects," all of which made it easier for people to rationalize discrimination, enslavement, and torture.

The same strategic manipulation of language surrounds our furry friends. Let's take a look at how we talk about animals, and try to make a few adjustments. By using more specific, and more *accurate* words, we can foster their well-being instead of creating the feeling that they're just here for human exploitation.

TOSS OUT THE "IT" WORD. When it comes to describing a woman as an "it girl" it's generally considered favorable; she's someone with natural appeal. It's also normal to ask, "Is *it* a boy or a girl?" with no demeaning consequences. However, when it comes to describing animals, using the word "it" alienates them from us. Rather than being the "someone" that they are, they become the "some*thing*" we can eat. When referring to a cow, pig, bird, fish, or any other animal, try to use the words *she* or *he*, and *her* or *his*, even if you're not certain of the gender. Doing so helps dispel the perverse idea that animals are things we can use and abuse, and will instead enforce the fact that animals are sentient beings, deserving of protection, just like you and me.

TAKE OUT THE "FOOD" NAME, AND REPLACE IT WITH THE NAME OF THE ANIMAL. Bacon, foie gras, ham, pork chops, veal, and steak are all examples of palatable names that people have created to describe animal bits and pieces used for food. Try replacing the assigned "food name" with that of the animal, for example, if someone asks you if you'd like some bacon, you might want to politely reply that you don't eat pigs. "Foie gras" sounds beautiful, as do most French words, but it's really just the engorged fatty liver of a force-fed duck. Who wants to eat *that*? In England and Ireland, "Black Pudding" is very popular, but if you think it's a chocolate treat, as I did, you're in for a big surprise. It's actually boiled pigs' blood that's mixed with fat, then sealed in a casing, aka skin. If you say it like it is, unveiling the truth, you'll likely inspire folks to eat *less* animal products and consume *more* plants. And that's always a good thing. Just give a little bit of thought to your audience though, as someone like super set-in-her-ways "Aunt Marge" might just get crankier, and that's the last thing you need. Whereas your college buddy might say, "Hey, I never thought about it like that. Good point!" Feel it out, and do what's best.

Changing the name of food can be *very* powerful; just ask the California Prune

Board. They petitioned the FDA to change "prunes" to "dried plums" because most folks associate prunes with elderly people who need help with their bowel movements. No joke. If you take a look at the grocery store shelf, you'll find the name "dried plums" has replaced "prunes" on all of their packaging, despite being the same product. According to the California Prune Board, "dried plums" evokes a positive feeling of "fresh fruit goodness."[4] Sales are up, and everyone's back to feeling good about the fruit that helps you poop. Many vegans simply take this same idea, and reverse it to help the consumption of animal products go *down*. If you don't sugarcoat the truth when it comes to eating animals, you'll help folks understand *exactly* what they're eating, enabling them to make healthier choices.

TRY NOT TO INSULT PEOPLE, BUT IF YOU MUST, LEAVE THE ANIMALS OUT OF IT. "You filthy, pig!" and "You're so pigheaded!" are just two examples of phrases containing the word *pig* that are used to insult someone. Pigs actually just roll around in the mud to stay cool (they're *very* smart!) and I've never met a stubborn pig (only sweet ones who enjoy tummy rubs).[5] There are so many ugly phrases that need to be retired. If we stop saying them, they'll go away. Do your best to be kind, and express yourself in language that's both respectful of people *and* the animals.

REPLACE IDIOMS THAT IMPLY HARM TO ANIMALS WITH NEW ONES THAT STILL GET THE POINT ACROSS. People blurt out so many idioms without giving them a second thought, but if you take a beat to listen to the words, you might be shocked to hear what you're actually saying. "I killed two birds with one stone!" is a great example. People say it so proudly, but if you stop and think about it, why on earth would someone be happy about throwing a rock into the air, and killing two birds flying by? Anyone with even half a heart would feel horrible as they fell to the ground dead. And how's about "Who let the cat out of the bag?" Geez, how is that a *bad* thing? If I found a cat trapped in a bag, I'd let her out, too, wouldn't you? Just give some thought as to what you're saying, i.e., "packed like sardines" and simply make the phrase kinder by replacing a word or two, such as "packed like cloves in a garlic bulb" or "packed like pickles."

Here are a few more common sayings to avoid, and adjust. Have some fun and create your own compassionate versions!

"Running around like a chicken with its head cut off"

"On a wild goose chase"

"No use beating a dead horse"

"There's more than one way to skin a cat"

"Open a can of worms"

HERE ARE A FEW EXTRA TIDBITS TO MULL OVER WHEN IT COMES TO USING LANGUAGE AS A TOOL TO PROMOTE COMPASSION:

ᑐ A healthy vegan diet is one of abundance, not restriction. Thankfully, no one is forcing you to go vegan with only a pile of sprouts to eat. So when folks give you that long "poor you" face and ask, "Aww, you can't eat eggs?" remember, it's not that you can't eat them, it's that you choose not to. Do your best to make sure your response reflects the healthy dietary choice you've made, rather than a dismal punishment they assume you've been sentenced to. Let your health and happiness shine!

ᑐ Being polite goes a long way. Calling non-vegans "corpse munchers" or other pejorative terms can shut down a productive conversation about being vegan before it's even begun. It's possible to be both effective and kind while talking about all issues involving wellness, the environment, and animals. Remember, you'll "attract" more flies with "agave" than you will with vinegar. (Notice I didn't catch any flies, nor use any honey. Wink.) Strive to be respectful of other vegans as well, including those who may see things differently than you do. We've all arrived here on different paths, with unique experiences along the way—so it's only natural that vegans don't always see eye-to-eye when it comes to inspiring change. There is no perfect, fail-proof blueprint for advocacy work; different situations require different strategies. What works for one person, might not work for another. Just try to keep an open mind and a warm heart when interacting with those who see things a bit differently. Healthy discourse is productive, so chat it up. I tend to learn a lot from those I disagree with. However, hostility not only dilutes your message, it will sap your precious energy, too; better to save and spend it elsewhere.

ᑐ Commonality keeps the door open and the conversation going. When I write about being vegan, I tend to stick to a focused message that conveys an urgency to help improve worldwide health, the environment, and animals. I'm passionate about issues surrounding religion, politics, and other hot topics, too, but these subjects can be divisive and detract from the subject at hand if I jumble up everything all at once. It's not that we shouldn't speak openly about other issues, please do; after all, silence is the voice of complicity. Just know that sometimes people tune others out if they don't agree with an opinion concerning a subject that's dear to their hearts, and before you know it, they're pissed, and they're gone. It's human nature to feel most comfortable with those you can relate to, and that's why I try to be likable and approachable to my audience when I write, not just to those who think exactly as I do. I pick up my soapbox and take it elsewhere when it's time to be vocal about everything beyond being vegan. One can argue that all issues concerning injustice are related, but based on my own experience, I've found that bringing up a few hot-button subjects while talking about being vegan inevitably makes some folks a little cranky, and others raging mad. So do your best to stay focused, using words and topics that create a conversation that's inviting to ensure it reaches the largest audience possible.

Now lets kick it up a notch, for those with a little extra energy to spare!

3. *Here are a few ideas for inspiring compassion in your community. If any float your vegan boat, spring out of that recliner, and set sail!*

Organize a peaceful demonstration in your town to educate the public about any health, environmental, or animal issue that you feel deserves attention. Just be sure to check with your local city hall to see if there are any laws or municipal ordinances you should be aware of. Although your freedom of speech and freedom to assemble are protected, there are laws that regulate the time, place, and manner in which you express yourself. If you'd rather attend one that's already being planned, many animal, environment, and health-related, non-profit websites offer newsletters that you can sign up for to keep you in the loop of activities happening near you. This summer I took my husband, my best friend, and my god-daughter to a Mercy for Animals demonstration where we held signs along the sidewalk in front of McDonald's, politely alerting the public to the horrifically cruel treatment of animals by Foster Farms, Tyson Foods, and Gordon Food Service. A former McDonald's Chicken McNuggets supplier, under contract with Tyson, was filmed stabbing birds with spiked clubs and breaking their necks by standing on their heads and pulling their bodies.[6] Thanks to the relentless efforts of animal advocates, the supplier was convicted of animal cruelty. The penalties weren't stiff enough, but at least we're moving forward when it comes to justice for animals. Public demonstrations can be extremely educational and effective. A little

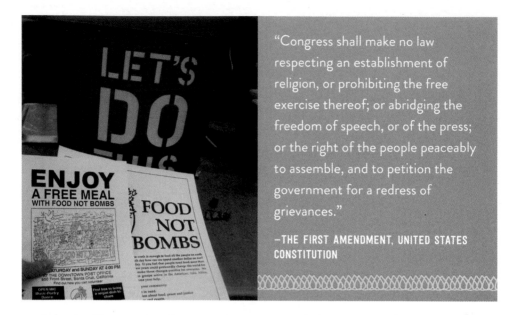

"Congress shall make no law respecting an establishment of religion, or prohibiting the free exercise thereof; or abridging the freedom of speech, or of the press; or the right of the people peaceably to assemble, and to petition the government for a redress of grievances."

—THE FIRST AMENDMENT, UNITED STATES CONSTITUTION

info here, a little info there, and before you know it, there's a heck of a lot of info out there, and all that knowledge provides the power to change the world. Most people really do want to do the right thing; they just need to know the "why" and the "how," and after reading this book, you'll be more than ready to get out there and teach them.

‿ Bring vegan food to share at work, school, and other community events. Surprise your coworkers, fellow students, or any gathering of community members with a plate of homemade vegan cookies, or better yet, those healthy date cashew balls from Day 14. Or perhaps a bowl of vegan meatballs with a marinara dipping sauce, or a little vegan nut cheese and crackers spread; whatever is easy for you to whip up! If you're leaving them on a table, fold an index card in half, write the words "It's Vegan: Enjoy!" and place it beside the goodies. Tasty treats invariably lead to a little vegan chitchat, giving you the opportunity to plant a few more seeds of compassion.

‿ Participate in Humane Lobby Day, organized by the Humane Society of the United States. After a few hours of preparation, you'll get to speak face-to-face with your elected officials and encourage them to vote for, or against, bills that impact the welfare of animals. That's what I did on my fiftieth birthday and I loved it! We urged state officials to vote against a bill that would increase the inhumane killing of wild pigs, and against another that would allow for the sale and trade of crocodile and alligator body parts. We also asked that they vote for a bill that would prohibit the use of second-generation anticoagulant rodenticides: poisons that people feed to rats and other little furry friends, who are then consumed by other animals (dogs, owls, pigs, squirrels, golden eagles, etc.), who in turn also die. These anticoagulants make the body unable to clot blood, so the animals bleed to death. Just when you think you've heard it all, right? Educating legislators about important issues so they can make smart choices when it comes time to vote is one of my very favorite things to do. It's so empowering. You'll exit the meetings feeling like a vegan rock star wondering whose door you can knock on next.

HOW TO HANDLE THE "MMMM BACON!" DUDE

As a newbie vegan, it's only a matter of time before you run into the infamous "Mmmm Bacon!" dude, and let me tell you, she or he can be quite cantankerous! That's OK, though, I've got your back. Just remember to pick your battles wisely; you don't need to show up to every argument you're invited to. However, should you decide to make a grand entrance and engage with the lovelies, I've created a little cheat sheet just for you.

They may think they're pressing your hot button, but with these replies, they'll find you're just cool as a cucumber, with a sharp mind and a patient, loving heart.

BUTTON #1

THE "MMMM, BACON!" DUDE: *Don't you know, humans have been eating animals for thousands of years!?*

THE CALM AND INFORMATIVE VEGAN: *Yes, that's true, but just because something has been done for a very long time doesn't make it right. Think of other atrocities that have occurred over a long period of time, such as African Americans being forced to be slaves, or women being denied the right to vote. Just because something occurs for a very long time doesn't make it acceptable.*

BREAKING VEGAN NEWS

If you want to stay in the loop on vegan news hot off the press, just create a "Google Alert" by going to www.google.com/alerts and plug in the term "vegan." Every day you'll get an e-mail with a list of the top vegan news stories across the world. Or, you can create an alert for something more specific that may interest you, such as "Animal Law," "Vegan Health," or "SeaWorld Closes." (It *will* happen one day!) I look forward to the list every evening!

BUTTON #2

THE "MMMM, BACON!" DUDE: *Well, to each his own. I respect your eating choices, so you should respect mine!*

THE CALM AND INFORMATIVE VEGAN: *Respect for each other's choices is great, unless your actions impinge on the well-being of others. Would you respect someone's choice to beat a dog? Or to abuse their spouse? What the animals endure to become your meal is just as painful. You might choose to harm others, but a compassionate person will never "respect" your decision to do so.*

BUTTON #3

THE "MMMM, BACON!" DUDE: *But we're carnivores, dammit. Look at our canine teeth!*

THE CALM AND INFORMATIVE VEGAN: *Have you ever checked out the canines on a Hippopotamus? They have the largest canines of any land animal, up to 16 inches long. And guess what? They don't eat meat. Neither do a lot of other mammals with canines and I'm pretty sure the last time you ate a steak, you used a knife and fork.*

BUTTON #4

THE "MMMM, BACON!" DUDE: *Other animals eat animals, so there's nothing wrong with humans eating animals.*

THE CALM AND INFORMATIVE VEGAN: *Well, except we have a choice not to, and we know better. If you're going to use the excuse that lions eat other animals, are you going to sniff someone else's butt when you meet them? Lions do that, too. Or are you just going to pick one trait that a lion has and use that as your excuse to eat animals? We don't need to eat other animals to live a happy, healthy life. Unfortunately, some animals, such as lions, do.*

BUTTON #5

THE "MMMM, BACON!" DUDE: *But I've always eaten animals. It's natural and instinctual.*

THE CALM AND INFORMATIVE VEGAN: *Really? Always? In the words of Fit for Life author Harvey Diamond, "You put a baby in a crib with an apple and a rabbit. If it eats the rabbit and plays with the apple, I'll buy you a new car." Our desire to eat animals is conditioned by those around us, not by instinct.*

BUTTON #6

THE "MMMM, BACON!" DUDE: *But if we stop eating them, farm animals will all die and go extinct!*

THE CALM AND INFORMATIVE VEGAN: *Wow, I didn't know you were suddenly worried about their well-being. You're eating them to save them? Hmmm . . . I'm pretty sure a farm animal* would rather take her chances eating grass in the wild than remain captive and abused on a factory farm, wouldn't you? As for their population numbers, they would no longer be force-bred, allowing nature to take its course, as it should. And since factory farm animals require so much grain, which takes so much land to grow, if we stop eating animals, we wouldn't be destroying so much wildlife habitat. The number of farm animals would naturally go down, but other animals would likely flourish again.

BUTTON #7

THE "MMMM, BACON!" DUDE: *OK, fine. I changed my mind. If we stop eating farm animals, they will overrun the earth! We have to eat them, or there will be billions of cows, pigs, lambs, and chickens everywhere!*

THE CALM AND INFORMATIVE VEGAN: *Wow, that's quite a mighty switch-a-roo. We both know that the world wouldn't go vegan overnight. Although it would be the most compassionate course of events, it's just not going to happen. Factory farm owners would simply end the force-breeding of animals, causing the farm animal population to gradually decline, which would give our ecosystem a fighting chance to return to a natural balance.*

BUTTON #8

THE "MMMM, BACON!" DUDE: *Well, I only eat what I can shoot, and I use every part of the animal!*

THE CALM AND INFORMATIVE VEGAN: *Do you know who else uses every part of the animal? The animal. Those "parts" don't belong to you, they belong to the animal. An animal in the wild wants to live just as much as you and I do. And their parents, children, or companions who are left behind want them to live as well. You don't need to hunt to live a happy, healthy life, no matter how many animal parts you use.*

BUTTON #9

THE "MMMM, BACON!" DUDE: *Ha! Another judgmental vegan!*

THE CALM AND INFORMATIVE VEGAN: *Yes, I do judge others; don't you? If someone is a murderer, we judge them to be mean. If someone volunteers to help others, we judge them to be kind. To judge is simply to evaluate someone by their actions. That's normal; people do it every day. In fact, you just "judged" that I'm judgmental. Fancy that.*

BUTTON #10

THE "MMMM, BACON!" DUDE: *"There you go! A typical self-righteous vegan. You think you're better than everyone else, don't cha?*

THE CALM AND INFORMATIVE VEGAN: *Actually, it's quite the opposite. Vegans don't think they're better than anyone else, that's why we're vegan. We think we're equal to others, and that's why we don't harm them. Unlike those who kill and eat animals and their by-products, we think animals are entitled to live out their lives free from harm, as they see fit. Being vegan is all about equality, not about being "above" or "better" than anyone else.*

LAST SHOT BUTTON #11

THE "MMMM, BACON!" DUDE: *Mmmm, Bacon!!*

THE CALM AND INFORMATIVE VEGAN: (Declines the invitation to engage and politely walks away.)

Checklist

☐ Did you select a few simple things you can do to inspire others to become more compassionate?

☐ Did you figure out a kinder way to express yourself without insulting people or animals?

☐ Did you think about a yummy vegan treat you could share with your coworkers or friends?

☐ Did you drink enough water today?

Thought FOR THE Day

Remember, it's progress, not perfection.
You've got this, kiddo!

DAY 21

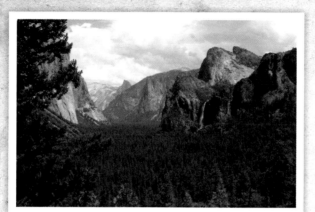

Vegan for the **WIN!**

GOAL FOR THE DAY: Learn how to pep yourself up when the world seems hopeless and you feel like no one cares or understands. It's time to learn a little bit about how far we've come and why the future looks so bright. Know in your heart that *everyone's* going vegan, baby!

My next-door neighbor is a fisherman, and I smell the dead fish every time he comes in from a haul. The man down the street raises lambs and turkeys to eat, and as the holidays approach, I watch the number of animals dwindle. I do my best not to count. Other than my husband, my entire family eats animal products—and lots of them, too.

And just like you, I'm bombarded by billboards, TV commercials, radio ads, magazine covers, and fast-food restaurant signs urging everyone else to do the same. It's enough to make you wish you could just nestle in bed with your slipper socks, a blankie, and a batch of warm vegan cookies, and shut the sadness out for the rest of your life. This is why I sometimes casually refer to being vegan as having the "disease of compassion." It's fun, it's delicious, and it's easy, but dammit, does it hurt sometimes. Worrying about the world's health and happiness is a heavy load to carry. If the less-than-compassionate actions of others bring you down, I want you to know: you're not alone. And listen up, I've got some great news for you. If you're ever feeling blue, I know how to turn that vegan frown upside down. So chin up, buttercup, the glass is *more* than half full; it's about to overflow!

Cue the trumpets and fanfare, folks! We're on the cusp of a paradigm shift, and I'm darn tootin' excited about it. And I'm not just tossing around "paradigm shift" as a catchy buzz phrase here. It's really happening, in the biggest, most wonderful way. We're living in a period of great upheaval, when existing ideas are replaced with radically new ones, because the anomalies we've been witnessing over countless decades can no longer be explained away. And that's exactly how great paradigm shifts occur, so enjoy the ride.

HISTORY IS ON OUR SIDE

Thousands of years ago, Greek astronomer Claudius Ptolemy believed Earth was at the center of the universe. Thanks to gravity, anything someone dropped from the air fell toward Earth. They didn't have telescopes back then, so with only rudimentary observations, it's no surprise folks thought Earth was the center of their entire world. But as observations became clearer and data more precise, Ptolemy's findings became shaky. Folks began to see planets seemingly moving forwards and backwards, which didn't make any sense if they all revolved around *us*. Instead of people changing their beliefs, though, scientists simply adjusted their diagrams and mathematical formulas to keep the geocentric believers happy. Bottom line? People's minds were made up: everything revolved around our planet, so scientists dutifully accommodated their false belief.

Flash forward a few thousand years to the mid-sixteenth century, and you'll find Renaissance astronomer and mathematician Nicolaus Copernicus seeing things in a whole new way. Copernicus believed the Sun was the center of the universe, but despite writing an entire book proving this was so, he was too scared to publish it for fear of scorn. People were, and arguably still are, used to being the most important beings, at the center of everything, and for the most part, *rebel against change* even if it evolves from solid facts (sound familiar?). The revelation that we're simply passengers on a planet that rotates around the sun, no different than all the other planets, was a tough pill to swallow. (Earth? No more important than the *other* planets? Say it ain't so!) Copernicus's work, *On the Revolutions of the Heavenly Bodies*, illustrating that Earth revolves around the Sun, wasn't published until the year of his death, decades after he developed his heliocentric theory. The book was forcefully removed from circulation, but not before Galileo Galilei managed to read a copy (thank goodness!), only to find himself slapped with an injunction forbidding him from teaching or defending heliocentrism. People fought tooth and nail to maintain their traditional views. So much so that Galileo was put on trial, convicted of heresy, and imprisoned under house arrest for the rest of his life, simply because he agreed with Copernicus! They both knew, *as we all know*, Earth *does indeed* revolve around the sun.

All of the adjustments to data, threats of imprisonment, and banned books, however frequent or widespread, could not stop this paradigm shift, or any others, from occurring. *When it comes to laws of nature, in the end, truth always prevails, and this should give you some comfort.* Humankind may be powerful, but we are *not* omnipotent.

Paradigm shifts have happened numerous times in our history. Einstein's theory of relativity replaced Newtonian physics in a likewise manner, and there's the crazy drama surrounding three thousand years of bloodletting, which was eventually replaced by modern medicine. Yes, it's true; doctors used to cut people open and drain their blood because they thought it healed them of just about everything, even pneumonia. They pressed little brass boxes with spring-loaded blades against patients' bodies, and they used leeches, too.[1] Bloodletting wasn't just practiced by fringe doctors—it was widespread. In the 1830s, *5 to 6 million* leeches per year were used in France alone.[2] It comes as no surprise that many patients died because, well, having your jugular slit to heal you is quite simply very hazardous, wouldn't you agree? And yet somehow doctors practiced the wacky treatment, and repeatedly *rationalized* it, for thousands of years, just like scientists rationalized the Sun rotating around Earth.

So what does all this history trivia have to do with you and me, and our desire to create a better world? It illustrates that time, truth, and change march on, with or without everyone's blessing. Anomalies that occur time after time, that can no longer be explained away, coupled with a magnificent "tipping point" that's quickly approaching, are creating an unstoppable and exciting dynamic. Fueled by solid research, compassion, and common sense, *the entire world is going vegan*. The shift is happening before our very eyes, right here and right now!

HEALTH

Our modern-day "bloodletters" keep clamoring that we must do one thing, while clearly research and facts teach us to do otherwise. Over the years we've been told we *must* eat animals for protein; we *must* drink milk for calcium; we *must* consume fish for omegas; but none of these statements is true. All of these claims have been made, over and over, and yet despite all of the twists and turns of research and media blasts, the truth just won't go away. We don't need to eat animals or their by-products, to be healthy! I'm not convinced the meat and dairy industries even believe their own assertions anymore. As they say, you can't wake up someone who's only *pretending* to be asleep. They may be greedy, but they're not stupid; they know what's going on. As do the masses.

People are changing their diet, and fast. They want to be healthy and they're making smart choices to ensure that they will. Just look at what happened when the World Health Organization announced that processed meats are indeed carcinogenic, placing them into the same category occupied by cigarettes and asbestos. Within just two weeks, sausage and bacon sales plummeted by over $4 million dollars in England alone.[3] That's not because meat suddenly didn't taste good anymore, it's because people don't want to die. There's a reason why McDonald's is closing more restaurants in the United States than it's opening—shutting the doors on seven hundred locations throughout the world.[4] The appetite for wellness is surpassing that for cheap, greasy food. Take Unilever, owner of Hellman's Mayonnaise: It dropped its "unfair competition" lawsuit against Hampton Creek and their eggless "mayo," then a few months later wowed the crowd with Unilever's other company—Ben and Jerry's—timely announcement that due to *popular demand*, it's creating a new cholesterol-free ice cream line with "no animal products of any kind, including eggs, dairy, or honey."[5] Unilever decided to create its *own* vegan mayo, too! It's called Best Foods Carefully Crafted Dressing & Sandwich Spread. They're not dummies. If you can't beat those leading the way to a more compassionate and sustainable world, stop bickering and just join 'em!

And folks aren't just flocking to vegan food at the stores; they're seeking all things vegan in droves on social media, too. Pinterest, which is more popular among U.S. adults than Twitter, announced that "Vegan Recipes" was one of the "Top 10" most-searched terms in 2015.[6,7] And when vegan- and vegetarian-related content was tracked across mainstream social media for ninety days, it revealed a whopping 4.3 *million* mentions, surpassing even Coca Cola's 4.1 million mark.[8] The overwhelming interest in the once unfamiliar word, *vegan*, shouldn't come as a shock; the positive association between "vegan" and "wellness" has been in the making for a while. After all, when's the last time someone went to the doctor to treat chronic heart disease or cancer—the leading causes of death—and was told they're dying because they didn't eat enough animal products? "Well, Fred, that's what happens when you don't eat enough meat, eggs, and dairy," scolded Dr. Jones. Nope. No one says that. Today, it's laughable. Can you feel the *shift*?

ANIMALS

Over the years, people have repeatedly made false claims to justify the use and abuse of animals, too. Misguided folks have promoted the odd belief that animals are simply like "clocks," incapable of reason, judgment, or pain, clear back to Descartes's ponderings in the 1600s and beyond. Because animals couldn't express themselves in a language people understood, it was assumed that they weren't aware of anything at all.[9] Today this belief sounds crazy, yet at the time, it was repeatedly rationalized. Thankfully, the truth finally emerged, and is accepted. Animals do indeed feel pain, just like humans do; after all, we're animals, too. When's the last time you took a dog or a cat in for surgery and the veterinarian said, "I'll save you a few bucks and skip the anesthesia; after all, animals don't feel pain"? No one says that. But folks *are* saying, and doing, a heck of a lot that affirms we're moving towards a kinder, more compassionate world. Here's a few examples:

The last medical school in the U.S. still using live animals to teach students surgical skills just joined nearly two hundred other medical schools and ended the practice. Feld Entertainment, owner of Ringling Brothers, announced that after 144 years, it's finally retiring its elephants, while many cities have banned animal circuses altogether.[10] In response to the public outrage over the killing of Cecil the lion, more than a dozen major airlines halted the transport of wildlife "trophies," quickly followed by the United States Fish and Wildlife Service's decision to give African lions protection under the Endangered Species Act.[11] After six hundred years of bloodlust, bullfighting in Barcelona has come to an end.[12] While here in the U.S., the military announced a halt to the use of live animals in military training, and the National Institutes of Health (NIH) is retiring all of its chimpanzees from biomedical research and sending them off to a sanctuary.[13] With the Senate's recent passage of the Frank R. Lautenberg Chemical Safety for the 21st Century Act—legislation that finally *requires* that alternatives to animal tests be considered and used—we've embarked on a road that will likely lead to the end of cosmetic testing on animals as well. And although it's far from idyllic, Nestlé, the largest food company in the world, is switching to cage-free eggs. This falls on the heels of Panera, Starbucks, Kellogg's, General Mills, Dunkin' Donuts, Taco Bell, and McDonald's all pledging to do the same. Is it to cut costs? Improve flavor? Be healthier? Nope. According to Nestlé, the move is in response to consumer demand, and their "commitment to the health, care, and welfare of animals raised for food."[14] It's happening. Can you feel the *shift*?

ENVIRONMENTAL POLLUTION

In the 1950s, family farms in the United States began to transition into Concentrated Animal Feeding Operations (CAFOs): aka factory farms. CAFOs produce over a billion tons of waste each year, which is 130 times more poop than the *entire* U.S. human population poops out.[15] Although we have treatment plants for human waste, none exists for the animals, but it's got to go somewhere, right? Sadly, it's often liquefied and then blast into the air over cropland, spreading viruses, bacteria, antibiotics, and heavy metals.[16] Or it sits stagnant in enormous toxic manure lagoons, where it often leaks or bursts after being flooded, drenching neighboring soil and groundwater. Accompanying the millions of gallons of piss and shit are pathogens such as *E. coli*, growth hormones, cleaning chemicals, blood, stillborn animals, hair, pus, antibiotic syringes, vomit, random body parts, and silage waste from the feed.[17] Just last summer a father and son died simply by inhaling the fumes at a CAFO manure pit in Iowa. The stench from

ENVIRONMENTAL CONSEQUENCES: THE HIGH PRICE OF EATING ANIMALS, DAIRY, EGGS, AND FISH[19]

- Cows produce 150 billion gallons of methane per day.
- Five percent of water consumed in the U.S. is by private homes. Fifty-five percent of water consumed in the U.S. is for animal agriculture.
- Animals used for food cover 45% of the earth's total land.
- Animal agriculture is the leading cause of species extinction, ocean dead zones, water pollution, and habitat destruction.
- One-third of the planet is "desertified," with "livestock" as the leading driver.
- It takes almost 900 gallons of water to produce 1 pound of cheese.
- For every 1 pound of fish caught, up to 5 pounds of unintended marine species are caught and discarded as by-kill.
- Scientists estimate as many as 650,000 whales, dolphins, and seals are killed every year by fishing vessels.

the poisonous mix of hydrogen sulfide, methane, ammonia, carbon dioxide, and volatile compounds can kill you within just a few seconds; it's *that* toxic.[18] Similar deaths have occurred in Wisconsin and Virginia, too.

Some may think, "Well that sure sucks for those who live near—or work on—factory farms," and indeed it does. However, the pollution doesn't stay put; it's a carte blanche world traveler. The environmental devastation caused by Big Ag spreads far beyond the immediate soil, water table, and air—the runoff finds its way to streams and rivers, too. The Chesapeake Bay is just one example of over four hundred "dead zones" where runoff from these toxins has taken a catastrophic toll. Anyone interested in picking up the estimated $19 billion dollar tab for cleanup?[20] Folks are still bickering over who should pay for it. Keep in mind, that's just the price tag for *one* location. The dead zone in the Gulf of Mexico is 5,052 square miles: nearly the size of Connecticut.[21] And in Iowa, manure-scented rivers lead to lakes so toxic that officials have been forced to post warnings advising swimmers to avoid splashing around in the E coli.[22]

The fish in the Potomac fair a bit better—they're still alive, but I wouldn't say they're doing well. Researchers who studied a sample of male smallmouth bass found that 85 percent were growing eggs inside their testicles.[23] It comes as no surprise that hormones washed downstream in factory farm waste are suspect.[24] And this is not an isolated incident.[25] We also know that raising animals for food pollutes our environment more than the entire transportation sector combined, and that's not just cars and trucks; it includes planes, trains, and ships, too! Like I said, that Big Mac costs a heck of a lot more than what you dole out at the counter. Check out the list of Environmental Consequences on the previous page for a taste of what else that cheeseburger does to our planet. Although folks will always argue over numbers, there's no debating the fact that eating animal products harms our environment, worldwide, in a *very* big way. The truth is out, and it's not pretty. And most important, it can no longer be explained away.

Those toxins may be spewing, but supersized change is near, my dear. A few things have lined up quite nicely in the past several years. Thanks to the incredible work of doctors, educators, scientists, lawyers, filmmakers, and the relentless effort of advocates across the world, we now have fantastic data and documentation that smashes the lies we've been fed regarding our health and the world around us. You've read a few solid tidbits in this book, but I've only shared the tip of the iceberg.

It's also well documented that in order to achieve great change, we must protest what we oppose while building alternatives that enable us to create the world we wish to see.[26] You don't need everyone to rise up and oppose the "old ways"—just *enough* so that they can no longer be ignored. Or as Founding Father Samuel Adams put it, "It does not require a majority to prevail, but rather an irate, tireless minority keen to set brush fires in people's minds," and it's true. After studying every nonviolent movement to overthrow the government or regain territory over the last one hundred years, renowned political scientist Dr. Erica Chenoweth found that *every* nonviolent resistance movement was successful if the amount of people who were actively involved was 3.5% or greater. That's it: just 3.5% of the population! Once they hit that mark, victory was assured, each and every time. Folks tend to join in to create change once a "tipping point" is reached where actions are perceived as social norms. Although we like to think we're independent, humans tend to follow the crowd.

Dr. Chenoweth noted something else, too: those who want change need to come from a wide segment of society, so the opposition can't target one pocket. It upsets their strategy when the minority becomes part of the whole. I know of vegan politicians, soldiers, musicians, nurses, educators, millionaires, ballet dancers, students, Olympians, lawyers, baristas, sheesh . . . need I go on? What section of the population *doesn't* have any vegans these days? Heck, even non-vegans are joining in to help vegans. After twenty-five years at the golden arches, McDonald's president and CEO Don Thompson just jumped ship to join the board of directors at 100 percent plant-based Beyond Meat.[27] Can you feel the *shift?*

As for the two necessary elements for change—it's pretty evident that lots of folks, including myself (and hopefully you!), are protesting what we oppose in a variety of ways (some big, some small, *all* are important!). What's super awesome is now, *finally*, the alternative "system" for our beautiful and healthy new world is being built—and *fast!* You want a plant-based doctor? There's a database full of them—there's even a vegan medical center![28] Need a vegan interior designer? They exist, too! Your kids want a school with 100 percent vegan food, at every meal, every day? It's out there. You long for a new Ferrari with vegan leather seats? Not a problem. Well, getting a new Ferarri may be a problem, but at least their new premium Mycro Prestige vegan leather won't be! BMW, Mercedes-Benz, Lexus, and Tesla now offer non-leather seats, too! You want vegan meals in outer space? Say *what?*! Yeah, that's right. No biggie. That's what NASA is preparing for astronauts on their two-and-one-half-year voyage to Mars in 2030. They've created over one hundred vegan recipes so far, including vegan pizza.[29] I kid you not. So if you decide to go to Mars, you're all set! Is this *really* all happening? Pinch me!

As you've read over the past 21 days, vegan everything is booming! Mintel tracks global market spending across thirty-four countries, and according to their 2016 food

WHAT'S SO COOL ABOUT A PLANT-BASED SCHOOL? EVERYTHING!

Last summer I had the opportunity to explore MUSE, a Southern California school that only serves 100 percent plant-based food—and let me tell ya, it rocks! Innovative sisters Suzy Amis Cameron and Rebecca Amis founded the school to inspire "students, teachers, staff and community to live sustainably in the classroom, at work and at home." Not only is the food 100 percent vegan, they do their best to ensure it's primarily local and organic, too. Upon arrival, Jeff King, the school's head, invited me to hop on a golf cart for a little ride, and boy, was I in for a treat! Jeff zipped me up a steep dirt road to their organic garden nestled on a hilltop with spectacular views, where they grow and harvest fruits and veggies to complement the school food. Any leftovers from the meals are placed into the compost, and then go back to the earth where they belong. So simple, clean, and healthy!

The pre-K to twelfth-grade school has two ecofriendly campuses, where they encourage students to follow their passions while providing a nurturing environment in which to do so. How cool is that? Five giant thirty-three-foot-tall sunflowers, with fourteen petals made from solar panels, adorn the school! Brainchild (or *flower child*?) of film director James Cameron, the sunflowers are designed to move with the sun just like real flowers do, enabling them to meet 75 to 90 percent of the school's energy needs. I'm sensing a blueprint for the future here, folks. Um, can I be a kid again, *please*? I'm ready for class! www.museschool.org

and drink report, new protein sources are now appealing to the "everyday consumer, foreshadowing a profoundly changed marketplace in which what was formerly 'alternative' could take over the mainstream." Yep, that's right. Vegan food is quickly becoming the norm, not the exception. It won't be too long before it's more difficult to find a restaurant to please a "meat" eater than one that satisfies a vegan.

If you're *still* bummed that Hunter Hank and Bacon Bob will never change, listen up. Think of anyone who still eats or abuses animals in any way. Where will they be in one hundred years? The same place as you and I. Every single one of them, and it won't be here. As Max Planck said, "A new scientific truth does not triumph by convincing its opponents and making them see the light, but rather because its opponents eventually die, and a new generation grows up that is familiar with it."[30] Out goes those who cause pain, misery, and destruction, and born are those who foster compassion, as they are embraced and nurtured by the kindness that unfolds anew in the world each day. If there's any bright side to death, this is it.

You know, it wasn't too long ago that ads featured babies suckling soda bottles, and doctors recommended cigarettes on TV.[31] Six-year-old kids were as familiar with Old Joe Camel as they were with Mickey Mouse.[32] Magazine ads urged women to douche with Lysol, and "DDT is Good For Me" promos claimed the now-banned toxin made homes "healthier." My, oh *my*, how things have changed, just within the past several decades. Are you ready for the next few? I know I am. They're going to be "*vegantastic!*"

AND ON THAT NOTE, I LEAVE YOU WITH THREE LITTLE REMINDERS:

- ☐ Remember, you can't be a perfect vegan, so just do your very best and keep moving forward.

- ☐ Strive to become a *healthy* vegan by eating lots of fresh, whole fruits, veggies, seeds, nuts, beans, and legumes. Remember: Health is wealth!

- ☐ And last, remember to relax now and then. Inhale the good. Exhale the bad. And always keep that chin up, buttercup! I need you, and the entire world does, too!

Now go whip up some yummy vegan food, wiggle that booty around a bit, and let that healthy, happy glow of yours shine a beacon of light and love for others to follow. And as you close this book, may you go about your way bursting with inspiration and steadfast determination, just as I did when that friendly stranger closed my little car door twenty-eight years ago. It's a whole new world, my warmhearted friend. Enjoy!

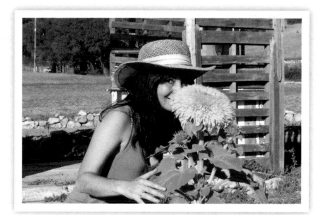

Acknowledgments

If I were to thank all of the friendly folks who have been following *My Vegan Journal* over the past few years, the names alone would fill more pages than there are in this book. I trust you know who you are, and I thank *all* of you for making me excited to roll out of bed and turn on my computer each morning. Chatting with you about health, the environment, and animals has provided me with more inspiration and joy than you'll ever know. And best of all: You give me hope.

Bushels of gratitude to my literary agent, Steve Troha, for sending me an e-mail in 2014, with the simple subject line: "Literary Agent." It provided a writer's fairy-tale moment that will nestle in my heart forever. Without Steve, this book wouldn't exist. And to literary agent, Dado Derviskadic, who, along with Steve, gave me tremendous guidance and a foolproof road map to successfully wade through the lengthy process of transforming an idea in the mind into a proposal in hand. They are so darn helpful and smart.

Much appreciation to my fabulous editor and steadfast cheerleader, Michael Flamini at St. Martin's Press, Macmillan, who indulged me with an abundance of freedom to express myself without reserve. Michael even tried out new vegan cuisine along the way. Made me so happy! Here's to making every meal "a small celebration!" And I'm grateful for associate editor Vicki Lame, too, who made sure everything moved along just as it should. And thank you to the writing world's unsung heroes who work behind the scenes in the marketing, publicity, design, and production departments: Leah Stewart,

Annie Hulkower, Crystal Ben, Donna Sinsgalli Noetzel, Eric C. Meyer, Eric Gladstone, Jessica Preeg, and Brant Janeway.

Thank you to my incredibly enthusiastic friends and family, and especially to my best friend, Becky Carroll, who just happens to be the best wife, nurse, and mother, too. I met Becky while she was working at my veterinarian's office decades ago, and she's been a pillar of strength and inspiration ever since.

A heartfelt thanks to Dan Matthews, Bruce Friedrich, Heather Moore, Rebecca Amis, Jeff King, Alka Chandra, Lisa Lange, Kathy Guillermo, Gene Baur, Miyoko Schinner, Jasmin Singer, Joyce Tischler, Nicole Pallotta, Beth Krauss, Leanne Mai-ly Hilgart, Ellie Laks, Kim Sturla, Sid Garza-Hillman, Dr. Neal Barnard, Dr. Mehmet and Lisa Oz, Moby, and Pamela Anderson for their kind help in so many ways.

Hugs and kisses to my supportive husband, Brandon, who not only went vegan after we were wed, but supplied me with plenty of coffee and sweets to keep me awake into the night while writing. I'm pretty sure I owe him a few back and foot rubs—and a double serving of Sunday crepes.

And last, my heart overflows with appreciation for the tireless efforts of advocates across the globe who could easily use their skills and smarts to live a quiet life in luxury, yet choose instead to spend their days in the trenches fighting the good fight for animals *and* people. And to the photographers who document with their own eyes what most of us can barely stomach to read. May your brilliant minds and hearts of gold continue to spread comfort, wellness, and justice throughout the world.

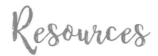

Resources

Swing by and say "Hi!"

Blog: *MyVeganJournal.com*
Pinterest: www.pinterest.com/myveganjournal
Twitter: www.twitter.com/myveganjournal
Facebook: Facebook.com/myveganjournal

Recommended Reading

The Animal Activist Handbook: Maximizing our Positive Impact in Today's World, by Matt Ball and Bruce Friedrich

Animal Liberation by Peter Singer

Breaking the Food Seduction: The Hidden Reasons Behind Food Cravings—And 7 Steps to End Them Naturally by Neal D. Barnard, MD

The China Study: The Most Comprehensive Study of Nutrition Ever Conducted And the Startling Implications for Diet, Weight Loss, And Long-term Health, by T. Colin Campbell, PhD and Thomas M. Campbell

Diet for a New America: How Your Food Choices Affect Your Health, Happiness and the Future of Life on Earth by John Robbins

Eat & Run: My Unlikely Journey to Ultramarathon Greatness by Scott Jurek

Eating Animals by Jonathan Safran Foer

The Engine 2 Diet: The Texas Firefighter's 28-Day Save-Your-Life Plan that Lowers Cholesterol and Burns Away the Pounds by Rip Esselstyn

The Food Revolution: How Your Diet Can Help Save Your Life and The World, by John Robbins

Forks Over Knives: The Planted-Based Way to Health, T. Colin Campbell, PhD and Caldwell B. Esselstyne, Jr., MD

Finding Ultra: Rejecting Middle Age, Becoming One of the World's Fittest Men, and Discovering Myself by Rich Roll

How Not to Die: Discover the Foods Scientifically Proven to Prevent and Reverse Disease by Michael Greger, MD

Living the Farm Sanctuary Life: The Ultimate Guide to Eating Mindfully, Living Longer, and Feeling Better Every Day by Gene Baur

Mad Cowboy: Plain Truth from the Cattle Rancher Who Won't Eat Meat by Howard F. Lyman

Making Kind Choices: Everyday Ways to Enhance Your Life Through Earth- and Animal-Friendly Living by Ingrid Newkirk

Meathooked: The History and Science of Our 2.5 Million Year Obsession with Meat by Marta Zaraska

Meatonomics: How the Rigged Economics of Meat and Dairy Make You Consume Too Much—and How to Eat Better, Live Longer, and Spend Smarter by David Robinson Simon

No Meat Athlete: Run on Plants and Discover Your Fittest, Fastest, Happiest Self, by Matt Frazier with Matthew Ruscigno MPH, RD

Prevent and Reverse Heart Disease: The Revolutionary, Scientifically Proven, Nutrition-Based Cure by Caldwell B. Esselstyn Jr., MD

Proteinaholic: How Our Obsession with Meat Is Killing Us and What We Can Do About It by Garth Davis, MD

21-Day Weight Loss Kickstart: Boost Metabolism, Lower Cholesterol, and Dramatically Improve Your Health by Neal D. Barnard, MD

What a Fish Knows: The Inner Lives of Our Underwater Cousins by Jonathan Balcombe

Whole: Rethinking the Science of Nutrition by T. Colin Campbell, PhD

Children's Books

Bambi, a Life in the Woods by Felix Salten

Charlotte's Web by E. B. White

The Giving Tree, by Shel Silverstein

The Lorax by Dr. Seuss

Our Farm: By the Animals of Farm Sanctuary by Maya Gottfried

Steven the Vegan by Dan Bodenstein

That's Why We Don't Eat Animals by Ruby Roth

'Twas The Night Before Thanksgiving by Dav Pilkey

Vegan is Love: Having Heart and Taking Action by Ruby Roth

V Is for Vegan: The ABCs of Being Kind by Ruby Roth

Recommended Viewing

Babe

Blackfish

Charlotte's Web

The Cove

Cowspiracy: The Sustainability Secret

Crazy Sexy Cancer

Diet For a New America

Earthlings

Fast Food Nation

Fat, Sick & Nearly Dead

Food Inc.

Forks Over Knives

Ghost in the Machine

Live and Let Live
Peaceable Kingdom: The Journey Home
PlantPure Nation
Racing Extinction
Speciesism: The Movie
Supersize Me
Tyke Elephant Outlaw
Unity
Vanishing of the Bees
Vegucated

Cookbooks

I don't use cookbooks very often; I'm more of a "figure-it-out-as-you-go, season-to-taste, and have-fun" type of cook when it comes to vegan cuisine. And there are far too many fantastic vegan cookbooks to choose from, so I'm leaving it up to you as to which ones to read. There are *so* many diverse and interesting types of cookbooks out there. There are gluten-free vegan, raw vegan, one-bowl vegan, slow-cooker vegan cookbooks—oh man, I could go on and on! Just go to the library, your local bookstore, or browse around online. If you need a cookbook, I have no doubt you'll find one that's perfect for you. Just remember, as you're starting off: keep it *simple*!

Cruelty-Free Cosmetics Info

(Cruelty-free icons on cosmetics mean they're not tested on animals, but they may still contain animal ingredients, so always double-check.)
www.crueltyfreeconsumer.com
www.drugstore.com/crueltyfree
http://features.peta.org/cruelty-free-company-search
www.leapingbunny.com
www.peta.org/living/beauty/order-cruelty-free-shopping-guide
www.vitacost.com/crueltyfree

Animal Sanctuaries

For a list of animal sanctuaries that never breed animals, nor use them for commercial purposes, visit the Global Federation of Animal Sanctuaries (GRAS): http://www.sanctuaryfederation.org/gfas

ARIZONA
Whisper's Sanctuary

CALIFORNIA
Animal Place Sanctuary
Farm Sanctuary
The Gentle Barn
Happy Hen Chicken Rescue
Harvest Home Animal Sanctuary
PreetiRang Sanctuary

COLORADO
Peaceful Prairie Sanctuary

FLORIDA
Kindred Spirits Sanctuary
Rooterville

HAWAII
Leilani Farm Sanctuary

INDIANA
Uplands Peak Sanctuary

KENTUCKY
Home at Last Animal Sanctuary

MARYLAND
Poplar Spring Animal Sanctuary

MASSACHUSETTS
Maple Farm Sanctuary
Sunny Meadow Sanctuary

MICHIGAN
Sasha Farm

MINNESOTA
Chicken Run Rescue

NEW JERSEY
For the Animals Sanctuary

NEW MEXICO
Kindred Spirits Animal Sanctuary

NEW YORK
Catskill Animal Sanctuary
Farm Sanctuary
Woodstock Farm Animal Sanctuary

NORTH CAROLINA
Carolina Waterfowl Rescue

OHIO
Happy Trails Farm Animal Sanctuary
Sunrise Animal Sanctuary

OREGON
Green Acres Farm Sanctuary
Lighthouse Farm Sanctuary
Out to Pasture Sanctuary
Sanctuary One
Wildwood Farm Sanctuary

PENNSYLVANIA
Chenoa Manor

TENNESSEE
The Gentle Barn

TEXAS
Cleveland Amory Black Beauty Ranch
Rowdy Girl Sanctuary

VERMONT
Vine Sanctuary

VIRGINIA
United Poultry Concerns

WASHINGTON
Baahaus Animal Rescue Group
Pasado's Safe Haven
Pigs Peace Sanctuary
River's Wish Animal Sanctuary

WEST VIRGINIA
Pigs Animal Sanctuary

WISCONSIN
Heartland Farm Sanctuary

Animal-Free Circuses

Bindlestiff Family Cirkus: www.bindlestiff.org
Circus Center: www.circuscenter.org
Circus Finelli: www.circusfinelli.com
Circus Luminous: www.wisefoolnewmexico.org
Circus of the Kids: www.circusofthekids.com
Circus Vargas: www.circusvargas.com
Cirque du Soleil: www.cirquedusoleil.com
Cirque Éloize: www.cirque-eloize.com
Cirque Plume: www.cirqueplume.com
Flying Fruit Fly Circus: www.fruitflycircus.com.au
Flying High Circus: www.circus.fsu.edu
The Great All-American Youth Circus
    www.ycircus.org
Gregangelo & Velocity Circus Troupe: www.
    gregangelo.com
Hiccup Circus: www.hawaiispace.com/hiccup.php
Imperial Circus: www.worldentertainment.net/
    family-entertainment/the-imperial-circus
Les Colporteurs www.colporteurs.fdp@wanadoo.fr
Les 7 dights de la main (7 Fingers Circus):
    www.7doigts.com/en/the-company
New Shanghai Circus www.acrobatsofchina.com
Swamp Circus www.swampcircus.com

Cool Vegan Stuff

Animal Legal Defense Fund: a great place to find
    events, campaigns, and cases related to animal
    law: www.aldf.org
Animal Place's Humane Eating Wallet Guide:
    AnimalPlace.org
Annual Ranking of Vegan Food on College
    Campuses: VeganReportCard.com
Barnard Medical Center (100% Vegan): http://
    www.pcrm.org/barnardmedical
Coalition for Healthy School Food: www.
    healthyschoolfood.org
Counting Animals: CountingAnimals.com;
    provides stats on animals killed for food

Daily Video from Dr. Greger (100% plant-based
    nutrition): NutritionFacts.org
Eat Drink Politics: EatDrinkPolitics.com
EcoScraps: www.ecoscraps.com; organic compost
    and garden soils made from fruit and veggie
    "food waste." No animal by-products
FDA Recall Alerts (sign up to know when there's a
    recall): www.fda.gov/Safety/Recalls/default.htm
The Good Food Institute www.gfi.org
Havahart: Cruelty-free Animal Traps to Safely
    Move Animals: http://www.havahart.com
Mercy for Animals http://www.chooseveg.com/vsg;
    free Vegetarian Starter Guide:
PETA's free Vegan Starter Kit: http://www.peta.
    org/living/food/free-vegan-starter-kit
Plant-based Diet Articles by Dr. Neal Barnard:
    pcrm.org
Plant-based Doctors Database: plantbaseddoctors.
    org
Post Punk Kitchen Forum: (vegan discussion
    board) http://forum.theppk.com
Palm Oil Investigations: www.palmoilinvestigations.
    com (Information re: palm oil and its
    devistating impact on animals and the
    rainforests)
Shannon Scott Design: www.shannonscottdesign.
    com/ssd.asp (vegan interior design)
Studio Can Can: www.studiocan-can.co.uk (vegan
    interior design)
T Colin Campbell Center for Nutrition Studies:
    www.nutritionstudies.org
True North Health Center (100% plant based):
    www.healthpromoting.com
Vegan Dog Food and "Breathbones." www.V-Dog.
    com
Vegan Meetup Groups for fun and support (over
    1,500 groups across the world!):
www.meetup.com/topics/vegan
Veg Voyages: www.vegvoyages.com 100% vegan
    travel adventures
WhaleSENSE Whale Watching: whalesense.org

Vegan Travel Blogs

Bounding Over Our Steps
The Healthy Voyager
Indefinite Adventure
Justin Plus Lauren
Mindful Wanderlust
Mostly Amelie
Travel & Tofu
Vegan in Brighton
Vegan Miam
Vegan Nom Noms
Vegan World Trekker
Will Travel for Vegan Food

RAW VEGAN BLOGS

FullyRaw www.fullyraw.com
Rachael's Raw Food www.rachaelsrawfood.com
Raw. Vegan. Not Gross www.imlauramiller.com
This Rawsome Vegan Life www.thisrawsomeveganlife.com

VEGAN YOUTUBE CHANNELS

Eco-Vegan Gal
Fully Raw Kristina
Happy Healthy Vegan
Jason Wrobel
Kalel
Laura Miller on Tastemade
PlantbasedAthlete
Raw. Vegan. Not Gross.
The Sweetest Vegan
The Vegan Zombie
Vegan Black Metal Chef
VegSource

VEGAN PODCASTS

Food For Thought, Colleen Patrick-Goudreau
Main Street Vegan, Victoria Moran
No Meat Athlete, Matt Frazier
Our Hen House, Mariann Sullivan and Jasmin Singer
Rich Roll Podcast

HEALTH CHARITIES THAT ONLY FUND NON-ANIMAL RESEARCH

Avon Foundation for Women
Birth Defect Research for Children
Cancer Support Community
Children's Oncology Group
Dr. Susan Love Research Foundation
Gateway for Cancer Research
International Association for Suicide Prevention
Organization for Autism Research

VEGAN MAIL-ORDER and STORES

The following companies sell only animal-free products.

ALTERNATIVE OUTFITTERS
26 Tamalpais Drive, Corte Madera, CA 94925
(415) 924-6100
E-mail: **CustomerCare@AlternativeOutfitters.com**
Website: **www.alternativeoutfitters.com**
This vegan boutique and online store offers footwear, handbags, accessories (including watch and luggage tags), and much more.

ANIMAL PLACE'S VEGAN REPUBLIC
1624 University Ave, Berkeley, CA 94703
(510) 280-5778
Website: www.veganrepublicstore.org
A vegan boutique with buttons, T-shirts, stickers, and food, etc.

ARTISAN GEAR
PO Box 205, Gold Hill, OR 97525
(888) 499-4367 or (541) 855-5468
E-mail: **sales@artisangear.com**
Website: **www.artisangear.com**
Artisan Gear produces a line of classic/casual bags, wallets and accessories (watch bands, toiletry bags, etc.) from hemp canvas. You can order products online or visit their website to find stores that sell their items.

BEYOND SKIN
59 Lansdowne Place, Hove, East Sussex BN3 1FL
E-mail: **info@beyondskin.co.uk**
Website: **www.beyondskin.co.uk**
Here you'll find "luxury" shoes—including bridal shoes—handmade in England.

BOURGEOIS BOHEME
Unit 22, Acklam Workspace, 10 Acklam Road, London, England W10 5QZ
Tel: 011-44-20-8045-4338
E-mail: **info@bboheme.com**
Website: **www.bboheme.com**
This vegan boutique offers unique women's and men's footwear, bags, wallets, black faux leather gloves, belts, plus much more. You can also order online.

BRAVE GENTLE MAN
Website: **www.bravegentleman.com**
Shoes, boots, and belts for men, plus more.

CALICO DRAGON
(941) 928-3121
E-mail: **candy@calicodragonbags.com**
Website: **www.calicodragonbags.com**
Purses, clutches, handbags, wallets, and more.

COUCH
2502 N. Palm Dr., Ste. 1, Signal Hill, CA 90755
(562) 595-6965
Website: **www.couchguitarstraps.com**
This online site specializes in vegan guitar straps. They also sell camera straps, wallets, and belts.

CRI DE COEUR
Website: **www.cridecoeur.myshopify.com**
Find high-end vegan shoes, bags, and more at this online store.

THE ETHICAL MAN
Website: **www.theethicalman.com**
Online store offering wallets, belts, and more.

ETHICAL WARES
Caegwyn, Temple Bar, Felinfach, Ceredigion, SA48 7SA, Wales, United Kingdom
Tel: 011-44-1570 471155; Fax: 011-44-1570 471166

E-mail: **vegans@ethicalwares.com**
Website: **www.ethicalwares.com**
This company sells shoes and belts. Shoe styles include hiking boots, steel-toe safety boots, dress shoes, etc.

ETHIQUE NOUVEAU
317 W. 48th St., Minneapolis, MN 5541
(612) 822-6161
Website: **www.ethiquenouveau.com**
Vegan store offering bags, wallets, belts, and more.

GOOD GUYS DON'T WEAR LEATHER
Website: **www.goodguys.bigcartel.com**
Online store offering unique unisex shoes designed in Paris and made in Portugal including derby shoes, desert boots, and cowboy boots.

GRAPE CAT
PO Box 72, Pipersville, PA 18947
E-mail: **support@grapecat.com**
Website: **www.grapecat.com**
Offers purses, men's and women's wallets, and more.

GUNAS
4630 Center Blvd., Ste. 1005, Long Island City, NY 11109
(917) 544-9454
Website: **www.gunasthebrand.com**
Website offering all types of bags for men and women.

HERBIVORE CLOTHING
1211 SE Stark St., Portland, OR 97214
503) 281-TOFU
E-mail: TK
Website: **www.herbivoreclothing.com**
Store and online site offering wallets, purses, belts, T-shirts, etc.

JAAN J.
Chula Vista, CA 91912
Website: **www.jaanj.com**
Online company sells vegan ties in an assortment of styles and colors. Recipient of PETA's Proggy Award.

LUCA CHIARA
13 West 38th St., New York, NY 10003
E-mail: **customercare@lucachiara.com**
Website: **www.lucachiara.com**
Storefront and online store offering vegan shoes for men and women, as well as bags, wallets, iPad cases, and passport cases for men and women.

MATT & NAT
(888) 586-2636
E-mail: **info@mattandnat.com**
Website: **www.mattandnat.com**
Unique bags including wallets, shoulder bags, laptop carriers, briefcases, overnighters, and totes.

MOOSHOES
78 Orchard St., New York, NY 10002
(212) 254-6512
3116 Sunset Blvd., Los Angeles, CA 90026
(323) 741-8090
E-mail: **info@mooshoes.com**
Website: **www.mooshoes.com**
Though shoes can be purchased online, customers are encouraged to walk in and try shoes on. MooShoes offers brands such as Vegan Wares, Vegetarian Shoes, and Ethical Wares. They also sell bags, wallets, belts, and faux leather jackets.

NICE SHOES
3568 Fraser St., Vancouver, BC V5V 4C4 Canada
(604) 558-3000
Website: **www.gotniceshoes.com**
Canadian shop offering men's and women's shoes, boots, belts, bags, wallets, guitar straps, and more.

NO HARM
(860) 577-8724
Website: **www.noharm.com**
Men's dress shoes and boots. Offices in U.S. and UK.

NOAH SHOES BOUTIQUE
Tel: 011-49-09391-504-169
Website: **www.noah-shop.com**
German store and online shop offering vegan shoes, boots, sandals, bags, and belts made in Italy.

OLSENHAUS
E-mail: **orders@olsenhaus.com**
Website: **www.olsenhaus.com**
Online shop offering shoes for men, women, and kids.

OLY VEGAN
313 5th Ave. SE, Ste. A, Olympia, OR 98501
(800) 340-1200; Fax: (301) 816-8955
Website: **www.olyvegan.tumblr.com**
This store carries shoes, clothing, bags, and more.

OXFORD HANDBAGS
E-mail: **Kathys@oxfordhandbags.com**
Website: **www.oxfordhandbags.com**
Online shop offering eco-friendly bags and wallets.

PAMMIES
Website: **www.pammieslife.com**
Pamela Anderson's clothing line, including vegan boots.

PANGEA VEGAN PRODUCTS
2381 Lewis Ave., Rockville, MD 20851
(800) 340-1200 or (301) 816-8955
E-mail: **info@veganstore.com**
Website: **www.veganstore.com**
This store and online company carries shoes, clothing, wallets, belts, bags, personal care products, and food. Pangea is the producer of the No Bull line.

SAVE THE DUCK USA
Award-winning high-end vegan down jackets for adults and children.
Website: www.savetheduckusa.com

Susan Nichole
8605 Santa Monica Blvd. #35905, Los Angeles, CA 90069
E-mail: service@susannichole.com
Website: www.susannichole.com
Offers unique non-leather handbags and wallets.

VEGAN CHIC
440 South Bentley, Los Angeles, CA 90049
(866) 91-VEGAN or (818) 235-4709
Website: www.veganchic.com
This online store offers a wide range of shoes and bags, as well as belts and wallets. They carry kids' shoes, too.

THE VEGAN COLLECTION
PO Box 811971, Los Angeles, CA 90081
Website: www.thevegancollection.com
This online vegan store offers wallets and belts.

VEGANESSENTIALS
1701 Pearl St., Unit 8, Waukesha, WI 53186
(866) 88-VEGAN or (262) 574-7761
E-mail: questions@veganessentials.com
Website: www.veganessentials.com
Vegan Essentials is a mail-order company and retail shop offering goods such as shoes, wallets, belts, etc.

VEGAN HAVEN
5270 B University Way NE, Seattle, WA 98105
(206) 523-9060
Website: www.veganhaven.org
This vegan store is located at a Pig Sanctuary. They offer belts, wallets, and much more.

VEGANLINE
2 Avenue Gds, London, England SW14 8BP
E-mail: soundsearchers.co.uk
Website: www.veganline.com
Stylish shoes, boots, dress shoes, jackets, and belts.

VEGANSTORE.CO.UK
Vegan Store Ltd., PO Box 110, Rottingdean, Brighton BN51 9AZ United Kingdom
E-mail: sales@veganstore.co.uk
Website: www.veganstore.co.uk
Online shop carrying boots, shoes, etc. They're a licensed distributor of No Bull leather alternatives.

VEGAN WARES
78 Smith St., Collingwood, 3066 VIC Australia
Tel.: 61-3-9417-0230
E-mail: veganw@veganwares.com
Website: www.veganwares.com
They offer shoes, boots, briefcases, wallets, and more.

VEGETARIAN SHOES
12 Gardner St., Brighton, East Sussex, BN1 1UP United Kingdom
Telephone: 011-44-1273 691913
E-mail: information@vegetarian-shoes.co.uk
Website: www.vegetarian-shoes.co.uk
Synthetic leather and synthetic suede shoes, hiking boots, work boots, sandals, "leather" jackets, and belts.

THE VEGETARIAN SITE
PO Box 222, Glastonbury, CT 06033
(860) 519-1918
E-mail: shopping@thevegetariansite.com
Website: www.thevegetariansite.com
The Vegetarian Site has an online vegan store filled with clothing, footwear, wallets, belts, bags, and "leather" gloves.

WILLS LONDON
Floor 3, 207 Regent Street, London, W1B 3HH
E-mail: will@wills-vegan-shoes.com
Website: www.wills-vegan-shoes.com
High-end vegan shoes and accessories for men, women, and children.

CATALOGS, COMPANIES, & STORES WITH LEATHER ALTERNATIVES

The following catalogs, companies, and stores carry some non-leather products, but also many that are not animal-free. Check the merchandise to make sure it is non-leather. This is a partial listing of catalogs/stores with synthetic options.

DR. MARTENS
1-800-810-6673
Website: www.drmartens.com
Several vegan options available; just search the word vegan and you'll see them!

EARTH
(877) 372-2814
Website: www.earthbrands.com
Earth offers a line of vegan shoes including shoes, sandals, and boots. Search the word vegan.

FOOTWEAR, ETC.
273 N. Mathilda Ave., Sunnyvale, CA 94086
(800) 720-0572
Website: www.footwearetc.com
Search the word vegan to find women's and men's shoes and sandals.

GREEN SHOES
The Old Chapel, 26A Cross St., Moretonhampstead, TQ13 8NL, United Kingdom
Tel: 011-44-1647 440735
Website: www.greenshoes.co.uk

Vegan line of handmade men's, women's, and children's shoes, boots, and sandals. They also make bags and belts.

LOVE IS MIGHTY
619) 537-6053
Website: **loveismighty.com**
Unique women's shoes made by tribal woman in India.

MODCLOTH
Website: **www.modcloth.com**
Hundreds of unique vintage inspired vegan clothes, shoes, and accessories. Search the term "vegan" on website.

PAYLESS SHOE SOURCE
Website: **www.payless.com**
Wide selection of non-leather, synthetic shoes available in men's, women's, and children's styles. Call (877) 474-6379 for a store in your area.

PLANETSHOES.COM
(888) 818-SHOE (7463)
E-mail: **info@planetshoes.com**
Website: **www.planetshoes.com**
This online store offers a line of vegan women's and men's casual shoes, boots, sandals, bags, etc. Search the word vegan.

REI
REI, Sumner, WA 98352-0001
(800) 426-4840
Website: **www.rei.com**
Search under vegan for shoes, boots, and sandals. Also sell non-leather belts and watch bands.

ROAD RUNNER SPORTS
(800) 743-3206
Website: **www.roadrunnersports.com**
Search under vegan for running shoes and sandals.

SPECK PRODUCTS
Website: **www.speckproducts.com**
Online store offering vegan protective covers for your Nook Touch, Kindle, iPhone, and more.

STELLA MCCARTNEY
Website: **www.stellamccartney.com**
Online store offering unique non-leather handbags and shoes.

TOMS
Website: **www.toms.com**
Search under the word vegan on this online store and you'll find shoes.

TOUGH TRAVELER
(800) GO-TOUGH
Website: **www.toughtraveler.com**
Offers baby carriers, backpacks, briefcases, laptop bags, camera, bags, hiking packs, luggage, cd disk and player waist pack, cell phone case, etc. Most are vegan; however, indicate "no leather" under comments in order.

ZAPPOS.COM
(800) 927-7671
Website: **www.zappos.com**
Search under the word vegan on this website and a long list of sandals and casual, formal, athletic, and other shoes will appear. They carry shoes for men, women, and children.

ATHLETIC SHOES
There are leather alternatives in most shoe styles.
Women's and Men's Athletic Shoes
Asics: (800) 678-9435: *Several synthetic shoes; call to find out about a certain shoe.*
Converse: (888) 792-3307: *Chuck Taylor All-Stars, high-top and low-top, come in many styles, colors, and fabrics. They also have canvas One Stars.*
Keds: (800) 680-0966: *Canvas oxfords and slip-ons in a variety of colors and patterns.*
New Balance: (800) 253-7463: *Several running shoes made with synthetic uppers. Call for a catalog.*
Payless Shoe Source: (877) 474-6379: *Many athletic shoes made with synthetic materials.*
Saucony: (800) 282-6575: *They have lots of vegan shoes, including the "Jazz Low Pro Vegan" in many colors.*
Vans: (855) 909-8267: *Styles include canvas shoes. Call for stores in your area.*

DRESS SHOES
Women's and Men's Dress Shoes
Men and women can find non-leather dress shoes at the **All-Vegan Stores** listed above, or at **Payless, Shoe Source, or Target.**

HIKING BOOTS
Ethical Wares: *Weald, Ranger, Trekking styles, and more.*
Hiking Boots: *Jess at VeganOutdoorAdventures.com has a nice list!*
Pangea: *Men's Wanderlust Hiking Boot.*
Vegetarian Shoes: *Offers several hiking boots.*
Wicked Hemp: *Hiking boot made from hemp.*

WORK BOOTS
Ethical Wares: *Safety Boot with a steel toe.*
Lacrosse Boots: *Several styles of rubber boots: insulated, non-insulated, and steel toe. Available from large retailers. Call (888) 323-2668 for information.*
Vegan Essentials: *Offers steel-toe boots.*

Veganline: *Offers safety boots and shoes.*
Vegetarian Shoes: *Safety boots with steel-toe caps.*

WHERE DO I FIND...

Ballet Shoes

Cynthia King Dance Studio *offers the CKDS ballet slipper with canvas uppers and synthetic leather soles in adult and children's sizes and various colors. Call (718) 437-0101 or visit* **www.cynthiakingdance.com.**

Baseball Gloves

Carpenter Trading Company *offers custom-made vegan gloves. Visit* **www.carpentertrade.com.**

Biking Gloves

Aerostich Rider Wearhouse *offers vegan riding gloves good for all seasons at* **www.aerostich.com**
Galtani *offers vegan cycling gloves at* **www.galtani.bigcartel.com**
Garneau *offers vegan cycling gloves at* **www.louisgarneau.com**

Bowling Shoes

Dexter Shoes *offers some bowling shoes made from 100% synthetics. Visit* **www.dextershoes.com.**

Briefcases

Luggageonline.com *offers non-leather briefcases.*
Mattandnat.com *offers non-leather briefcases.*
Tough Traveler: *See* **www.toughtraveler.com**

Camera Straps

Couch *offers a wide variety of camera straps.*

Dance Shoes

Very Fine Shoes *offers a wide variety of custom-made vegan dance shoes. Visit* **www.veryfineshoes.com** *and go to vegan shoes.*

Gloves

The Vegetarian site *and* **Vegetarian Shoes** *offer vegan "leather" gloves.*

Guitar Straps

Couch *offers a wide variety of handmade straps.*
Pangea *offers a guitar strap without the leather ends.*
Splaff Flops *offers guitar straps.*
Vegan Wares *offers guitar straps.*

Hand Drums

www.rhythmhousedrums.com: *Search under the vegan category and drums that have non-leather heads.*

Heelys

Shoes.com: *Search under the word Heelys and you'll find varieties that are non-leather.*

Ice Skates

Bauer Pro Shop *offers many non-leather Bauer hockey skates at* **bauer.hockeygiant.com**

Motorcycle Gear

Cycleport *offers synthetic motorcycle apparel including the Motoport Racing Glove. See* **www.motoport.com**

GetGeared *offers motorcycle gloves. Search under the word vegan at* **www.getgeared.co.uk**
Motoliberty *sells several styles of non-leather motorcycle jackets. Visit* **www.motoliberty.com**
Motonation *has several varieties of non-leather Sidi motorcycle boots. See* **www.motonation.com**

Musical Instrument Cases

Tough Traveler *See* **www.toughtraveler.com**

Rock Climbing Shoes

Evolv Sports and Design *offers a number of vegan rock climbing shoes. Visit* **www.evolvsports.com**

Snow Boots/Snowboarding Boots

Burton Snowboards: *You'll find several types of non-leather snow boots at* **www.burton.com**
Sole Technology (owns "Thirty Two") *offers several non-leather snow boots for men and women. See* **www.thirtytwo.com**

Speed Skates

Riedell Divine Quad Speed Skates: *You'll find these vegan speed skates at* **www.lowpriceskates.com**

Synthetic Leather Manufacturer

Ecolorica: *For information on this Italian companyv visit* **www.ecolorica.com** *or e-mail* **ecolorica@ecolorica.com**
Willow Tex: *Visit* **www.izitleather.com** *or call (815) 399-4048 for information on their ecologically friendly vegan leather alternative. It comes in several colors.*

Tool Belts

Nailers, Inc.: *Visit* **www.nailersinc.com** *or call (619) 562-2215 for their non-leather tool belts, nail bags, and knee pads, made from Dupont's Cordura fabric.*

Watches with Non-leather Bands

Alternative Outfitters *carries watches with non-leather bands. See* **www.alternativeoutfitters.com**
There are also lots of non-leather bands on **www.amazon.com.**

Shopping list compiled with the help and permission of Vegetarian Resource Group: www.vrg.org

Notes

My Road to Vegan

1. https://www.youtube.com/
watch?v=uQCe4qEexjc accessed 12/5/15.

Setting a Date

1. http://time.com/money/3648918/ways-
to-make-your-new-years-resolutions-stick/
accessed 1/2/15.
2. http://lifehacker.com/5921478/shhh-
keeping-quiet-may-help-you-achieve-your-
goals accessed 1/2/15.
3. http://articles.latimes.com/2012/nov/17/
health/la-he-five-questions-salley-20121117
accessed 1/2/15.
4. http://www.rd.com/health/healthy-eating/
becoming-vegan-tips/ accessed 1/2/15.

The 21 Days to Vegan Roadmap

1. https://research.kpchr.org/News/News-
Archive/Post/343/CHR-Study-Finds-
Keeping-Food-Diaries-Doubles-Weight-Loss
accessed 9/2/15.
2. http://www.jasonmraz.com/journal/2012/
plant-based/ accessed 9/1/15.
3. https://www.nhlbi.nih.gov/files/docs/public/
sleep/healthy_sleep.pdf accessed 9/1/15.
4. http://journalsleep.org/ViewAbstract.
aspx?pid=29022 accessed 9/1/15.
5. http://www.thelancet.com/journals/lancet/
article/PIIS0140-6736(11)60749-6/abstract
accessed 9/1/15.
6. http://www.cdc.gov/foodborneburden/2011-
foodborne-estimates.html accessed 9/1/15.
7. http://www.cdc.gov/foodsafety/foodborne-
germs.html accessed 9/1/15.

Day 1: Finding Your Muse

1. http://www.unep.org/climatechange/
News/PressRelease/tabid/416/
language/en-US/Default.
aspx?DocumentId=628&ArticleId=6595
accessed 9/1/15.
2. *The China Study*, T Colin Campbell, PhD and
Thomas M. Campbell II, pg. 7.
3. *Jane Velez-Mitchell Brings Vegan Meal for
Anderson*, https://www.youtube.com/
watch?v=RU995xSNlBE accessed 12/5/15.
4. *Earthlings*, https://www.youtube.com/
watch?v=GVE6eZCJZv8 accessed 6/25/16.

5. *The China Study*, T Colin Campbell, PhD and
Thomas M. Campbell II, pg. 7.
6. http://www.toprntobsn.com/veganism/
accessed 10/4/15.

Day 2: Creepy Crawlies in Your Food, Oh My!

1. http://www.tropicana.com/products/pure-
premium/healthy-heart/ accessed 8/1/15
2. http://www.fda.gov/ForConsumers/
ConsumerUpdates/ucm433555.htm accessed
6/25/16.
3. https://www.govtrack.us/congress/bills/111/
hr2086/text accessed 10/8/15.
4. http://www.businessinsider.com/facts-about-
natural-and-artificial-flavors-2014-1 accessed
8/1/15.
5. https://www.publicintegrity.
org/2015/04/14/17112/why-fda-doesnt-
really-know-whats-your-food accessed 9/1/15.

Day 3: Finding Your Vegan Oasis

1. https://www.nal.usda.gov/afsic/community-
supported-agriculture accessed 9/24/15.
2. http://www.nbcbayarea.com/investigations/
USDA-Inspections-Offer-Glimpse-into-
the-Supply-Chain-for-Whole-Foods-New-
Rabbit-Meat-Pilot-Program-304500531.html
accessed 9/24/15.
3. http://www.courthousenews.
com/2015/09/22/peta-calls-out-whole-
foods-on-meat.htm accessed 9/24/15.
4. http://www.ewg.org/research/bisphenol
accessed 9/24/15.
5. https://snaped.fns.usda.gov/nutrition-through-
seasons/seasonal-produce accessed 9/24/15.

Day 4: Let's Get Nutty

1. http://www.ers.usda.gov/media/1118789/
err149.pdf accessed 8/18/15.
2. https://www.hsph.harvard.edu/
nutritionsource/calcium-full-story/#calcium-
from-milk accessed 8/18/15.
3. Ganmaa D, Sato A. The possible role of female
sex hormones in milk from pregnant cows
in the development of breast, ovarian, and
corpus uteri cancers. Med Hypotheses. 2005;
65:1028–37.
4. Yang M, Kenfield SA, Van Blarigan EL, et al.
Dairy intake after prostate cancer diagnosis in
relation to disease-specific and total mortality.
Int J Cancer. Published online May 20, 2015.

5. http://www.pcrm.org/health/diets/vsk/ vegetarian-starter-kit-protein 8/17/15.
6. http://www.soyinfocenter.com/HSS/white_ wave.php, 8/17/15.
7. *Steve Demos White Wave – Selling Without Selling Out*, YouTube, http://www. soyinfocenter.com/HSS/white_wave.php accessed 8/17/15.
8. *Milk cows and production by State and region (Annual)*, http://www.ers.usda.gov/data-products/dairy-data.aspx accessed 8/18/15.
9. http://www.epa.gov/oecaagct/ag101/ dairyphases.html accessed 8/18/15.
10. https://timedotcom.files.wordpress. com/2015/03/ucm435759.pdf accessed 8/18/15.
11. http://time.com/3738069/fda-dairy-farmers-antibiotics-milk/ accessed 8/18/15.
12. http://www.whfoods.com/genpage. php?tname=foodspice&dbid=99 accessed 8/19/15.
13. https://www.hsph.harvard.edu/ nutritionsource/what-should-you-eat/ calcium-and-milk/ accessed 8/18/15.
14. http://www.pcrm.org/health/health-topics/ calcium-and-strong-bones accessed 4/18/15.
15. http://www.medscape.com/ viewarticle/461898 accessed 12/7/15.
16. http://www.pcrm.org/health/diets/vsk/ vegetarian-starter-kit-calcium accessed 12/7/15.

Day 5: Eggs Make Babies, Not Breakfast

1. http://nutritiondata.self.com/facts/fast-foods-generic/8051/2 accessed 8/21/15.
2. http://www.eggnutritioncenter.org/egg-101/ accessed 6/28/16.
3. https://circ.ahajournals.org/content/ early/2014/12/18/CIR.0000000000000152. full.pdf accessed 8/21/15.
4. http://awic.nal.usda.gov/government-and-professional-resources/federal-laws/humane-methods-slaughter-act accessed 8/24/15.
5. http://blog.humanesociety.org/ wayne/2014/04/this-isnt-chicken-little-talk-about-usdas-poultry-slaughter-rules.html accessed 8/22/15.
6. http://www.humanesociety.org/issues/ slaughter accessed 8/21/15.
7. https://www.washingtonpost.com/ politics/usda-plan-to-speed-up-poultry-processing-lines-could-increase-risk-of-bird-abuse/2013/10/29/aeeffe1e-3b2e-11e3-b6a9-da62c264f40e_story.html 8/23/15.

8. http://uepcertified.com/wp-content/ uploads/2015/08/UEP-Animal-Welfare-Guidelines-20141.pdf accessed 6/28/16.
9. http://www.huffingtonpost.com/bruce-friedrich/eggs-from-caged-hens_b_2458525. html accessed 8/24/15.
10. http://openjurist.org/570/f2d/157/national-commission-on-egg-nutrition-v-federal-trade-commission accessed 8/21/15.
11. Ibid. 8/21/15.
12. http://usda.mannlib.cornell.edu/ usda/nass/ChicEggs//2010s/2015/ ChicEggs-08-21-2015.pdf accessed 9/1/15.
13. http://www.bizjournals.com/sanfrancisco/ blog/2015/09/hampton-creek-just-mayo-fda-eggs-unilever-lawsuit.html accessed 9/5/15.
14. https://www.theguardian.com/ business/2015/sep/06/usda-american-egg-board-paid-bloggers-hampton-creek accessed 9/5/15.
15. http://www.eatdrinkpolitics. com/2015/09/02/hampton-creek-targeted-by-usda-controlled-egg-industry-program/ accessed 9/5/15.
16. https://www.youtube.com/watch?v=eM-JsyyfSmE accessed 8/23/15.
17. https://www.yahoo.com/style/classic-eggless-mayonnaise-from-homemade-vegan-127214966481.html accessed 8/25/15.
18. https://en.wikipedia.org/wiki/Aquafaba accessed 8/25/15.
19. http://food52.com/recipes/32483-vegan-eggnog accessed 8/25/15.
20. https://en.wikipedia.org/wiki/Bird%27s_ Custard accessed 8/26/15.
21. http://www.humanesociety.org/issues/ confinement_farm/facts/cage-free_vs_ battery-cage.html accessed 8/24/15.
22. http://animalethics.org.uk/i-ch7-2-chickens. html accessed 8/24/15.
23. http://www.humanesociety.org/issues/ confinement_farm/facts/guide_egg_labels. html accessed 8/25/15.

Day 6: I Smell Something Fishy

1. http://www.huffingtonpost.com/ bruce-friedrich/fish-are-smart-and-of-cou_b_5545914.html accessed 8/29/15.
2. *Eating Animals* by Jonathan Safran Foer, pg. 65, 1st Edition, Little, Brown and Company, 2009.
3. Dunayer, Joan, "Fish: Sensitivity Beyond the Captor's Grasp," The Animals' Agenda, July/ August 1991, pp. 12–18.

4. *Healthy Eating for Life to Prevent and Treat Diabetes*, Neal Barnard, M.D., pg. 38, 1st Edition, John Wiley & Sons, 2002.

5. *The Plantpower Way: Whole Food Plant-Based Recipes and Guidance for The Whole Family*, by Rich Roll, pg. 14, Avery, 1st Edition, 2015.

6. https://nccih.nih.gov/health/omega3/introduction.htm accessed 9/1/15.

7. http://www.slate.com/articles/health_and_science/medical_examiner/2014/08/does_fish_oil_prevent_heart_disease_original_danish_eskimo_diet_study_was.html, 9/1/15.

8. http://www.cspinet.org/new/200811251.html accessed 9/1/15.

9. *On Food and Cooking: The Science and Lore of the Kitchen*, Harold McGee, pg. 184 Scribner, 1st revised edition, 2004.

10. http://www.ecfr.gov/cgi-bin/text-idx?c=ecfr&sid=0bfba9505f9e71f6ad1b482c1fc1c99a&rgn=div5&view=text&node=7:3.1.1.1.7&idno=7#sg7.3.60_1133.sg1 accessed 9/2/15.

11. http://www.teamuse.com/article_110701.html accessed 9/2/15.

12. http://www.foodandwaterwatch.org/insight/factory-fish-farming, accessed 9/2/15.

13. Ibid.

14. http://ncleg.net/Library/studies/2007/st11669.pdf accessed 9/2/14

15. https://www.foodandwaterwatch.org/sites/default/files/factory_fed_fish_report_july_2012.pdf accessed 9/2/15.

16. *On Food and Cooking: The Science and Lore of the Kitchen*, Harold McGee, pg. 516 Scribner, 1st revised edition, 2004.

17. http://classics.mit.edu/Hippocrates/ulcers.4.4.html accessed 9/1/15.

18. http://www.aicr.org/foods-that-fight-cancer/flaxseed.html#research accessed 9/2/15.

19. http://www.nytimes.com/2005/04/10/dining/stores-say-wild-salmon-but-tests-say-farm-bred.html?_r=0 accessed 9/5/15.

20. http://www.ncbi.nlm.nih.gov/pmc/articles/PMC1691351/ accessed 9/3/15.

Day 7: Mystery Meat

1. http://www.adaptt.org/killcounter.html accessed 9/3/15.

2. http://www.huffingtonpost.com/bruce-friedrich/meatonomics-the-bizarree_b_3853414.html accessed 9/3/15.

3. *On Food and Cooking: The Science and Lore of the Kitchen*, Harold McGee, pg. 119 Scribner, 1st revised edition, 2004.

4. Ibid.

5. https://www.drmcdougall.com/misc/2012nl/

6. http://www.ers.usda.gov/data-products/farm-income-and-wealth-statistics/annual-cash-receipts-by-commodity.aspx#P067767e8fa1d45149cb08450513a22a2_3_16iT0R0x0 accessed 12/7/15.

7. Ibid.

8. http://www.huffingtonpost.com/elliott-negin/eat-your-fruits-and-veggi_b_3715132.html accessed 9/5/15.

9. http://www.whale.to/a/light.html accessed 9/4/15.

10. https://farm.ewg.org/region.php accessed 9/5/15.

11. http://cbo.gov/sites/default/files/cbofiles/attachments/hr2642LucasLtr.pdf accessed 9/4/15.

12. http://www.washingtonpost.com/news/wonkblog/wp/2014/01/28/the-950-billion-farm-bill-in-one-chart/ accessed 9/4/15.

13. http://thehill.com/policy/finance/196856-lawmakers-wont-have-to-disclose-crop-insurance-subsidies-under accessed 9/6/15.

14. https://meatonomics.com/2013/08/15/each-time-mcdonalds-sells-a-big-mac-were-out-7/ accessed 9/6/15.

15. http://nutrition.mcdonalds.com/getnutrition/ingredientslist.pdf 9/4/15.

16. *The China Study*, T. Colin Campbell, PhD and Thomas M. Campbell II, pg. 7, 1st Paperback Edition, Benbella Books, 2006.

17. *On Food and Cooking: The Science and Lore of the Kitchen*, Harold McGee, pg. 468 Scribner, 1st revised edition, 2004.

18. *Soy Oh Soy, Is It Really Bad for You?*, David Schardt, Nutrition Action Health Newsletter, Center for Science in the Public Interest, September 2014.

19. http://www.ncbi.nlm.nih.gov/pubmed/18558591 accessed 9/4/15.

20. Ibid.

21. https://www.youtube.com/watch?v=ZwX9Ll19cX0 *CNN Report: Secret of long life in Okinawa*, accessed 9/1/15.

22. http://www.japantimes.co.jp/news/2015/09/11/national/japans-centenarian-population-tops-60000-first-time/ accessed 9/30/15.

23. http://www.nongmoproject.org/find-non-gmo/search-participating-products/?catID=2139569536 accessed 9/30/15.

24. http://www.humanesociety.org/issues/confinement_farm/facts/gestation_crates.html accessed 12/5/15.

25. *Eating Animals*, Jonathan Safran Foer, pg. 186, 1st Edition, Little, Brown and Company, 2009.

26. Ibid. pg. 187.
27. http://www.huffingtonpost.com/ paul-shapiro/on-farms-not-all- cruelty-_b_5960710.html accessed 12/5/15.
28. http://www.fao.org/docrep/003/X6909E/ x6909e09.htm#b7-Determining%20 insensibility%20at%20slaughter accessed 8/24/15.
29. http://www.consumerfed.org/pdfs/CFA- COOL-poll-press-release-May-2013.pdf accessed 12/28/15.

Day 8: But I Love Cheese Too Much...

1. http://www.vegsource.com/talk/veganism/ messages/980048.html accessed 9/1/15.
2. http://www.veggieboards.com/forum/23- product-reviews/7534-galaxy-soymage-vegan- cheese.html accessed 9/1/15.
3. https://www.google.com/ trends/explore#q=vegan%20 cheese&cmpt=q&tz=Etc%2FGMT%2B7 (Data from January 2006 compared to January 2016) accessed 2/25/16.
4. http://www.pcrm.org/health/diets/ffl/ newsletter/breaking-the-cheese-addiction- step-3-cleansing-the accessed 9/5/15.
5. http://www.americasdairyland.com/dairy/ milk/milk-facts accessed 6/30/16.

Day 9: Fast, Cheap, and Easy!

1. http://www.pcrm.org/health/diets/vegdiets/ how-can-i-get-enough-protein-the-protein- myth accessed 9/3/15.
2. Ibid.
3. https://www.nlm.nih.gov/medlineplus/ency/ article/002442.htm accessed 9/3/15.
4. http://www.inc.com/magazine/20090601/ fresh-from-prison-a-brother-rejoins-his- family-business.html accessed 9/3/15.
5. http://www.foodnavigator-usa.com/ Manufacturers/Flowers-Foods-To-Acquire- Dave-s-Killer-Bread, acccessed 9/3/15.
6. On Food and Cooking: The Science and Lore of the Kitchen, Harold McGee, pg. 772 Scribner, 1st revised edition, 2004.
7. https://www.pastemagazine.com/ articles/2015/09/8-popular-cooking-oils-to- avoid-and-why.html accessed 9/13/15.
8. The Vegetarian Flavor Bible, Karen Page, pg. 338. Little, Brown and Company, 1st Edition, 2014.
9. http://www.fns.usda.gov/wic/wic- food- packages-regulatory-requirements- wic- eligible-foods#JUICE%20 (Women%20 and%20Children) accessed 9/10/15.

10. http://www.foodnotbombs.net/story.html, accessed 9/1/15.

Day 10: Culinary "Arts"

1. Understanding Nutrition, Whitney/Rolphs, pg. 379, Wadsworth Cengage Learning, Student Edition, 2011.
2. http://www.ncbi.nlm.nih.gov/pmc/articles/ PMC3249911/ accessed 9/1/15.
3. Ibid.
4. How to Make Natural Food Coloring - Concentrated Color Recipe https://www. youtube.com/watch?v=Q0dhvWA5iq4 accessed 9/1/15.

Day 11: Because Bunnies Don't Have Tear Ducts

1. http://www.scientificamerican.com/article/ cosmetics-animal-testing/ accessed 9/3/15.
2. http://www.humanesociety.org/issues/ cosmetic_testing/qa/questions_answers.html accessed 10/4/15.
3. http://www.fda.gov/cosmetics/labeling/ ucm2005202.htm accessed 10/4/15.
4. http://www.hsi.org/issues/becrueltyfree/ facts/infographic/en/, 10/4/15.
5. Civic Impulse. (2015). H.R. 4148—113th Congress: Humane Cosmetics Act. Retrieved from https://www.govtrack.us/congress/ bills/113/hr4148, accessed 10/4/15.
6. The O'Jays—For The Love of Money (Audio). https://www.youtube.com/watch?v=GXE_ n2q08Yw accessed 10/4/15.
7. U.S. Code § 2132, United States Animal Welfare Act.
8. http://www.wetnwildbeauty.com/faq accessed 9/3/15.
9. From an email sent to me via customer service on 10/4/15.
10. http://occmakeup.com/pages/faq1.html accessed 10/4/15.
11. Inside Amy Schumer, Girl You Don't Need Makeup. https://www.youtube.com/ watch?v=fyeTJVU4wVo, accessed 10/4/15.

Day 12: I Spy with My Vegan Eye

1. http://www.oprah.com/world/tips-for- buying-an-eco-friendly-mattress accessed 10/5/15.

Day 13: The Skeletons in Your Closet

1. http://www.businessinsider.com/r-peta- animal-cruelty-video-prompts-probe-by- apparel-maker-patagonia-2015-8 accessed 10/1/15.

2. http://www.animalsaustralia.org/issues/mulesing.php accessed 6/30/16.
3. http://kb.rspca.org.au/what-are-the-animal-welfare-issues-with-shearing-of-sheep_603.html accessed 10/1/15.
4. http://www.dictionary.com/browse/caterpillar accessed 10/1/15.
5. http://www.silk-road.com/artl/silkhistory.shtml accessed 10/1/15.
6. http://www.merriam-webster.com/dictionary/schizophrenia accessed 10/1/15.
7. http://qz.com/578941/bangladeshs-nightmarish-leather-industry-makes-the-case-for-vegan-products/ accessed 12/22/15.
8. http://www.theguardian.com/world/shortcuts/2013/dec/16/angora-production-ethical-peta-video-chinese-rabbits accessed 10/1/15.
9. http://www.peta.org/blog/robert-redfords-still-got-it-as-long-as-it-isnt-made-of-angora accessed 10/6/15.
10. *Alicia Silverstone Helps Uncover the Cruelty of Down*, YouTube Video https://www.youtube.com/watch?v=vTfZiVi6Kdo accessed 10/1/15.
11. http://www.humanesociety.org/assets/pdfs/fur/investigation_century_21.pdf accessed 10/1/15.
12. http://www.careforthewild.com/what-we-do/campaigns/previous-campaigns/fighting-the-fur-trade accessed 12/1/15.
13. http://www.humanesociety.org/assets/pdfs/fur/investigation_century_21.pdf accessed 10/1/15.
14. http://www.today.com/money/rossen-reports-some-faux-fur-sold-stores-comes-real-animals-1D80374119 accessed 10/1/15.
15. http://journals.plos.org/plosone/article?id=10.1371/journal.pone.0083615 accessed 10/1/15.
16. http://the.honoluluadvertiser.com/article/2003/Jan/19/ln/ln07a.html accessed 10/1/15.

Day 14: Excuse Me, Waiter, There's a Fish in My Beer!

1. https://www.bonnydoonvineyard.com/about/ingredient-labeling accessed 9/1/15.
2. http://www.spiegel.de/international/germany/oktoberfest-organizers-introduce-vegan-food-options-a-924929.html accessed 9/1/15.
3. https://en.wikipedia.org/wiki/Reinheitsgebot accessed 9/1/15.
4. http://nynow.org/post/meat-drenched-oktoberfest-warms-vegans accessed 9/1/15.
5. http://www.smh.com.au/nsw/local-hunters-keen-to-begin-national-parks-trial-20140118-311l5.html accessed 9/1/15.
6. http://www.whitetailsunlimited.com accessed 9/1/15.

Day 15: Keeping the Happy in the Holiday

1. www.vegansociety.com/resources/recipes/special-occasions accessed 10/2/15.
2. https://munchies.vice.com/en/videos/how-to-make-a-vegan-christmas-dinner accessed 10/2/15.

Day 16: Vegan Wanderlust

1. http://www.businessinsider.com/kfcs-huge-advantage-over-chick-fil-a-2015-9 accessed 9/2/15.
2. http://www.kfc.com/nutrition accessed 9/1/15.
3. https://www.tacobell.com/faq accessed 9/1/15.
4. https://denver.cbslocal.com/2012/11/29/yelp-reviews-go-through-filter-some-claim-isnt-fair/ accessed 10/2/15.
5. http://www.pcrm.org/health/reports/2015-airport-food-review accessed 1/2/16.
6. Ibid.
7. https://www.vegansociety.com/shop/books/vegan-passport accessed 10/2/15.
8. Note: Phrases are according to the Google Translate Search Engine. Readers should confirm for accuracy, as dialects can vary.

Day 17: Now, *That's* Entertainment!

1. http://www.stopcircussuffering.com/circus-bans/ accessed 10/1/15.
2. http://www.bornfreeusa.org/b4a3_circuses_and_shows.php accessed 10/1/15.
3. http://aldf.org/blog/5-things-you-didnt-know-about-the-carriage-horse-industry/ accessed 10/1/15.
4. www.bornfree.org.uk/campaigns/zoo-check/captive-whales-dolphins/global, accessed 10/1/15.
5. www.aldf.org/cases-campaigns/features/rodeo-facts-the-case-against-rodeos accessed 10/1/15.
6. www.peta.org/issues/animals-in-entertainment/cruel-sports/rodeos accessed 10/1/15.

Day 18: Adopt, Don't Stop

1. https://vmacs.vmth.ucdavis.edu/userpages/beh/feline_behavior/spay.html accessed 12/5/15.
2. http://www.aldf.org/blog/meet-national-justice-for-animals-weeks-mascot-teagan accessed 10/1/15.
3. http://www.slate.com/blogs/xx_factor/2015/04/15/most_domestic_violence_shelters_don_t_take_pets_a_new_bill_can_help_change.html accessed 10/1/15.
4. http://www.ncbi.nlm.nih.gov/pubmed/17420515 accessed 10/1/15.
5. http://ericandpeety.com/about-eric-o-grey/ accessed 6/1/16.
6. http://www.peta.org/issues/companion-animal-issues/cruel-practices/dog-hot-car/ accessed 10/1/15.

Day 19: Vegan 911! Tips and Tricks to Stay on the Vegan Wagon

1. http://www.pnas.org/content/113/15/4146.full accessed 6/1/16.

Day 20: Planting Seeds of Compassion

1. http://www.usatoday.com/story/news/2015/10/14/social-media-posts-constituents-grab-congresss-attention-report-says/73831114 accessed 10/14/15.
2. http://www.humanesociety.org/issues/eating/facts/meatless_monday_toolkits.html accessed 10/14/15.
3. http://www.peta.org/living/food/free-vegan-starter-kit/ accessed 10/15/15.
4. http://www.californiadriedplums.org/press-room/2000/6/you-won-t-have-prunes-to-kick-around-anymore accessed 10/1/15.
5. http://www.seeker.com/iq-tests-suggest-pigs-are-smart-as-dogs-chimps-1769934406.html accessed 12/5/15.
6. http://www.mfablog.org/abby-the-abused-chicken-tours-70-cities-to accessed 12/5/15.

Day 21: Vegan for the WIN!

1. https://www.youtube.com/watch?v=TZNVEfGjjNQ accessed 12/5/15.
2. http://www.bcmj.org/premise/history-bloodletting accessed 12/5/15.
3. http://www.thetimes.co.uk/tto/business/industries/retailing/article4621808.ece accessed 12/5/15.
4. http://www.usatoday.com/story/money/business/2015/06/18/mcdonalds-shrinking-in-us/28920223/ accessed 12/5/15.

5. http://www.benjerry.com/flavors/non-dairy accessed 12/15/15.
6. https://blog.pinterest.com/en/what-world-are-people-searching accessed 12/7/15.
7. http://www.businessinsider.com/study-more-us-adults-use-pinterest-than-twitter-2013-12 accessed 12/7/15.
8. http://www.foodnavigator-usa.com/Markets/Vegan-is-going-mainstream-trend-data-suggests accessed 12/15/15.
9. *Animal Rights, Human Wrongs: An Introduction to Moral Philosophy*, Tom Reagan, pg. 34. Rowman & Littlefield Publishers, 2003.
10. http://news.nationalgeographic.com/2015/09/150916-ringling-circus-elephants-florida-center accessed 12/5/15.
11. https://www.federalregister.gov/articles/2015/12/23/2015-31958/endangered-and-threatened-wildlife-and-plants-listing-two-lion-subspecies#h-8 accessed 12/23/15.
12. https://www.theguardian.com/world/2011/sep/25/last-bullfight-in-barcelona accessed 12/5/15.
13. http://www.nature.com/news/nih-to-retire-all-research-chimpanzees-1.18817 accessed 12/5/15.
14. http://www.nestleusa.com/media/pressreleases/nestle-usa-announces-cage-free-eggs accessed 12/22/15.
15. http://www.cdc.gov/nceh/ehs/docs/understanding_cafos_nalboh.pdf accessed 12/5/15.
16. http://www.gao.gov/archive/1999/rc99205.pdf accessed 12/5/15.
17. Eating Animals, Jonathan Safran Foer, pg. 176, 1st Edition, Little, Brown and Company, 2009.
18. http://www.desmoinesregister.com/story/money/agriculture/2015/07/28/iowa-father-son-die-manure-pit-fumes/30809037 accessed 12/5/15.
19. http://www.cowspiracy.com/facts/stats used with permission of *Cowspiracy*, accessed 12/5/15.
20. Karl Blankenship, "Analysis Puts Bay Cleanup Tab at $19 Billion," Alliance for the Chesapeake Bay, *Bay Journal*, December 2002.
21. https://www.washingtonpost.com/national/health-science/large-dead-zone-signals-continued-problems-for-the-chesapeake-bay/2014/08/31/1e0c2024-2fc2-11e4-9b98-848790384093_story.html accessed 12/5/15.

22. http://www.desmoinesregister.com/story/news/local/2015/08/16/local-algae-iowa-city-dangers/31818937 accessed 12/5/15.

23. http://www.pressherald.com/2015/12/26/study-finds-chemicals-may-be-affecting-maine-bass accessed 12/26/15.

24. http://www.planetexperts.com/why-are-male-fish-growing-eggs-in-their-testicles-in-north-carolina accessed 12/26/15.

25. Ibid.

26. https://www.popularresistance.org/history-teaches-that-we-have-the-power-to-transform-the-nation-heres-how/ accessed12/15/15.

27. http://finance.yahoo.com/news/mcvegan-former-mcdonalds-ceo-joining-164723685.html accessed 12/15/15.

28. http://www.pcrm.org/barnardmedical accessed 12/15/15.

29. http://abcnews.go.com/blogs/lifestyle/2012/07/scientists-explore-better-menu-options-for-mars-trip accessed 12/15/15.

30. Thomas Kuhn, *The Structure of Scientific Revolutions*, pg. 151, 3rd Edition, University of Chicago Press, 1996.

31. http://www.collectorsweekly.com/articles/the-top-10-most-dangerous-ads accessed 12/15/15.

32. http://www.nytimes.com/1991/12/11/us/smoking-among-children-is-linked-to-cartoon-camel-in-advertisements.html accessed 12/15/15.

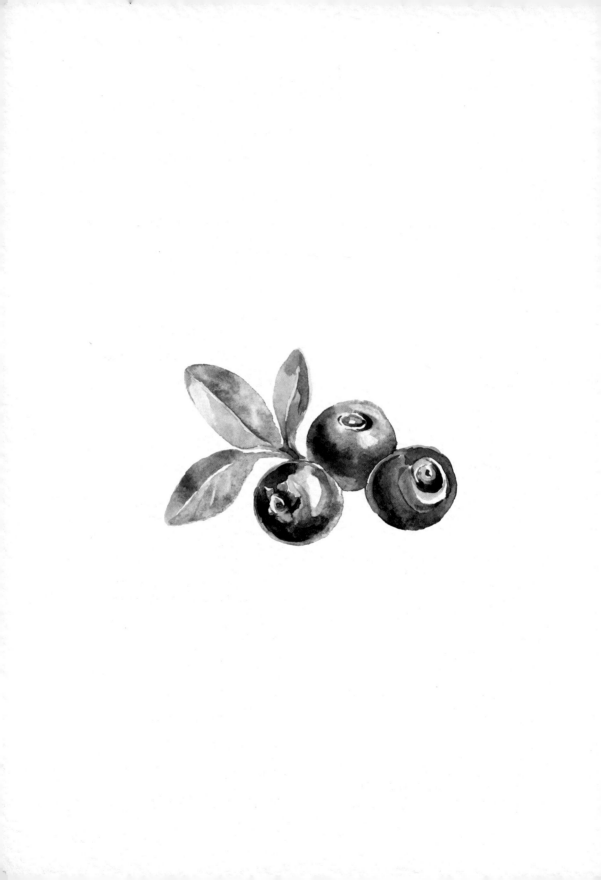

Index

abuse:
    of animals, 247–48
    domestic, 248
activism, 259–70
Adams, Samuel, 277
ADAPTT, 102
additives, 52
adopting a companion animal, 249
airlines, 275
airports, 231–32
albumin, 44
alcoholic beverages, 40, 140, 205–10
almond butter, 129
    Healthy Snack-Attack Cookies, 166
Almond Milk, Easy, 76
Alvarado Street Bakery, 137
American Egg Board (AEB), 84, 85
amino acids, 128
Amis, Rebecca, 279
Amy's Drive Thru, 228
anchovies, 46, 97
Anderson, Kip, 34
angora, 199–200
Animal Place, 236
animal products, 8
    in cosmetics, 180, 181
    separating from non-animal products in your
      kitchen, 39–54
    two schools of thought on avoiding small
      amounts of, 40–41
animals, 275
    abuse of, 247–48
    companion, see companion animals
    compassion for, see compassion
    food names for, 262
    language and, 261–64
    spending mindful time with, 36
animal sanctuaries, 236
antibiotics, 71, 96
anticoagulant rodenticides, 267
antioxidants, 150–51
Antonio, Luiz, 94
Approaching the Natural: A Health Manifesto
    (Garza-Hillman), 232–33
aquafaba, 86, 220
    Easy Meringue Bites, 221
aquariums, 235, 236, 238–39
aquatic ecotours, 238
armchair activism, 259–60
asking questions about food, 41–42, 230–31
Atwood, Margaret, 15

Aveda, 187
avocado, 136, 141
    Kale, Avocado, and Bean Pasta Salad, 167

bacon, 262, 274
    vegan, 109
bananas:
    Healthy Snack-Attack Cookies, 166
    My Sweet Bah Nah Nas, 53
Barnard, Neal, 65
Barnivore, 206
Baskin-Robbins Ice Cream, 30
bathroom cleaners, 191
beans:
    antioxidants in, 151
    Black Bean Beet Burgers, 162–63
    Eggplant Seitan Chili, 157
    Kale, Avocado, and Bean Pasta Salad, 167
    protein in, 129
    Three Sisters Chili, 169
    see also chickpeas
beautiful meals, 147–76
beef, 118
beer, 40, 105–10
beerfests, 206–7
bees, 8
beeswax, 181
beets, 154
    Black Bean Beet Burgers, 162–63
    Farmers' Market Soup, 164–65
    holiday, 217
Ben & Jerry's, 274
berries, 154
    strawberries, 142
    Sweet Sunday French Crepes, 170–71
    Valentine's Day Chocolate-Dipped Strawber-
      ries, 220
Bialik, Mayim, 31
Big Ag, 103–4, 277
Big Bang Theory, The, 31
Big Lots, 131–32
bike rides, 238
Bircher-Benner, Maximilian, 135
Bird, Alfred, 87
Black Bean Beet Burgers, 162–63
Blackfish, 238
black pudding, 262
blankets, 190
Block, John, 103
bloodletting, 273
blood tests, 32–33, 68–69, 72, 74

bone, jewelry made from, 203
bone health, 73, 74
Bonnie Doon Winery, 206
books, 33–34, 257–58, 260
BPA, 59
Brand, Russell, 34–35
bread, 42–43, 137–38
breakfast and brunch:
    Easy Peasy Pancakes, 158
    My Overnight Oats, 135
    My Vegan Breakfast Scramble, 88
    scrambles, 87–90
    smoothies, 134–35
    Sweet Sunday French Crepes, 170–71
    toast, 136
brown sugar, 142
Buddha Bowls, 255
bullfighting, 209, 275
bumper stickers, 261
buns, 163
burgers, vegan, 107–8
    Black Bean Beet Burgers, 162–63
    buns for, 163
    Eggplant Hummus Veggie Burger Wrap, 168
Butterfield Foods Company, 85
butterflies, 198

cabbage, 155
    Krautfleckerl, 159
caffeine, 73
calcium, 72, 73, 116, 274
California Prune Board, 262–63
Cameron, James, 30, 34, 279
Cameron, Suzy Amis, 30, 34, 279
cancer, 35, 68, 99, 151, 275
candy, 46
capers, 141
career, 24–25
carmine, 40, 44, 45, 181
carpets, 190–91
Carr, Kris, 23, 34
carrageenan, 72
Carter, David, 135
casein, caseinate, 44, 49, 123
cashew milk, 72
cashews, 129
    Easy Cashew Date Balls, 215
    Soft-Crusted Cashew Cheese, 125
    Vegan Parmesan Cheese, 174
casomorphines, 123
castoreum, 40, 44
caterpillars, 197–98
cats, 201, 245–50
Cecil the lion, 275
Center for Disease Control, 27
champagne, 208

Charlemagne, 99
cheap, fast, and easy meals, 127–46
cheese, 123–24
cheese, vegan, 119–26
    homemade nut cheese, 124–25
    nutritional yeast and, 124
    Soft-Crusted Cashew Cheese, 125
    Vegan Parmesan Cheese, 174
chemical additives, 52
Chenoweth, Erica, 278
cherries, 154
Chesapeake Bay, 277
chia seeds, 94
chicken, vegan, 109
Chicken Pot Pie, KFC, 224–26
chickens, 6, 102
    eggs and, 2, 80–83
chickpeas (garbanzo beans), 86
    aquafaba, 86, 220
    Easy Meringue Bites, 221
    Eggplant Hummus Veggie Burger Wrap, 168
    Homemade Collard Rolls, 172
    No Tuna Salad Sandwich, 99
    Sun-Dried Tomato-Kalamata Hummus, 222
chili:
    Eggplant Seitan Chili, 157
    Three Sisters Chili, 169
chimpanzees, 275
China, 201
    angora from, 199–200
    cosmetics and, 186–87
    down from, 200
chocolate, 46–47, 151, 219
    Valentine's Day Chocolate-Dipped Strawber-
    ries, 220
cholesterol, 69, 81, 107
chorizo, vegan, 109–10
circuses, 235–37, 275
citrus, 140
    Zucchini Noodles with Citrus Peanut Sauce,
    175
clean food, 27
cleaning products, 189–94
    cruelty-free and vegan, 193–94
clothing, 195–204
    angora, 199–200
    down, 200
    fur, 200–201
    jewelry, 202–3
    leather, 198–99
    silk, 197–98
    wool, 196–97
cochineal, 44, 45
coconut palm sugar, 142
coffee, 74–75
coffee shops, 74, 75, 260

Collard Rolls, Homemade, 172
colors, 150–55
    contrasting, 150
comforters, 190
community, 25
    planting seeds of compassion in, 259–70
    sharing vegan food with, 266
Community Supported Agriculture (CSAs), 57
companion animals, 245–50
    adopting, 249
    spaying and neutering, 246–47
Compass Group, 85
compassion, 2, 30–31, 272
    language and, 261–64
    planting seeds of, 259–70
Concentrated Animal Feeding Operations (CAFOs;
    factory farms), 2, 70–71, 83, 276
condiments, 256
Constitution, 266
convenience foods, vegan, 107
Cookies, Healthy Snack-Attack, 166
cooking at home, benefits of, 26–27
Copernicus, Nicolaus, 272–73
corn:
    Eggplant Seitan Chili, 157
    Three Sisters Chili, 169
cosmetics and toiletries:
    animal by-products in, 180, 181
    animal testing and, 177–81, 186, 260, 275
    China and, 186–87
    cruelty-free and free of animal ingredients,
        182–86
    expiration of, 187
    men's products, 186
    separating vegan and non-vegan, 177–88
    soap, 184
    sunscreens, 234
Costco, 60, 88
Coulombe, Joe, 58–59
coupons, 131
Cove, The, 238
cows and calves, 2, 8, 27, 29, 68–71, 102, 123
    calf roping, 240
Cowspiracy: The Sustainability Secret, 34, 257
crab, 97
Crazy Sexy Diet (Carr), 34
crepes, 79–80
    Sweet Sunday French Crepes, 170–71
crumbles, vegan, 108
culinary arts, 147–76
Cunningham, Marion, 176
curtains, 191
custard, 87
cysteine, 44, 46

Dahl, Dave, 137–38

Dahmer, Jeffrey, 248
dairy products, 30, 104, 274, 275
    "non-dairy" labels and, 48–49
    see also milk, dairy
Date Cashew Balls, Easy, 215
date sugar, 142
Dave's Killer Bread, 137–38, 163
dead zones, 277
Dean Foods, 69–70
decorations, 191
decorative pillows, 191
demonstrations, peaceful, 265–66
Demos, Steve, 69
Descartes, René, 275
desserts, see sweets
diabetes, 35
Diamond, Harvey, 268
DiCaprio, Leonardo, 34
Diet for a New America (Robbins), 33
dining out, see restaurants
Dirty Dozen and Clean 15, 62
diseases, see health problems and diseases
dogs, 102, 201, 245–50
Dollar Store and Dollar Tree, 131, 231, 254
dolphins, 235–36, 239
domestic abuse, 248
Dominican University, 16
down, 200
Draize Test, 177–78
dressings, 139
    My Dressing, 139
    suggestions for making, 139–42
Dr. Seuss, 210
ducks, 200, 262
Duhamel, Meagan, 31
duvets, 190

Earth Day, 16
Earth Day Health Festival, 10
Earthlings, 34, 257
easy, fast, and cheap meals, 127–46
Easy Almond Milk, 76
Easy Cashew Date Balls, 215
Easy Meringue Bites, 221
Easy Peasy Pancakes, 158
Easy Tofu Veggie Stir Fry, 160
Easy Vegan Gravy, 214
Eating Animals (Foer), 257–58
EBT cards, 144
eggnog, 86–87
eggplant:
    Eggplant Hummus Veggie Burger Wrap, 168
    Eggplant Seitan Chili, 157
    Stovetop Ratatouille, 161
egg rolls, 87
eggs, 2, 40, 80–85, 275

baking and, 90
chalazae in, 80
chickens and, 2, 80–83
cholesterol in, 81
free range and cage free, 90–91, 275
turning egg-based meals into vegan ones, 79–92
Einstein, Albert, 273
elephants, 275
elephant seals, 239
e.l.f., 181, 186
entertainment, 235–44
aquariums, 235, 236, 238–39
bike rides, 238
circuses, 235–37, 275
farm animal sanctuaries, 236
horse-drawn carriage rides, 237–38
rodeos, 209, 236, 239–40
Veggie Festivals, 240–43
zoos and animal parks, 236
environment, 3, 30, 34
fish and shrimp farming and, 96
Environmental Working Group, 62, 185
Eskimo Diet, 95
Esseltyn, Caldwell, 35
estrogen, 73
ethnic grocery stores, 60–61
Eureka Bread, 137
events, bringing vegan food to, 266
exercise, 24, 73

factory farms, 2, 70–71, 83, 276
Farm Bill, 104
farm animal sanctuaries, 236
farmers' markets, 56–57
Farmers' Market Nutrition Program (FMNP), 144
Farmers' Market Soup, 164–65
Farm Sanctuary, 29, 236
fast, cheap, and easy meals, 127–46
fast-food, vegan, 107, 224–29
fat, body, 129
obesity, 30
fats:
animal, 30
healthy, 94
oils, 141
omega-3 and omega-6 fatty acids, 72, 94–95, 99, 274
saturated, 69, 73, 81
Federal Trade Commission (FTC), 58, 84
Feeding America, 145
Feld Entertainment, 275
fiber, 72, 99
films, 34–36, 235, 257, 260
Forks Over Knives, 30, 34–35
on ocean animals, 238
First Amendment, 266

fish, 46, 93–96, 274, 277
contaminated, 95–96
country of origin, 95–96
fish, veganizing meals that contain, 93–100
fish sticks, 96–97
No Tuna Salad Sandwich, 99
fishing, 236
fish oil, 95
flavor, 253, 256
flavors, natural, 40, 44, 48
flaxseeds, 94, 99, 129
Flower Foods, Inc., 137–38
Foer, Jonathan Safran, 257–58
foie gras, 262
Food and Drug Administration (FDA), 46–47, 49, 52, 71, 177, 178, 263
food banks, 143, 145
food-borne illnesses, 27
food co-ops, 57–58
Food 4 Less, 59
food labels, 41–49
country of origin on, 95–96, 118
see also ingredients
Food Not Bombs, 145
food politics, 41
food pyramid, 30, 103
food stamps, 144
Forks Over Knives, 30, 34–35
free radicals, 151
fresh produce delivery services, 57
Freston, Kathy, 34
Friedrich, Bruce, 40
From Farm to Fridge, 36, 102
frozen foods, 51, 130
fruit juice, 40–41, 46
fruits, 103, 104–5, 106, 130, 142
antioxidants in, 150–51
colors of, 150–55
frozen, 51, 130
slicing, 149–50
see also produce
Fukushima Daiichi radiation leak, 96
fur, 200–201
furniture, 190
future, envisioning, 32

Galileo Galilei, 273
Gandhi, Mahatma, 201
garbanzo beans (chickpeas), 86
aquafaba, 86, 220
Easy Meringue Bites, 221
Eggplant Hummus Veggie Burger Wrap, 168
Homemade Collard Rolls, 172
No Tuna Salad Sandwich, 99
Sun-Dried Tomato-Kalamata Hummus, 222
garlic, 56

Garza-Hillman, Sid, 232–33
Gates, Bill, 84
geese, 200
Gein, Ed, 198–99
gelatin, 39, 44
gellan gum, 72
Gentle Barn, 9, 236
gin, 209
glazes, 44, 46
global population, 30
glucose, 44
glycerides, 44
goals, 20–21
    for beers, wines, and liquors, 205–10
    for cats and dogs, 245–50
    for cheese, 119–26
    for clothing items, 195–204
    for compassion, 259–70
    for cosmetics, 177–88
    for egg-based meals, 79–92
    for entertainment, 235–44
    for fast, cheap, and easy meals, 127–46
    for finding inspiration, 29–38
    for fish dishes, 93–100
    for food shopping, 55–66
    for holidays, 211–22
    for household items and cleaners, 189–94
    for meals that look beautiful, 147–76
    for meat dishes, 101–18
    for milks, 67–78
    pepping yourself up, 271–80
    separating vegan and non-vegan food items,
        39–54
    staying on the vegan wagon, 251–58
    for travel, 223–34
Gollwitzer, Peter, 17
Good Food Institute, 40
Google Alerts, 267
goose down, 200
Grahm, Randall, 206
grains, 106
    antioxidants in, 151
    Farmers' Market Soup, 164–65
    protein in, 129
Gravy, Easy Vegan, 214
Grits, Tofu and, 142–43
Grocery Outlet, 59–60
grocery shopping, see shopping for food
grocery stores, 58–60, 131, 231
    ethnic, 60–61
    vegan, 61
Guinness, 207
Gulf of Mexico, 277

hair color, 187
hair salons, 187

hamburgers, 27
    McDonald's, 81, 105–6, 274, 277
Hampton Creek, 84–85, 86, 87, 274
Happy Cow, 229
Harvard's School of Public Health, 73, 74
Harvest Bowls, 255
health, 1–2, 21, 24–26, 35, 68–69, 106, 274–75
    benefits of a whole foods, plant-based diet, 33
    blood tests and, 32–33, 68–69, 72, 74
    diseases, 35
    medical checkup and, 32–33
health problems and diseases, 30, 35, 68, 151
    cancer, 35, 68, 99, 151, 275
    heart disease, 35, 65, 68, 72, 81, 84, 95, 99, 103,
        151, 275
    obesity, 30
    strokes, 81, 99
Healthy Snack-Attack Cookies, 166
heart disease, 35, 65, 68, 72, 81, 84, 95, 99, 103,
    151, 275
hemp milk, 72
hemp seeds, 129
Hill, Julia Butterfly, 31
Hippocrates, 99, 258
history, 272–73
Hodo Soy, 60, 115
holidays, 211–22
    Easy Cashew Date Balls, 215
    Easy Vegan Gravy, 214
    first as a vegan, 216
    holiday beers, 217
    Okinawan sweet potato, 217
    pomegranate seeds and greens, 150, 217–18
    premade options for, 213
    at someone else's home, 214–15
    sweets for, 218–19
    Vegan Whipped Cream, 218
home cooking, benefits of, 26–27
Homemade Collard Rolls, 172
Homemade Vegan Pantry (Schinner), 86
honey, 8, 44
Hormel Foods, 103
horse-drawn carriage rides, 237–38
hospitals, 261
hot dogs, vegan, 108
hotels, 230–31
household items and cleaners, 189–94, 260
Howard, Lisa, 141
Humane Lobby Day, 266
Humane Methods of Slaughter Act, 82, 91
Humane Society of the United States, 85, 266
hummus:
    Eggplant Hummus Veggie Burger Wrap, 168
    Homemade Collard Rolls, 172
    Sun-Dried Tomato-Kalamata Hummus, 222
hunting, 209, 236

ice cream, 30, 274
idioms, 263–64
ingredients, 26, 41–49, 72, 106
    unfamiliar, 252
In N Out, 227–28
inspiration:
    books, 33–34, 257–58, 260
    discovering and memorializing, 29–38
    envisioning the future, 32
    films, *see* films
    providing to others, 26–27
    reminders of, 36–37
    spending mindful time with animals, 36
insults and pejorative terms, 263, 264
iron, 116–17
isinglass, 40, 44, 207
Ivy, Joanne, 85

jackfruit, 173
Jacobs, Marc, 201
jambalaya, 97
Japan, 96, 113
jewelry, 202–3
journal, 20–22, 34
junk food, vegan, 107, 132–33, 254

Kabobs, Seitan Veggie, 160
Kaiser Permanente, 21, 33
Kalamata-Sun-dried Tomato Hummus, 222
Kale, Avocado, and Bean Pasta Salad, 167
KFC Chicken Pot Pie, 224–26
kidneys, 129
Kind Diet, The (Silverstone), 34
King, Jeff, 279
kitchen cleaning products, 191, 193–94
Krautfleckerl, 159
Kroger, 59

labels, 41–49
    country of origin on, 95–96, 118
    see also ingredients
lactose, 44, 68
Lahey, Lisa, 15
lampshades, 190
language, 261–64
lanolin, 46, 181
lard, 44
laundry products, 192, 193–94
L-cysteine, 44, 46
leather, 198–99
leeches, 273
legislation, 260, 266–67
legumes:
    antioxidants in, 151
    Farmers' Market Soup, 164–65
    lentils, 129

    see also beans
lentils, 129
    Farmers' Market Soup, 164–65
letters to the editor, 260
Levin, Susan, 142–43
library, 260
Light, Luise, 103
Li Ka-Shing, 84
lions, 275
liquors, beers, and wine, 40, 140, 205–10

makeup:
    going without, 185
    see also cosmetics and toiletries
maple syrup, 142
Marc Jacobs, 201
marine parks and aquariums, 235, 236, 238–39
martial arts matches, 239
mattresses, 190
mayonnaise, 86
McDonald's, 81, 105–6, 265, 274, 275, 277, 278
meals, week's worth of, 155–56
meat, 30, 65, 101–5, 274, 275
    country of origin on, 118
    food-borne illnesses and, 27
    McDonald's hamburgers, 81, 105–6, 274, 277
    processed, 274
meat dishes, veganizing, 101–18
    "meat" products, 107–10
    mushrooms in, 110–11
    seitan in, 111
    Simple Seitan, 112
    tempeh in, 115
    tofu in, *see* tofu
meatballs, vegan, 109
medical checkup, 32–33
Meet Your Meat, 36, 102
Mercy for Animals, 265
meringue, 86
    Easy Meringue Bites, 221
military, 275
milk, dairy, 11, 67–71, 274
    cows and, 2, 8, 27, 29, 68–71, 123
    switching out for plant-based milks, 67–78
milks, plant-based:
    Easy Almond Milk, 76
    making your own, 75–76
    nutrients in, 72
    in recipes, 212
    types of, 73
    switching out dairy for, 67–78
mind-set, 258
Mintel, 278
miso, 142
mixed martial arts (MMA) matches, 239
Miyoko's Kitchen, 121–22

"Mmmm Bacon" dude, dealing with, 267–70
molasses, 142
Monsanto, 96, 103
movement and exercise, 24, 73
movies, *see* films
Mraz, Jason, 24
muesli, 135
MUSE, 279
mushrooms, 110–11, 129
    Stovetop Ratatouille, 161
    Three Sisters Chili, 169
mustard, 140
    My Dressing, 139
My Dressing, 139
    Kale, Avocado, and Bean Pasta Salad, 167
MyFitnessPal.com, 72
My Overnight Oats, 135
My Sweet Bah Nah Nas, 53
My Vegan Breakfast Scramble, 88

National Commission on Egg Nutrition (NCEN),
    84
National Dairy Council, 10
National Institutes of Health (NIH), 24, 95, 275
Native Foods, 213–14
natural flavors, 40, 44, 48
Nestlé, 275
neutering and spaying, 246–47
Newton, Isaac, 273
New Year's Day, 16
Noble, Matt, 145
noodles:
    Zucchini Noodles with Citrus Peanut Sauce,
    175
    see also pasta
No Tuna Salad Sandwich, 99
nut cheese, homemade, 124–25
    Soft-Crusted Cashew Cheese, 125
nut milks, *see* milks, plant-based
nutritional yeast, 88, 124
    Vegan Parmesan Cheese, 174
nuts:
    antioxidants in, 151
    in dressings and marinades, 141
    protein in, 129

oat milk, 72
oats, 129, 151
    Healthy Snack-Attack Cookies, 166
    My Overnight Oats, 135
    overnight, 136
Obama, Barack, 104
obesity, 30
Obsessive Compulsive Cosmetics, 181
oceans, 238–39
oils, 141

Oktoberfests, 206–7
olives, 141
    Sun-Dried Tomato-Kalamata Hummus, 222
omega-3 and omega-6 fatty acids, 72, 94–95, 99,
    274
omelets, 87–88
online shopping, 61–62
On the Revolutions of the Heavenly Bodies (Co-
    pernicus), 273
orange juice, 40–41, 46
orcas, 235, 239
organic produce, 26, 62
Oxford University, 257

Pallotta, Nicole, 247
pamphlets, 261
Pancakes, Easy Peasy, 158
pantry:
    emptying, 44
    vegan essentials for, 50
paradigm shifts, 272–73
pasta, 86
    Kale, Avocado, and Bean Pasta Salad, 167
    Krautfleckerl, 159
Patagonia, 197
Paul Mitchell, 186, 187
peanut butter, 129, 141
    Healthy Snack-Attack Cookies, 166
    Zucchini Noodles with Citrus Peanut Sauce,
    175
peanuts, 39
pearls, 202
peas, 129
pejorative terms and insults, 263, 264
People for the Ethical Treatment of Animals
    (PETA), 11, 70, 179, 180, 212, 237
pepping yourself up, 271–80
pepsin, 44
pets, *see* companion animals
Phoenix, Joaquin, 34
Physician's Committee for Responsible Medicine,
    11, 142, 231–32
Piedras Blancas, 239
pigs, 102, 116, 262, 263
pillows, 190
    decorative, 191
Pinterest, 274
pizza, 173
Planck, Max, 279–80
planning ahead, 254
    travel and, 229–31
    week's worth of meals, 155–56
plates, 148
Polenta (Grits), Tofu and, 142–43
politeness, 264
pomegranate seeds and greens, 150, 217–18

population, 30
pork, 118, 262
Potomac River, 277
presentation, 147–76
Price Loss Coverage (PLC) Program, 104
priorities, 255
Proceedings of the National Academy of Sciences (PNAS), 257
processed foods, 106, 107, 254
    meats, 274
produce:
    delivery services for, 57
    organic, 26, 62
    price of, 130
    seasonal, 61, 63–64
    see also fruits; vegetables
proportions, 26
protein, 45, 68–69, 72, 73, 99, 128–29, 274
    amino acids in, 128
    amount in plant foods, 128–29
    amount needed, 128
    kidneys and, 129
prunes, 262–63
Ptolemy, Claudius, 272
public assistance programs, 143–44

questions about food, asking, 41–42, 230–31
quinoa, 129
    Farmers' Market Soup, 164–65

rabbit fur, 201
    angora, 199–200
rabbits, 102
    cosmetic testing on, 177–78
raccoon dogs, 201
radiation, 96
Rainbowls, 255
Ralph's, 59
Ratatouille, Stovetop, 161
rats, rodenticides and, 267
recipes:
    Black Bean Beet Burgers, 162–63
    Easy Almond Milk, 76
    Easy Cashew Date Balls, 215
    Easy Meringue Bites, 221
    Easy Peasy Pancakes, 158
    Easy Tofu Veggie Stir Fry, 160
    Easy Vegan Gravy, 214
    Eggplant Hummus Veggie Burger Wrap, 168
    Eggplant Seitan Chili, 157
    Farmers' Market Soup, 164–65
    Healthy Snack-Attack Cookies, 166
    Homemade Collard Rolls, 172
    Kale, Avocado, and Bean Pasta Salad, 167
    Krautfleckerl, 159
    My Dressing, 139

My Overnight Oats, 135
My Sweet Bah Nah Nas, 53
My Vegan Breakfast Scramble, 88
No Tuna Salad Sandwich, 99
Seitan Veggie Kabobs, 160
Simple Seitan, 112
Soft-Crusted Cashew Cheese, 125
Stovetop Ratatouille, 161
Sun-Dried Tomato-Kalamata Hummus, 222
Sweet Potato Split Pea Soup, 117
Sweet Sunday French Crepes, 170–71
Three Sisters Chili, 169
Tofu and Grits, 142–43
Valentine's Day Chocolate-Dipped Strawberries, 220
Vegan Parmesan Cheese, 174
Vegan Whipped Cream, 218
Zucchini Noodles with Citrus Peanut Sauce, 175
recipes, complicated, 351–52
Redford, Robert, 200
refrigerator:
    emptying, 44
    vegan ideas for, 51
relationships, 24
reminders, 36–37
rennet, 44
respect, 264
restaurants, 230, 260
    fast-food, 224–29
    food-borne illnesses and, 27
ribs, vegan, 108
rice, 129
    Farmers' Market Soup, 164–65
Ringling Brothers, 237, 275
Robbins, John, 30, 33
rodenticides, 267
rodeos, 209, 236, 239–40
Roessel, Joël, 86
Roosevelt, Franklin D., 104
Roth, Ruby, 16
rugs, 190–91
rum, 209

salad dressings, 139
    My Dressing, 139
    suggestions for making, 139–42
salads, 138
    Kale, Avocado, and Bean Pasta Salad, 167
Salley, John, 17, 209
salmon, 97
sandwiches, 136
scallops, 97
Schinner, Miyoko, 86
schools, 261
    MUSE, 279

Schumer, Amy, 185
Schweitzer, Albert, 100
scrambles, breakfast, 87–90
    My Vegan Breakfast Scramble, 88
sea life sanctuaries, 238
seals, elephant, 239
seasonal eating, 61, 63–64
seaweed, 96, 97, 98, 120, 141
seeds:
    in dressings and marinades, 141
    protein in, 129
seitan, 111
    Eggplant Seitan Chili, 157
    Seitan Veggie Kabobs, 160
    Simple Seitan, 112
sesame seeds, 129, 141
Shannon, Annie, 107
shapes, food, 149
shaving products, 186
sheep, 196–97
shellac, 44, 46
shells, 203
shopping for food, 42, 55–66
    delivery services and, 57
    at farmers' markets, 56–57
    at food co-ops, 57–58
    at grocery stores, see grocery stores
    money-saving strategies for, 130–32
    online, 61–62
    plant-based milks, 72
    seasonal eating and, 61, 63–64
shrimp, 96, 97
silk, 197–98
Silk soy milk, 69
Silverstone, Alicia, 34
Simmons, Russell, 32
Simple Seitan, 112
Sinclair, Upton, 85
sleep, 24
smoothies, breakfast, 134–35
Snack-Attack Cookies, Healthy, 166
SNAP supplemental nutrition assistance program, 144
snorkeling, 238, 239
soap, 184
social media, 25, 260–61, 274
sodas, 73
sodium, 73
sodium caseinate, 44
sodium tallowate, 184
Soft-Crusted Cashew Cheese, 125
solitude, 25
Sonic, 40
soups:
    Farmers' Market Soup, 164–65
    miso, 142

Sweet Potato Split Pea Soup, 117
soybeans:
    miso, 142
    tempeh, 115
    tofu, see tofu
Soymage, 119–20
soy milk, 69, 72, 113
spaying and neutering, 246–47
Speciesism, 257
spinach, 129
Split Pea Sweet Potato Soup, 117
Sprouts Market, 131
Standard American Diet (SAD), 30, 104, 107, 226, 253
Stanford Inn, 232–33
Starbucks, 45, 275
stearic acid, stearate, 45
Steve-O, 31
Steyer, Tom, 84
Stir Fry, Easy Tofu Veggie, 160
Stone, Biz, 29
Stovetop Ratatouille, 161
strawberries, 142
    Valentine's Day Chocolate-Dipped Strawberries, 220
strokes, 81, 99
stuffing, 213
sugar, 47–48, 69, 129, 142
    lactose, 44, 68
Sun-Dried Tomato-Kalamata Hummus, 222
sunscreens, 234
sushi, 97
sweeteners, 48, 142
    honey, 8, 44
    sugar, see sugar
sweet potatoes:
    Okinawan, 217
    Sweet Potato Split Pea Soup, 117
sweets, 130
    Easy Cashew Date Balls, 215
    Easy Meringue Bites, 221
    Healthy Snack-Attack Cookies, 166
    holiday, 218–21
    My Sweet Bah Nah Nas, 53
    Valentine's Day Chocolate-Dipped Strawberries, 220
    Vegan Whipped Cream, 218
Sweet Sunday French Crepes, 170–71

Taco Bell, 226–27, 275
tacos, 173
tahini, 141
tallow, 45, 184
Target, 131, 181
tea, 96, 151
Teagan, 247–48

television shows, 260
tempeh, 115
Tetrick, Josh, 84, 85
Thompson, Don, 278
Three Sisters Chili, 169
throw rugs, 190–91
tipping points, 273, 278
toast, breakfast, 136
tofu, 74, 113–15
    dressing, 141
    Easy Tofu Veggie Stir Fry, 160
    how it's made, 114
    My Vegan Breakfast Scramble, 88
    Tofu and Grits, 142–43
    types of, 114
tomatoes and tomato sauce:
    Eggplant Seitan Chili, 157
    Kale, Avocado, and Bean Pasta Salad, 167
    Stovetop Ratatouille, 161
    Sun-Dried Tomato-Kalamata Hummus, 222
    Three Sisters Chili, 169
    Zucchini Noodles with Citrus Peanut Sauce,
      175
Toronto Vegetarian Food Bank, 145
Trader Joe's (TJ's), 58–59, 86, 87, 88, 121, 173, 184,
    207, 231
travel, 223–34
    airports and, 231–32
    fast-food and, 224–29
    planning in advance, 229–31
    translations of "plant foods only, please," 233
    see also entertainment
t-shirts, 261
Tuna Salad Sandwich, vegan, 99
turmeric, 88

Unilever, 85, 86, 274
Union of Concerned Scientists, 103
United Egg Producers, 83
United Nations, 30, 102
United States Department of Agriculture (USDA),
    30, 47, 56, 68, 80, 82, 84, 85, 90–91, 95, 103,
    104
University of California Davis, 246

Valentine's Day, 16, 219
    Chocolate-Dipped Strawberries, 220
variety, 151
veal, 8, 71, 262
vegan, coining of word, 76
vegan grocery stores, 61
Veganissimo, A to Z (Proctor and Thomsen), 45
Veganist (Freston), 34
vegan lifestyle:
    100 percent, 22–23, 40, 46
    affordability of, 27–28, 254–55

announcing adoption of, 16–17
author's adoption of, 5–11
compassion and, see compassion
as complicated, 251–52
dealing with common problems and staying on
    the wagon, 251–58
as difficult, 256
environment and, see environment
flavors and, 253, 256
health and, see health
mind-set and, 258
mistakes and, 23
obstacles to, 37–38, 252
outside forces and, 252
reasons for adopting, 1–3, 21
setting a date for adopting, 13–16
transitioning too quickly to, 253–54
two schools of thought on avoiding small
    amounts of animal products, 40–41
vegan lifestyle, 21-day plan for adopting, 19–28
    Day 1, 29–38
    Day 2, 39–54
    Day 3, 55–66
    Day 4, 67–78
    Day 5, 79–92
    Day 6, 93–100
    Day 7, 101–18
    Day 8, 119–26
    Day 9, 127–46
    Day 10, 147–76
    Day 11, 177–88
    Day 12, 189–94
    Day 13, 195–204
    Day 14, 205–10
    Day 15, 211–23
    Day 16, 223–34
    Day 17, 235–44
    Day 18, 245–50
    Day 19, 251–58
    Day 20, 259–70
    Day 21, 271–80
    goals in, see goals
    journal in, 20–22, 34
    planning in, 22
    progress in, 21
Vegan Parmesan Cheese, 174
Vegan Starter Kits, 261
Vegan Whipped Cream, 218
vegetables, 103, 104–5
    antioxidants in, 150–51
    colors of, 150–55
    Easy Tofu Veggie Stir Fry, 160
    Eggplant Hummus Veggie Burger Wrap, 168
    Farmers' Market Soup, 164–65
    frozen, 51, 130
    Homemade Collard Rolls, 172

protein in, 129
   Seitan Veggie Kabobs, 160
   slicing, 149–50
   see also produce
vegetarianism, 2, 7, 227
Veggie Festivals, 240–43
Velez-Mitchell, Jane, 31
vinegar, 140
vitamins:
   A, 73
   B_{12}, 72
   C, 116
   D, 40–41, 45, 46, 74, 116, 185
   E, 72
vodka, 209

walnuts, 72, 94, 151
water, 253
Watson, Donald, 76
weekends, 16
week's worth of meals, 155–56
weight, 30, 68
Wet *n* Wild, 181, 186
whey, 45
White Wave Foods, 69–70

Whitetails Unlimited, 209
Whole Foods Market (WFM), 58, 85, 131, 141,
   173, 213
WIC (Women, Infants, and Children) program,
   143–44
wildlife "trophies," 275
wine, 40, 140, 205–10
Wonder Bread, 138
wool, 196–97
words, choosing, 261–64
work, 24–25
World Health Organization, 274
Wrap, Eggplant Hummus Veggie Burger, 168

yeast, nutritional, 88, 124
   Vegan Parmesan Cheese, 174
Yourofsky, Gary, 257

zoos and animal parks, 236
   aquariums, 235, 236, 238–39
zucchini:
   Stovetop Ratatouille, 161
   Three Sisters Chili, 169
   Zucchini Noodles with Citrus Peanut Sauce,
   175

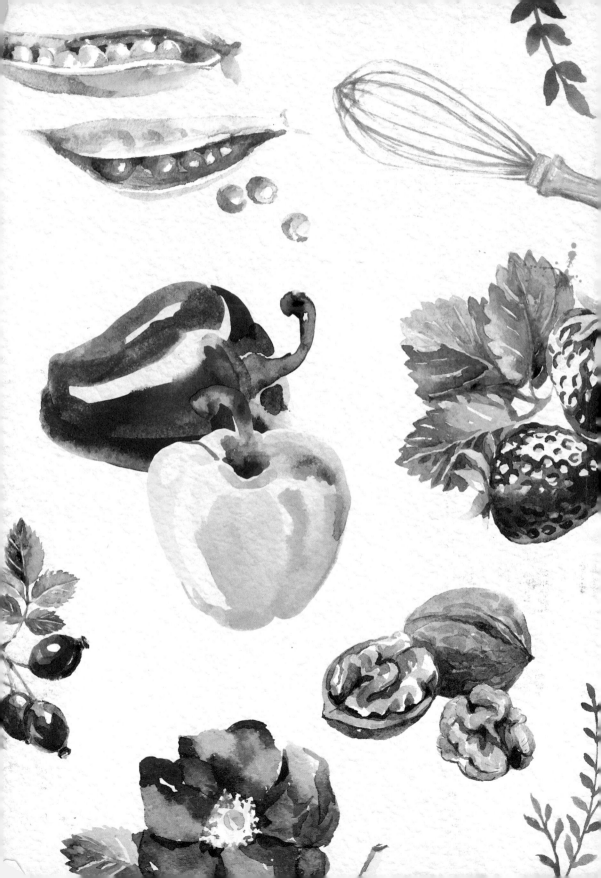